Cindy Haynes

nervous system

the nervous system

WILLIAM F. GANONG, MD

Professor of Physiology
Chairman, Department of Physiology
University of California
San Francisco, California

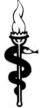

Los Altos, California   **LANGE Medical Publications**

International Standard Book Number: *0–87041–240–X*
Library of Congress Catalogue Card Number: *77–83652*

A Concise Medical Library for Practitioner and Student

The Nervous System $8.00

Current Medical Diagnosis & Treatment 1977 (annual revision). Edited by M.A. Krupp and M.J. Chatton. 1066 pp.	1977
Current Pediatric Diagnosis & Treatment, 4th ed. Edited by C.H. Kempe, H.K. Silver, and D. O'Brien. 1053 pp, *illus.*	1976
Current Surgical Diagnosis & Treatment, 3rd ed. Edited by J.E. Dunphy and L.W. Way. 1139 pp, *illus.*	1977
Current Obstetric & Gynecologic Diagnosis & Treatment. Edited by R.C. Benson. 911 pp, *illus.*	1976
Review of Physiological Chemistry, 16th ed. H.A. Harper, V.W. Rodwell, and P.A. Mayes. 681 pp, *illus.*	1977
Review of Medical Physiology, 8th ed. W.F. Ganong. 599 pp, *illus.*	1977
Review of Medical Microbiology, 12th ed. E. Jawetz, J.L. Melnick, and E.A. Adelberg. 542 pp, *illus.*	1976
Review of Medical Pharmacology, 5th ed. F.H. Meyers, E. Jawetz, and A. Goldfien. 740 pp, *illus.*	1976
Basic & Clinical Immunology. Edited by H.H. Fudenberg, D.P. Stites, J.L. Caldwell, and J.V. Wells. 653 pp, *illus.*	1976
Basic Histology, 2nd ed. L.C. Junqueira, J. Carneiro, and A.N. Contopoulos. 453 pp, *illus.*	1977
General Urology, 8th ed. D.R. Smith. 492 pp, *illus.*	1975
General Ophthalmology, 8th ed. D. Vaughan and T. Asbury. 379 pp, *illus.*	1977
Correlative Neuroanatomy & Functional Neurology, 16th ed. J.G. Chusid. 448 pp, *illus.*	1976
Principles of Clinical Electrocardiography, 9th ed. M.J. Goldman. 412 pp, *illus.*	1976
Handbook of Psychiatry, 3rd ed. Edited by P. Solomon and V.D. Patch. 706 pp.	1974
Handbook of Obstetrics & Gynecology, 6th ed. R.C. Benson. 772 pp, *illus.*	1977
Physician's Handbook, 18th ed. M.A. Krupp, N.J. Sweet, E. Jawetz, E.G. Biglieri, and R.L. Roe. 754 pp, *illus.*	1976
Handbook of Pediatrics, 12th ed. H.K. Silver, C.H. Kempe, and H.B. Bruyn. 723 pp, *illus.*	1977
Handbook of Poisoning: Diagnosis & Treatment, 9th ed. R.H. Dreisbach. About 520 pp.	1977

Lithographed in USA

Table of Contents

III. FUNCTIONS OF THE NERVOUS SYSTEM

Preface To
Review Of Medical Physiology,
Eighth Edition

This book is designed to provide a concise summary of mammalian and, particularly, of human physiology which medical students and others can supplement with readings in current texts, monographs, and reviews. Pertinent aspects of general and comparative physiology are also included. Summaries of relevant anatomic considerations will be found in each section, but this book is written primarily for those who have some knowledge of anatomy, chemistry, and biochemistry.

Examples from clinical medicine are given where pertinent to illustrate physiologic points. Physicians desiring to use this book as a review will find short discussions of important symptoms produced by disordered function in several sections.

It has not been possible to be complete and concise without also being dogmatic. I believe, however, that the conclusions presented without a detailed discussion of the experimental data on which they are based are those supported by the bulk of the currently available evidence. Much of this evidence can be found in the papers cited in the credit lines of the illustrations. Further discussions of particular subjects and information on subjects not considered in detail in this book can be found in the references listed at the end of each section. Information about serial review publications which provide up-to-date discussions of various physiologic subjects is included in the note on general references in the appendix.

In the interest of brevity and clarity, I have in most instances omitted the names of the many investigators whose work made possible the view of physiology presented here. This is in no way intended to slight their contributions, but including their names and specific references to original papers would greatly increase the length of this book.

I am greatly indebted to many individuals who helped in the preparation of this book. Those whom I wish especially to thank for their help with the Eighth Edition include Drs. Choh Hao Li, David Ramsay, Floyd Rector, Jr., and Isadore Edelman. I am also indebted to my wife, who labored long hours typing corrections, and to Annette Lowe and André Sala, who drew many of the illustrations. I also wish to thank all the students and others who took the time to write to me offering helpful criticisms and suggestions. Such comments are always welcome, and I solicit additional corrections and criticisms, which may be addressed to me at the Department of Physiology, University of California, San Francisco, California 94143, USA. Many associates and friends provided unpublished illustrative materials, and numerous authors and publishers generously granted permission to reproduce illustrations from other books and journals.

With the appearance of the eighth edition I am pleased to be able to announce that the following translations have been published: Portuguese (second edition), German (third edition), Italian (fifth edition), Spanish (fifth edition), Japanese (fourth edition), Polish, Czechoslovakian, Chinese, Greek, and Serbo-Croatian. French, Vietnamese, Iranian, and Turkish translations are under way. The book has also been recorded on tape for use by the blind.

San Francisco
June, 1977

William F. Ganong

Preface To
The Nervous System

For several years, a number of friends and associates have urged that the sections of *Review of Medical Physiology* that deal with the nervous system be made available as a separate book. Integrated courses in neuroscience are becoming increasingly common in colleges and professional schools, and some students are interested in obtaining a short text that deals with the nervous system and its function without obtaining a complete textbook of physiology.

The Nervous System should meet their needs. It is drawn from the eighth edition of *Review of Medical Physiology* and is made up primarily of slightly edited versions of Chapters 1–16 plus parts of Chapter 32, the Appendix, and the tabular material from the larger book. It deals primarily with the function of the nervous system, but it also contains information on the many aspects of brain anatomy, a variety of anatomic diagrams, and considerable data on neurochemistry and neuropharmacology. Therefore, it should be of use to students in integrated neuroscience courses and to others interested in reviewing the functions of the nervous system. Some clinical correlates are included, but few are considered in detail.

Individuals interested in a more exhaustive consideration of neuroanatomy and its application in the clinical practice of neurology are advised to consult *Correlative Neuroanatomy & Functional Neurology*, 16th edition, by Joseph G. Chusid, MD (Lange, 1976). More detailed information on neuroendocrine control mechanisms is available in *Review of Medical Physiology*, because, in addition to the information in the present text, that book includes a consideration of neural control in the section on each endocrine gland. The bigger text is also recommended for those interested in the broader picture of the interaction of the nervous system with the other systems in the body and in the role of neural function in the integration of their activity.

William F. Ganong, MD

San Francisco
August, 1977

I. Introduction
1...
Physiologic Principles

In unicellular organisms, all vital processes occur in a single cell. As the evolution of multicellular organisms has progressed, various cell groups have taken over particular functions. In higher animals and humans, the specialized cell groups include a gastrointestinal system to digest and absorb food, a respiratory system to take up O_2 and eliminate CO_2, a urinary system to remove wastes, a cardiovascular system to distribute food, O_2, and the products of metabolism, a reproductive system for perpetuating the species, and nervous and endocrine systems to coordinate and integrate the functions of the other systems. This book is concerned with the way the nervous system functions to effect this coordination and integration.

CELLULAR STRUCTURE & FUNCTION

Revolutionary advances in the understanding of cell structure and function have been made through the use of electron microscopy, x-ray diffraction, and the other technics of modern cellular and molecular biology. The specialization of the cells in the various organs of higher animals is very great, and no cell can be called "typical" of all cells in the body. However, a number of structures, or **organelles**, are common to most cells. These structures are shown in Fig 1–1.

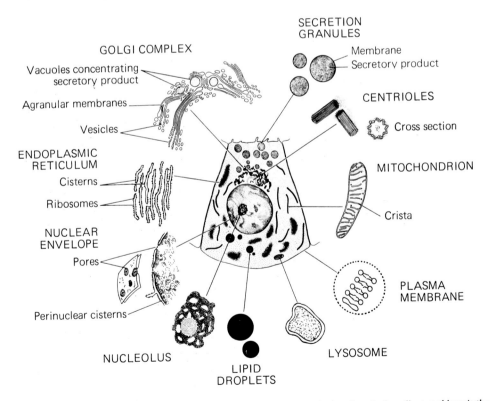

Figure 1–1. Ultrastructure of the common cell organelles and inclusions. The endoplasmic reticulum illustrated here is the granular type, with ribosomes attached to it. Some cells also contain tubes of membrane without ribosomes (agranular endoplasmic reticulum). The pores in the nuclear envelope are closed by a thin, homogeneous membrane. (Modified and reproduced, with permission, from Bloom & Fawcett: *A Textbook of Histology*, 10th ed. Saunders, 1975.)

1

Cell Membrane

The membrane which surrounds the cell is a remarkable structure. It is not only semipermeable, allowing some substances to pass through it and excluding others, but its permeability can be varied. It is generally referred to as the **plasma membrane**. The nucleus is also surrounded by a membrane, and the organelles are surrounded by or made up of membrane.

Although the chemical structure of membranes and their properties vary considerably from one location to another, they have certain common features. They are generally about 7.5 nm (75 Angstrom units) thick. They are made up primarily of protein and lipids, and the major lipids are phospholipids such as phosphatidyl choline and phosphatidyl ethanolamine. The chemistry of proteins and lipids is discussed in Chapter 17. The shape of the phospholipid molecule is roughly that of a clothespin (Fig 1–2). The head end of the molecule contains the phosphate portion, is positively charged, and is quite soluble in water (polar, or **hydrophilic**). The tails are quite insoluble (nonpolar or **hydrophobic**). In the membrane, the hydrophilic ends are exposed to the aqueous environment that bathes the exterior of the cells and the aqueous cytoplasm; the hydrophobic ends meet in the water-poor interior of the membrane.

There are many different proteins embedded in the membrane. They exist as separate globular units and stud the inside and outside of the membrane in a random array (Fig 1–2). Some are located in the inner surface of the membrane; some are located on the outer surface; and some extend through the membrane (**through and through proteins**). In general, the uncharged, hydrophobic portions of the protein molecules are located in the interior of the membrane and the charged, hydrophilic portions are located on the surfaces. Some of the proteins contain lipids (lipoproteins) and some carbohydrates (glycoproteins). Through and through glycoproteins with the carbohydrates attached to their outer ends function as receptors for hormones and neurotransmitters. Other proteins function as enzymes and probably as ion channels.

The protein structure—and particularly the enzyme content—of biologic membranes varies not only from cell to cell but also within the same cell. For example, plasma membranes contain relatively large quantities of magnesium adenosine triphosphatase, whereas monoamine oxidase is found in high concentration in the outer membranes of mitochondria. The membranes are dynamic structures, and their constituents are being constantly renewed at different rates. In addition, it is now clear that glycoproteins move laterally in the membrane. For example, membrane proteins that bind antibodies can aggregate in one or more spots on the membrane or spread diffusely over the surface. There is evidence that the lateral movement of components in the membrane is not random but is controlled by intracellular mechanisms that probably involve microfilaments and microbules (see below).

Underlying most cells is a thin fuzzy layer plus some fibrils that collectively make up the **basement membrane** or, more properly, the **basal lamina**. The material that makes up the basal lamina has been shown to be made up of a collagen derivative plus 2 glycoproteins.

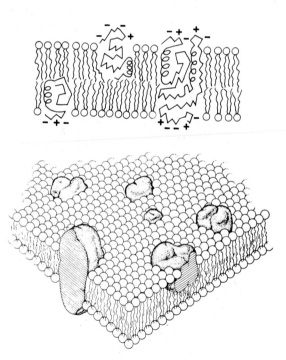

Figure 1–2. Biologic membrane. *Top:* Model of membrane structure. The phospholipid molecules each have 2 fatty acid chains (wavy lines) attached to a phosphate head (open circle). The proteins, indicated by the heavy lines, are partly in the a-helical configuration and partly folded, with the charged ends (+ and − signs) on the exterior or interior sides of the membrane. *Bottom:* Three-dimensional view of membrane. Proteins are shown as irregular shaded globules. (Reproduced, with permission, from Singer & Nicolson: The fluid mosaic model of the structure of cell membranes. Science 175:720, 1972. Copyright 1972 by the American Association for the Advancement of Science.)

Intercellular Connections

Most cells stop dividing and moving when they come in contact with other cells. This **contact inhibition**, which is deficient in cancer cells, indicates that cells must communicate with each other. The mechanisms responsible for this transfer of information are the subject of intensive research.

There are morphologically demonstrable connections between cells in tissues. Two types of connections are associated with cell-to-cell adhesion and maintenance of tissue strength and organization. One of these is the **tight junction**, in which the membranes of 2 cells become apposed and the outer layers of the membranes fuse. The other is the **adherens** type of junction in which there are various forms of membrane specialization but the 2 membranes are separated by a 15–35 nm space. A third junction, the **gap junction** or nexus, permits the direct transfer of ions and other small molecules between cells without traversing the extracellular space. The gap junction is characterized by a 2 nm space between the opposing membranes. This gap is filled with densely packed particles through each of which there appears to be a channel that connects the 2 cells. Thus, the junction permits rapid propagation of electrical potential changes from one cell to another.

Nucleus & Related Structures

A nucleus is present in all animal cells that divide. If a cell is cut in half, the anucleate portion eventually dies without dividing. The nucleus is made up in large part of the **chromosomes,** the structures in the nucleus which carry a complete blueprint for all the heritable species and individual characteristics of the animal. During cell division, the pairs of chromosomes become visible, but between cell divisions the irregular clumps of the dark material called **chromatin** are the only evidence of their presence. Each chromosome is made up of supporting protein and a giant molecule of **deoxyribonucleic acid (DNA).** The ultimate units of heredity are the **genes** on the chromosomes, and each gene is a portion of the DNA molecule.

During normal cell division by **mitosis,** the chromosomes duplicate themselves and then divide in such a way that each daughter cell receives a full complement **(diploid number)** of chromosomes. During their final maturation, germ cells undergo a division in which half the chromosomes go to each daughter cell. This reduction division, or **meiosis,** is actually a 2-stage process; but the important consideration is that, as a result of it, mature sperms and ova contain half the normal number (the **haploid number)** of chromosomes. When a sperm and ovum unite, the resultant cell **(zygote)** has a full (diploid) complement of chromosomes, one-half from the female parent and one-half from the male. The chemistry of DNA and the way the base chains of DNA split during mitosis and meiosis are discussed in other texts.

The nucleus of most cells contains a **nucleolus** (Fig 1–1), a patchwork of granules rich in **ribonucleic acid (RNA).** In some cells, the nucleus contains several of these structures. Nucleoli are most prominent and numerous in growing cells. The DNA in the nucleus serves as a template for the synthesis of RNA, which then moves to the cytoplasm, where it regulates the synthesis of proteins by the cell. The nucleolus is probably the site where the RNA found in the ribosomes (see below) is synthesized. Since the enzymes that control the metabolism of the cell are proteins, the synthesis of protein is the key to the control of the development of the cell. The chemistry of RNA and the subject of protein synthesis should be studied in greater detail in other texts.

The nucleus is surrounded by a **nuclear membrane,** or **envelope** (Fig 1–1). This membrane is double, and the spaces between the 2 folds are called **perinuclear cisterns.** The nuclear membrane is apparently quite permeable, since it permits passage of molecules as large as RNA from the nucleus to the cytoplasm. There are areas of discontinuity in the nuclear membrane, but these "pores" are closed by a thin, homogeneous membrane.

Endoplasmic Reticulum

The endoplasmic reticulum is a complex series of tubules in the cytoplasm of the cell (Fig 1–1). The tubule walls are made up of membrane. In **granular** endoplasmic reticulum, granules called **ribosomes** are attached to the cytoplasmic side of the membrane, whereas in **agranular** endoplasmic reticulum the granules are absent. Free ribosomes are also found in the cytoplasm. The ribosomes are about 15 nm in diameter. Each is made up of a large and a small subunit called, on the basis of their rates of sedimentation in the centrifuge, the 50 S and the 30 S subunits, respectively. Sometimes, 3–5 ribosomes are clumped together, forming **polyribosomes (polysomes).** The ribosomes contain about 65% RNA and 35% protein. They are the sites of protein synthesis. The ribosomes that are attached to the endoplasmic reticulum synthesize proteins such as hormones that are secreted by the cell. The polypeptide chains are extruded into the endoplasmic reticulum. The free ribosomes synthesize cytoplasmic proteins such as hemoglobin.

The agranular endoplasmic reticulum is the site of steroid synthesis in steroid-secreting cells and the site of detoxification processes in other cells. As the sarcoplasmic reticulum (see Chapter 3), it plays an important role in skeletal and cardiac muscle.

Golgi Complex

The Golgi complex is a collection of membranous tubules and vesicles. It is usually located near the nucleus, and is particularly prominent in actively secreting gland cells. Hormones and enzymes are stored in protein-secreting cells as membrane-enclosed **secretion granules,** and these granules are produced in the Golgi complex. Thus, the Golgi complex "packages" proteins. The complex is also the site of formation of lysosomes (see below), and it adds certain carbohydrates to proteins to form glycoproteins. These carbohydrate-containing proteins on the cell surface play important roles in the association of cells to form tissues.

Mitochondria

Although their morphology varies somewhat from cell to cell, each mitochondrion (Figs 1–1, 1–3) is in essence a sausage-shaped structure. It is made up of an outer membrane and an inner membrane that is folded to form shelves **(cristae).** The mitochondria are the power-generating units of the cell and are most plentiful and best developed in parts of cells where energy-requiring processes take place. The chemical reactions occurring in them are discussed in detail in textbooks of biochemistry. The outer membrane of each mitochondrion is studded with the enzymes concerned with biologic oxidations, providing raw materials for the reactions occurring inside the mitochondrion. The interior of the mitochondrion contains the enzymes con-

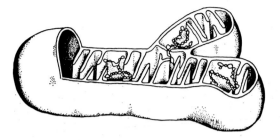

Figure 1–3. Cutaway drawing of a mitochondrion, showing the inner and outer membranes. The inner membrane is folded, forming shelves (cristae). The coiled structures represent possible arrangements of the mitochondrial DNA. Mitochondrial branching of the type shown here is not present in all cells. (Reproduced, with permission, from Nass: Mitochondrial DNA: Advances, problems and goals. Science 165:25, 1969. Copyright 1969 by the American Association for the Advancement of Science.)

Table 1–1. Some of the enzymes found in lysosomes and the cell components which are their substrates.

Enzyme	Substrate
Ribonuclease	RNA
Deoxyribonuclease	DNA
Phosphatase	Phosphate esters
Glycosidases	Complex carbohydrates: glycosides and polysaccharides
Aryl sulfatases	Sulfate esters
Collagenase	Proteins
Cathepsins	Proteins

cerned with the citric acid cycle and the respiratory chain enzymes by which the 2-carbon fragments produced by metabolism are burned to CO_2 and water. In this process electrons are transferred along the respiratory enzyme chain. Coupled with the electron transfer is **oxidative phosphorylation**, the synthesis of the high-energy phosphate compound, **adenosine triphosphate (ATP)**. This ubiquitous molecule is the principal energy source for energy-requiring actions in animals and plants. The inner membrane of the mitochondrion appears to be made up of repeating units, each of which contains a basepiece, a stalk, and a spherical headpiece. The basepieces contain the enzymes of the electron transfer chain, and the stalks and headpieces contain adenosine triphosphatase and other enzymes concerned with the synthesis and metabolism of ATP.

The mitochondria contain DNA and can synthesize protein. It now appears that the mitochondrial DNA represents a second genetic system in the cell. However, the mitochondrial DNA alone does not contain enough genetic information to code for all mitochondrial components, and the nuclear and mitochondrial genetic systems apparently interact in the formation of the protein systems in the mitochondria.

Lysosomes

In the cytoplasm of the cell, there are large, somewhat irregular structures surrounded by membrane which may contain fragments of other cell structures. These organelles are the **lysosomes**. Some of the granules of the granulocytic white blood cells are lysosomes. Each lysosome contains a variety of enzymes (Table 1–1) which would cause the destruction of most cellular components if the enzymes were not separated from the rest of the cell by the membrane of the lysosome.

The lysosomes function as a form of digestive system for the cell. Exogenous substances such as bacteria which become engulfed by the cell end up in membrane-lined vacuoles. A vacuole of this type (**phagocytic vacuole**) may merge with a lysosome, permitting the contents of the vacuole and the lysosome to mix within a common membrane. Some of the products of the "digestion" of the engulfed material are absorbed through the walls of the vacuole, and the remnants are dumped from the cell by rupture of the vacuole to the exterior of the cell. The lysosomes also engulf worn out components of the cell in which they are located, forming **autophagic vacuoles**. When a cell dies, lysosomal enzymes cause autolysis of the remnants. In vitamin A intoxication and certain other conditions, lysosomal enzymes are released to the exterior of the cell with resultant breakdown of intercellular material. There is evidence that in gout, phagocytes ingest uric acid crystals, and that such ingestion triggers the release of lysosomal enzymes which contribute to the inflammatory response in the joints. When one of the lysosomal enzymes is congenitally absent, the lysosomes become engorged with one of the materials they normally degrade. This eventually disrupts the cells that contain the defective lysosomes and leads to one of the **lysosomal storage diseases.** More than 25 such diseases have been described. They are generally rare, but they include such widely known disorders as Tay-Sachs disease.

Centrioles

In the cytoplasm of most cells there are 2 short cylinders called **centrioles**. The centrioles are located near the nucleus, and they are arranged so that they are at right angles to each other. Tubules in groups of 3 run longitudinally in the walls of the centriole (Fig 1–1). There are 9 of these triplets spaced at regular intervals around the circumference. **Cilia**, the hair-like motile processes which in higher animals extend from various types of epithelial cells, also have an array of 9 tubular structures in their walls, but they have in addition a pair of tubules in the center and there are 2 rather than 3 tubules in each of the 9 circumferential structures. The **basal granule**, on the other hand, which is the structure to which a cilium is anchored, has 9 circumferential triplets, like a centriole.

The centrioles seem to be concerned with the movement of the chromosomes during cell division. They duplicate themselves at the start of mitosis, and the pairs move apart to form the poles of the mitotic spindle. In multinucleate cells, there is a pair of centrioles near each nucleus.

Microtubules & Microfilaments

Many cells contain **microtubules**, long hollow structures about 25 nm in diameter, and **microfilaments**, solid fibers 4–6 nm in diameter. The microtubules and microfilaments are found in the mitotic spindles of dividing cells and are involved in the movement of the chromosomes. They are also involved in cell movement, in the processes which move secretion granules within cells, and in the movement of proteins within cell membranes. The structure of the microtubules is disrupted by the drug colchicine. The microtubules are made up of actin, the contractile protein in muscle (see Chapter 3), and the contractile protein myosin is also found in many kinds of cells. The function of the microfilaments is disrupted by cytochalasin, a compound secreted by certain fungi. Microtubules may make up the structures or "tracks" on which chromosomes and secretion granules move, and microfilaments may be responsible for the motion.

Secretion Granules

Secretion granules in cells which secrete proteins have been mentioned in the section on the Golgi complex. Typical examples include the granules of tropic hormones in the anterior lobe of the pituitary gland, the granules of renin in the juxtaglomerular cells of the kidney, and the granules of proteolytic enzyme precursors in the exocrine cells of the pancreas.

The proteins in these granules are synthesized in the endoplasmic reticulum, packaged into membrane-enclosed granules in the Golgi apparatus, and stored in the cytoplasm until they are extruded from the cell by exocytosis (see below).

Other Structures in Cells

If cells are homogenized and the resulting suspension is centrifuged, various cellular components can be isolated. The nuclei sediment first, followed by the mitochondria. High-speed centrifugation that generates forces of 100,000 times gravity or more causes a fraction made up of granules called the **microsomes** to sediment. This fraction includes the ribosomes, but it is not homogeneous and includes other granular material as well. The ribosomes and other components can be isolated from the microsomal fraction by further ultracentrifugation or other technics. One particle fraction isolated in this way contains oxidases capable of reducing O_2 to hydrogen peroxide and then to water. These particles have been called **peroxisomes**.

BODY FLUID COMPARTMENTS

Organization of the Body

The cells which make up the bodies of all but the simplest multicellular animals, both aquatic and terrestrial, exist in an "internal sea" of **extracellular fluid (ECF)** enclosed within the integument of the animal. From this fluid the cells take up O_2 and nutrients; into it, they discharge metabolic waste products. The ECF is more dilute than present-day sea water, but its composition closely resembles that of the primordial oceans in which, presumably, all life originated.

In animals with a closed vascular system, the ECF is divided into 2 components: the **interstitial fluid** and the circulating **blood plasma**. The plasma and the cellular elements of the blood, principally red blood cells, fill the vascular system, and together they constitute

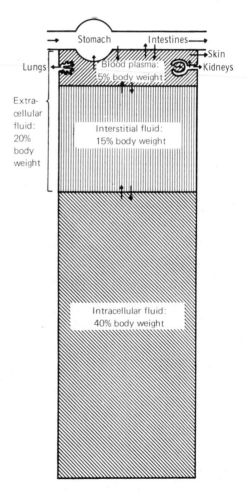

Figure 1–4. Body fluid compartments. Arrows represent fluid movement. Transcellular fluids, which constitute a very small percentage of total body fluids, are not shown. (Modified and reproduced, with permission, from Gamble: *Chemical Anatomy, Physiology, and Pathology of Extracellular Fluid,* 6th ed. Harvard Univ Press, 1954.)

the **total blood volume**. The interstitial fluid is that part of the ECF which is outside the vascular system, bathing the cells. The special fluids lumped together as transcellular fluids are discussed below. About a third of the **total body water (TBW)** is extracellular; the remaining two-thirds are intracellular (**intracellular fluid**).

Size of the Fluid Compartments

In the average young adult male, 18% of the body weight is protein and related substances, 7% is mineral, and 15% is fat. The remaining 60% is water. The distribution of this water is shown in Fig 1–4.

The intracellular component of the body water accounts for about 40% of body weight and the extracellular component about 20%. Approximately 25% of the extracellular component is in the vascular system (plasma = 5% of body weight), and 75% outside the blood vessels (interstitial fluid = 15% of body weight). The total blood volume is about 8% of body weight.

Measurement of Body Fluid Volumes

It is theoretically possible to measure the size of each of the body fluid compartments by injecting substances which will stay in only one compartment and then calculating the volume of fluid in which the test substance is distributed (the **volume of distribution** of the injected material). The volume of distribution is equal to the amount injected (minus any which has been removed from the body by metabolism or excretion during the time allowed for mixing) divided by the concentration of the substance in the sample. *Example:* 150 mg of sucrose are injected into a 70 kg man. The plasma sucrose level after mixing is 0.01 mg/ml, and 10 mg have been excreted or metabolized during the mixing period. The volume of distribution of the sucrose is

$$\frac{150 \text{ mg} - 10 \text{ mg}}{0.01 \text{ mg/ml}} = 14{,}000 \text{ ml}$$

Since 14,000 ml is the space in which the sucrose was distributed, it is also called the **sucrose space**.

Volumes of distribution can be calculated for any substance that can be injected into the body provided the concentration in the body fluids and the amount removed by excretion and metabolism can be accurately measured.

Although the principle involved in such measurements is simple, there are a number of complicating factors which must be considered. The material injected must be nontoxic, must mix evenly throughout the compartment being measured, must have no effect of its own on the distribution of water or other substances in the body, and must be unchanged by the body during the mixing period. It also should be relatively easy to measure.

Plasma Volume, Total Blood Volume, & Red Cell Volume

Plasma volume has been measured by using dyes which become bound to plasma protein—particularly Evans blue (T-1824). Plasma volume can also be measured by injecting serum albumin labeled with radioactive iodine. Suitable aliquots of the injected solution and plasma samples obtained after injection are counted in a scintillation counter. An average value is 3500 ml (5% of the body weight of a 70 kg man, assuming unit density).

If the plasma volume and the hematocrit are known, **total blood volume** can be calculated by multiplying the plasma volume by

$$\frac{100}{100 - \text{hematocrit}}$$

Example: The hematocrit is 38 and the plasma volume 3500 ml. The total blood volume is

$$3500 \times \frac{100}{100 - 38} = 5645 \text{ ml}$$

The **red cell volume** (volume occupied by all the circulating red cells in the body) can be determined by subtracting the plasma volume from the total blood volume. It may also be measured independently, by injecting tagged red blood cells and, after mixing has occurred, measuring the fraction of the red cells that is tagged. A commonly used tag is ^{51}Cr, a radioactive isotope of chromium which is attached to the cells by incubating them in a suitable chromium solution. Isotopes of iron and phosphorus (^{59}Fe and ^{32}P) and antigenic tagging have also been employed.

Extracellular Fluid Volume

The ECF volume is difficult to measure because the limits of this space are ill-defined and because few substances mix rapidly in all parts of the space while remaining exclusively extracellular. The lymph cannot be separated from the ECF, and is measured with it. Many substances enter the cerebrospinal fluid (CSF) slowly because of the blood-brain barrier (see Chapter 32). Equilibration is slow with joint fluid and aqueous humor and with the ECF in relatively avascular tissues such as dense connective tissue, cartilage, and some parts of bone. Substances which distribute in ECF appear in glandular secretions and in the contents of the gastrointestinal tract. Because they are not strictly part of the ECF, these fluids, as well as CSF, the fluids in the eye, and a few other special fluids, are called **transcellular fluids**. Their volume is relatively small.

Perhaps the most accurate measurement of ECF volume is that obtained by using inulin. Radioactive inulin has been prepared by substituting ^{14}C for one of the carbon atoms of the molecule; and when this material is used, inulin levels are easily determined by counting the samples with suitable radiation detectors. Mannitol and sucrose have also been used to measure ECF volume. Because chloride ions, for example, are largely extracellular in location, radioactive isotopes of chloride (^{36}Cl and ^{38}Cl) have been used for determination of ECF volume. However, some chloride is known to be intracellular. The same objection applies to ^{82}Br, which interchanges with chloride in the body. Other anions which have been used include sulfate, thiosulfate, thiocyanate, and ferrocyanide.

Careful measurement with each of these substances gives a range of values, which indicates that each has a slightly different volume of distribution. A generally accepted value for ECF volume is 20% of the body weight, or about 14 liters in a 70 kg man (3.5 liters = plasma; 10.5 liters = interstitial fluid).

Interstitial Fluid Volume

The interstitial fluid space cannot be measured directly since it is difficult to sample interstitial fluid and since substances which equilibrate in interstitial fluid also equilibrate in plasma. The volume of the interstitial fluid can be calculated by subtracting the plasma volume from the ECF volume. The ECF volume/intracellular fluid volume ratio is larger in infants and children than it is in adults, but the absolute volume of ECF in children is, of course, smaller than it is in adults. Therefore, dehydration develops more rapidly and is frequently more severe in children than in adults.

Intracellular Fluid Volume

The intracellular fluid volume cannot be measured directly, but it can be calculated by subtracting the ECF volume from the total body water (TBW). TBW can be measured by the same dilution principle used to measure the other body spaces. Deuterium oxide (D_2O, heavy water) is most frequently used. D_2O has properties which are slightly different from H_2O, but in equilibration experiments for measuring body water it gives accurate results. Tritium oxide and aminopyrine have also been used for this purpose.

The water content of lean body tissue is constant at $71-72$ ml/100 g of tissue, but since fat is relatively free of water the ratio of TBW to body weight varies with the amount of fat present. In young men, water constitutes about 60% of body weight. The values for women are somewhat lower. In both sexes the values tend to decrease with age (see Table 1−2).

Table 1−2. TBW (as percentage of body weight) in relation to age and sex.*

Age	Male	Female
10−18	59%	57%
18−40	61%	51%
40−60	55%	47%
Over 60	52%	46%

*Modified and reproduced, with permission, from Edelman & Liebman: Anatomy of body water and electrolytes. Am J Med 27:256, 1959.

UNITS FOR MEASURING CONCENTRATION OF SOLUTES

In considering the effects of various physiologically important substances and the interactions between them, the number of molecules, electrical charges, or particles of a substance per unit volume of a particular body fluid are often more meaningful than simply the weight of the substance per unit volume. For this reason, concentrations are frequently expressed in mols, equivalents, or osmols.

Mols

The mol is defined as the gram-molecular weight of a substance, ie, the molecular weight of the substance in grams. Each mol consists of approximately 6 $\times 10^{23}$ molecules. The millimol (mmol) is 1/1000 of a mol and the micromol (μmol) is 1/1,000,000 of a mol. Thus, 1 mol of NaCl = 23 + 35.5 g = 58.5 g, and 1 mmol = 58.5 mg.

Equivalents

The concept of electrical equivalence is important in physiology because many of the important solutes in the body are in the form of charged particles. One equivalent (Eq) is 1 mol of an ionized substance divided by its valence. One mol of NaCl dissociates into 1 Eq of Na^+ and 1 Eq of Cl^-. One Eq of Na^+ = 23 g/1 = 23 g; but 1 Eq of Ca^{++} = 40 g/2 = 20 g. The milliequivalent (mEq) is 1/1000 of an equivalent.

Electrical equivalence is not necessarily the same as chemical equivalence. A gram equivalent is that weight of a substance which is chemically equivalent to 8.000 g of oxygen. The normality (N) of a solution is the number of gram equivalents in 1 liter. A 1 N solution of hydrochloric acid contains 1 + 35.5 g/liter = 36.5 g/liter.

Osmols

When dealing with concentrations of osmotically active particles, the amounts of these particles are usually expressed in osmols. One osmol (Osm) equals the molecular weight of the substance in grams divided by the number of *freely moving particles* each molecule liberates in solution. The milliosmol (mOsm) is 1/1000 of 1 osmol. Osmosis is discussed in detail in a later section of this chapter.

The **osmolal concentration** of a substance in a fluid is measured by the degree to which it depresses the freezing point, 1 mol/liter of ideal solute depressing the freezing point 1.86° C. The number of mOsm/ liter in a solution equals the freezing point depression divided by 0.00186. The **osmolarity** is the number of osmols per liter of solution—eg, plasma—while the **osmolality** is the number of osmols per kg of solvent. Therefore, osmolarity is affected by the volume of the various solutes in the solution and the temperature, while the osmolality is not. Osmotically active substances in the body are dissolved in water, and the density of water is 1, so osmolal concentrations can be

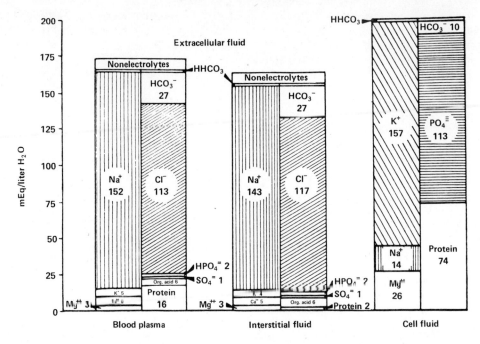

Figure 1–5. Electrolyte composition of human body fluids. Note that the values are in mEq/liter of water, not of body fluid. (Reproduced, with permission, from Leaf & Newburgh: *Significance of Body Fluids in Clinical Medicine,* 2nd ed. Thomas, 1955.)

expressed as Osm/liter of water. In this book, osmolal (rather than osmolar) concentrations are considered, and osmolality is expressed in mOsm/liter (of water).

COMPOSITION OF BODY FLUIDS

The distribution of electrolytes in the various compartments of the body fluid is shown in Fig 1–5. The figures for the intracellular phase ("cell fluid") are approximations. The composition of intracellular fluid varies somewhat depending upon the nature and function of the cell.

It is apparent from Fig 1–5 that electrolyte concentrations differ markedly in the various compartments. The most striking differences are the relatively low content of protein anions in interstitial fluid compared to intracellular fluid and plasma, and the fact that Na$^+$ and Cl$^-$ are largely extracellular, whereas most of the K$^+$ is intracellular.

FORCES PRODUCING MOVEMENT OF SUBSTANCES BETWEEN COMPARTMENTS

The differences in composition of the various body fluid compartments are due in large part to the nature of the barriers separating them. The membranes of the cells separate the interstitial fluid and intra-

cellular fluid, and the capillary wall separates the interstitial fluid from the plasma. The forces producing movement of water and other molecules across these barriers are diffusion, solvent drag, filtration, osmosis, active transport, and the processes of exocytosis and endocytosis.

Diffusion

Diffusion is the process by which a gas or a substance in solution expands, because of the motion of its particles, to fill all of the available volume. The particles (molecules or ions) of a substance dissolved in a solvent are in continuous random movement. In regions where they are abundant, they frequently collide. They therefore tend to spread from areas of high concentration to areas of low concentration until the concentration is uniform throughout the solution. Solute particles are, of course, moving both into and out of the area of high concentration; however, since more molecules move out than in, there is a **net flux** of the molecular species to the area of low concentration. The magnitude of the diffusing tendency from one area to another is proportionate to the difference in concentration of the substance in the 2 areas (the **concentration, or chemical gradient**). Diffusion of ions is also affected by their electrical charge. Whenever there is a difference in potential between 2 areas, positively charged ions move along this **electrical gradient** to the more negatively charged area; negatively charged ions move in the opposite direction.

In the body, diffusion occurs not only within fluid compartments but also from one compartment to another provided the barrier between the compartments is permeable to the diffusing substances. The diffusion rate of most solutes across the barriers is much slower than the diffusion rate in water, but diffusion is still a major force affecting the distribution of water and solutes.

Donnan Effect

When there is an ion on one side of a membrane that cannot diffuse through the membrane, the distribution of other ions to which the membrane is permeable is affected in a predictable way. For example, the negative charge of a nondiffusible anion hinders diffusion of the diffusible cations and favors diffusion of the diffusible anions. Consider the following situation:

$$
\begin{array}{c|c}
X & Y \\
\hline
K^+ & K^+ \\
Cl^- & Cl^- \\
Prot^- & \\
\end{array}
$$

in which the membrane (m) between compartments X and Y is impermeable to Prot⁻ but freely permeable to K⁺ and Cl⁻. Assume that the concentrations of the anions and of the cations on the 2 sides are initially equal. Cl⁻ tends to diffuse down its concentration gradient from Y to X and some K⁺ moves with the negatively charged Cl⁻. Therefore,

$$[K^+_X] > [K^+_Y] \text{ and } [Cl^-_X] < [Cl^-_Y]$$

Furthermore,

$$[K^+_X] + [Cl^-_X] + [Prot^-_X] > [K^+_Y] + [Cl^-_Y]$$

ie, there are more osmotically active particles on side X than on side Y.

Donnan and Gibbs showed that in the presence of a nondiffusible ion, the diffusible ions distribute themselves so that, at equilibrium, their concentration ratios are equal:

$$\frac{[K^+_X]}{[K^+_Y]} = \frac{[Cl^-_Y]}{[Cl^-_X]}$$

In the case of single cations and anions of the same valence, the product of the concentration of the diffusible ions on one side equals that on the other side. Thus,

$$[K^+_X]\ [Cl^-_X] = [K^+_Y]\ [Cl^-_Y]$$

Electrochemical neutrality would require that the sum of the anions on each side of the membrane equal the sum of the cations on that side. Neutrality is not achieved when the diffusible ions are distributed so that the product of their concentrations on the 2 sides of the membrane are equal. There is a slight excess of cations on side Y and a slight excess of anions on side X at equilibrium, and therefore a difference in electrical potential exists between X and Y. However, it should be emphasized that the difference between the number of anions and the number of cations on either side of the membrane is extremely small relative to the total numbers of anions and cations present.

The **Donnan effect** on the distribution of diffusible ions is of physiologic importance in the body because of the presence in cells and in plasma, but not in interstitial fluid, of large quantities of nondiffusible protein anions.

Solvent Drag

When solvent is moving in one direction (**bulk flow**), the solvent tends to drag along some molecules of solute. This force is called **solvent drag**. In most situations in the body, its effects are very small.

Filtration

Filtration is the process by which fluid is forced through a membrane or other barrier due to a difference in hydrostatic pressure on the 2 sides. The amount of fluid filtered in a given interval is proportionate to the difference in pressure and the surface area of the membrane. Molecules which are smaller in diameter than the pores of the membrane pass through with the fluid, and larger molecules are retained. Filtration of small molecules across the capillary walls occurs when the hydrostatic pressure in the vessels is greater than that in the extravascular tissues.

Osmosis

Osmosis is the movement of **solvent** molecules across a membrane into an area in which there is a higher concentration of a **solute** to which the membrane is impermeable. It is an immensely important factor in physiologic processes. The tendency for movement of solvent molecules to a region of greater solute concentration can be prevented by applying pressure to the more concentrated solution. The pressure necessary to prevent solvent migration is the **effective osmotic pressure** of the solution.

Osmotic pressure, like vapor pressure lowering, freezing point depression, and boiling point elevation, depends upon the number rather than the type of particles in a solution, ie, it is a fundamental colligative property of solutions. In effect, it is due to a reduction in the **activity** of the solvent molecules in a solution. The activity of a substance is its effective concentration as evaluated by its behavior in solution. When a solute is dissolved in a solvent, the activity of the solvent molecules is decreased. A homogeneous solution of a single substance has an osmotic pressure, but this pressure can be expressed—ie, the solution has an effective osmotic pressure—only when the solution is in contact with a more dilute solution across a membrane permeable to the solvent but not to the solute. In this situation, solvent molecules will diffuse from the area in which their activity is greater (the **dilute** solution) to the area in which their activity is less (the **concentrated** solution). Thus, if a 10% aqueous solution of glucose is placed in contact with distilled water across a membrane permeable to water but not to glucose, the

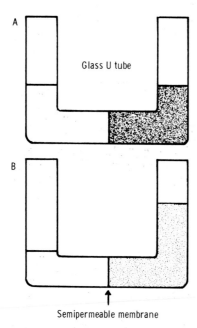

A

Glass U tube

B

↑
Semipermeable membrane

Figure 1–6. Demonstration of osmotic pressure. *A:* Immediately after adding a solution of glucose (shaded area) to the right arm of the U tube and an equal volume of water (clear space) to the other. *B:* After equilibration has taken place. The water has entered the glucose solution which has increased in volume and decreased in concentration.

volume of the glucose solution increases and its glucose concentration decreases as water molecules move into it from the water compartment (see Fig 1–6).

Osmotic pressure (P) is related to temperature and volume in the same way as the pressure of a gas:

$$P = \frac{nRT}{V}$$

where n is the number of particles, R the gas constant, T the absolute temperature, and V the volume. If T is held constant, it is clear that the osmotic pressure is proportionate to the number of particles in solution per unit volume of solution. If the solute is a nonionizing compound such as glucose, the osmotic pressure is a function of the number of glucose molecules present. If the solute ionizes and forms an **ideal** solution, each ion is an osmotically active particle. For example, NaCl would dissociate into Na^+ and Cl^- ions, so that each mol in solution would supply 2 Osm. One mol of Na_2SO_4 would dissociate into Na^+, Na^+, and $SO_4^=$, supplying 3 Osm. However, the body fluids are not ideal solutions, and although the dissociation of strong electrolytes is complete, the number of particles free to exert an osmotic effect is reduced due to interactions between the ions. Thus, it is actually the effective concentration, or activity in the body fluids, rather than the number of equivalents of an electrolyte in solution that determines its osmotic effect. This is

why, for example, 1 mmol/liter of NaCl in the body fluids contributes somewhat less than 2 mOsm/liter of osmotically active particles.

Osmolal Concentration of Plasma: Tonicity

The freezing point of normal human plasma averages −0.54° C, which corresponds to an osmolal concentration in plasma of 290 mOsm/liter. This is equivalent to an osmotic pressure of 7.3 atmospheres. The osmolality might be expected to be higher than this, because the sum of all the cation and anion equivalents in plasma is over 300. It is not this high because plasma is not an ideal solution, and ionic interactions reduce the number of particles free to exert an osmotic effect. Except when there has been insufficient time after a sudden change in composition for equilibration to occur, all fluid compartments of the body are apparently in or nearly in osmotic equilibrium. The term **tonicity** is used to describe the effective osmotic pressure of a solution relative to plasma. Solutions which have the same effective osmotic pressure as plasma are said to be **isotonic**; those with greater pressures are **hypertonic**; and those with lesser pressure are **hypotonic**. All solutions which are isosmotic with plasma—ie, have the same actual osmotic pressure or freezing point depression as plasma—would also be isotonic if it were not for the fact that some solutes diffuse into cells and others are metabolized. Thus, a 0.9% saline solution is isotonic because there is no net movement of the osmotically active particles in the solution into cells and the particles are not metabolized. However, urea diffuses rapidly into cells, so that the effective osmotic pressure drops when cells are suspended in an aqueous solution that initially contains 290 mOsm/liter of urea. Similarly, a 5% glucose solution is isotonic when initially infused intravenously, but glucose is metabolized, so the net effect is that of infusing a hypotonic solution.

It is important to note the relative contributions of the various plasma components to the total osmolal concentration of plasma. All but 20 of the 290 mOsm in each liter are contributed by Na^+ and its accompanying anions, principally Cl^- and HCO_3^-. Other cations and anions make a small contribution. Glucose normally makes a much smaller contribution—about 5 mOsm—because it does not dissociate and has a molecular weight of 180. The plasma proteins have a high molecular weight, so that, even though they are present in large quantities, they make a very small contribution to the plasma osmolality. The osmolal concentration of protein derivatives (other than electrolytes) is about 0.33 times the blood urea nitrogen (BUN), or approximately 6 mOsm/liter. Since plasma is not an ideal solution, the osmolality of the plasma can be estimated from the following formula:

Osmolality	=	2 [Na$^+$]	+	0.05 [Glucose]	+	0.33 [BUN]
(mOsm/liter)		(mEq/liter)		(mg/dl)		(mg/dl)

This formula is useful in evaluating patients as well as assessing the contributions of the various components to normal plasma osmolality. Hyperosmolality can cause coma.

Nonionic Diffusion

Some weak acids and bases are quite soluble in cell membranes in the undissociated form, whereas in the ionic form they cross membranes with difficulty. Consequently, molecules of the undissociated substance diffuse from one side of the membrane to the other and then dissociate, effectively moving ions from one side of the membrane to another. This phenomenon, which occurs in the gastrointestinal tract and kidneys, is called **nonionic diffusion.**

Carrier-Mediated Transport

In addition to moving across cell membranes by diffusion, osmosis, and the processes described above, ions and larger nonionized molecules are transported by carrier molecules in the membranes. When such **carrier-mediated transport** is from an area of greater concentration of the transported molecule to an area of lesser concentration, energy is not required and the process is called **facilitated diffusion.** In many instances, facilitated diffusion is regulated by hormones; eg, insulin increases the facilitated diffusion of glucose into muscle cells. When, on the other hand, the transport is from an area of lesser to an area of greater concentration, the process requires energy and is referred to as **active transport.** The energy is supplied by the metabolism of the cells, generally through adenosine triphosphate (APT). Active transport is of major importance throughout the body.

Transport of Proteins & Other Large Molecules

In certain situations proteins enter cells, and a number of hormones secreted by endocrine cells are proteins or large polypeptides. Proteins and other large molecules enter cells by the process of endocytosis, and proteins and polypeptides are secreted by exocytosis. These processes provide an explanation of how large molecules can enter and leave cells without disrupting cell membranes.

In **exocytosis,** which has also been called **reverse pinocytosis,** or **emeiocytosis** ("cell vomiting"), the membrane around a vacuole or secretion granule fuses with the cell membrane and the region of fusion breaks down, leaving the contents of the vacuole or secretion granule outside the cell and the cell membrane intact (Fig 1–7). This requires Ca^+ and energy.

Endocytosis is the reverse process. One form of endocytosis, called **phagocytosis** ("cell eating"), is the process by which bacteria, dead tissue, or other bits of material visible under the microscope are engulfed by cells such as the polymorphonuclear leukocytes of the blood. The material makes contact with the cell membrane, which then invaginates. The invagination is pinched off, leaving the engulfed material in the membrane-enclosed vacuole and the cell membrane intact. **Pinocytosis** ("cell drinking") is essentially the same process, the only difference being that the substances ingested are in solution and hence not visible under the microscope. In the cell, the membrane around a **pinocytic** or **phagocytic vacuole** may fuse with that of a lysosome, mixing the "digestive" enzymes in the lysosome with the contents of the vacuole. It has also been assumed that the membrane around vacuoles can be digested away, but the ultimate fate of the vacuoles is uncertain.

The rate of pinocytosis is greatly increased by substances called **inducers.** In mammalian cells, proteins such as albumins and globulins are potent inducers. Insulin apparently acts as an inducer in fat cells. There is evidence that pinocytosis, and, presumably, phagocytosis are active processes in the sense that they do not occur when the energy-producing processes in the cell are blocked.

It is apparent that exocytosis adds to the total amount of membrane in the cell, and, if membrane were not removed elsewhere at an equivalent rate, the cell would enlarge. However, removal of membrane occurs by endocytosis, and such exocytosis-endocytosis coupling maintains the cell at its normal size.

CELL MEMBRANE & RESTING MEMBRANE POTENTIALS

Ion Distribution Across Cell Membranes

The unique properties of the cell membranes are responsible for the differences in the composition of

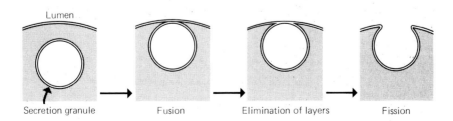

Figure 1–7. Exocytosis. In this process, the secretion granule moves up to the cell membrane and its membrane fuses with the cell membrane. The area of fusion then breaks down, leaving the contents of the granule outside of the cell. (Modified from Palade G: Intracellular aspects of the process of protein synthesis. Science 189:347, 1975.)

Table 1–3. Concentration of some ions inside and outside frog skeletal muscle cells.*

Ion	Concentration (mmol/liter H_2O)		Equilibrium Potential (mV)
	Inside Cell	Outside Cell	
Na^+	13.0	110.0	+55
K^+	138.0	2.5	−101
Cl^-	3.0	90.0	−86
Resting potential = −99 mV			

*Data from DeVoe: Principles of cell homeostasis. In: *Medical Physiology*, 13th ed. Vol 1. Mountcastle VB (editor). Mosby, 1974.

Table 1–5. Sizes of hydrated ions relative to $K^+ = 1.00$. The diameter of the hydrated K^+ is about 0.4 nm.*

Cl^-	0.96	CH_3COO^-	1.80
K^+	1.00	$SO_4^=$	1.84
Na^+	1.47	$H_2PO_4^-$	2.04
HCO_3^-	1.65	$HPO_4^=$	2.58

*Data from Eccles: *The Physiology of Nerve Cells.* Johns Hopkins Univ Press, 1957.

intracellular and interstitial fluid. Average values for the composition of intracellular fluid in humans are shown in Fig 1–5, and specific values for frog skeletal muscle are shown in Table 1–3.

Membrane Potentials

There is a potential difference across the membranes of most if not all cells, with the inside of the cells negative to the exterior. By convention, this **resting membrane potential** or **steady potential** is written with a minus sign, signifying that the inside is negative to the exterior. Its magnitude varies considerably from tissue to tissue, ranging from −10 to −100 mV.

Membrane Permeability

Cell membranes are practically impermeable to intracellular protein and other organic anions, which make up most of the intracellular anions and are usually represented by the symbol A^-. However, they are moderately permeable to Na^+, and rather freely permeable to K^+ and Cl^-. K^+ permeability is 50–100 times greater than Na^+ permeability. The permeability values listed in Table 1–4 for the cell membrane of frog skeletal muscle are representative. It should be noted that permeability of these ions in the membrane, although appreciable, is a fraction of their permeability in water.

Table 1–4. Permeability coefficients (P) for cell membrane of frog skeletal muscle. Values are equivalents diffusing through 1 sq cm of membrane under specified conditions and have the dimensions of cm/sec. For purposes of comparison, P_{K^+} in water is 10.*

P_{A^-}	~ 0
P_{Na^+}	2×10^{-8}
P_{K^+}	2×10^{-6}
P_{Cl^-}	4×10^{-6}

*Data from Hodgkin & Horowicz: The influence of potassium and chloride ions on the membrane potential of single muscle fibers. J Physiol 148:127, 1959.

The reason for the differences in the permeability of cell membranes to various small ions is unknown. It is tempting to speculate that the membranes contain pores and that the differences in permeability can be explained on the basis of ion size. Most nonjunctional cell membranes behave as if they contained pores approximately 0.7 nm in diameter. The sizes of some of the principal inorganic ions are listed in Table 1–5.

The ions in the body are hydrated, and although the atomic weight of potassium (39) is greater than that of sodium (23), the hydrated sodium ion, ie, Na^+ with its full complement of water, is larger than the hydrated potassium ion. Therefore, one might expect Na^+ to move through membranes with greater difficulty than K^+. However, the postulated membrane pores have not been visualized, and ions may traverse the membrane attached to carriers, or by some other method. Fortunately, an exact explanation of the way ions move passively across membranes is not necessary for an analysis of ion fluxes; for this purpose, the empirical data on ion permeability are sufficient.

Forces Acting on Ions

The forces acting across the cell membrane on each ion can be analyzed. Chloride ions are present in higher concentration in the ECF than in the cell interior, and they tend to diffuse along this **concentration gradient** into the cell. The interior of the cell is negative relative to the exterior, and chloride ions are pushed out of the cell along this **electrical gradient**. An equilibrium is reached at which Cl^- influx and Cl^- efflux are equal. The membrane potential at which this equilibrium exists is the **equilibrium potential**. Its magnitude can be calculated from the **Nernst equation**, as follows:

$$E_{Cl} = \frac{RT}{FZ_{Cl}} \ln \frac{[Cl_o^-]}{[Cl_i^-]}$$

Where E_{Cl} = equilibrium potential for Cl^-
R = gas constant
T = absolute temperature
F = the faraday (number of coulombs per mol of charge)
Z_{Cl} = valence of Cl^- (−1)
$[Cl_i^-]$ = Cl^- concentration inside the cell
$[Cl_o^-]$ = Cl^- concentration outside the cell

Converting from the natural log to the base 10 log and replacing some of the constants with numerical values, the equation becomes:

$$E_{Cl} = 61.5 \log \frac{[Cl_i^-]}{[Cl_o^-]} \text{ at } 37° \text{ C}$$

Note that in converting to the simplified expression, the concentration ratio is reversed because the minus 1 valence of Cl⁻ has been removed from the expression.

The equilibrium potential for Cl⁻ (E_{Cl}) can be calculated in this fashion for frog skeletal muscle fibers; using the data in Table 1–3, the calculated value is −86 mV. This figure is close to the experimentally measured resting membrane potential for these cells. It therefore seems likely that no forces other than those represented by the chemical and electrical gradients need be invoked to explain the distribution of Cl⁻ across the membrane.

A similar equilibrium potential can be calculated for K⁺.

$$E_K = \frac{RT}{FZ_K} \ln \frac{[K_o^+]}{[K_i^+]} = 61.5 \log \frac{[K_o^+]}{[K_i^+]} \text{ at } 37° \text{ C}$$

Where E_K = equilibrium potential for K⁺
　　　Z_K = valence of K⁺ (+1)
　　　$[K_i^+]$ = K⁺ concentration inside the cell
　　　$[K_o^+]$ = K⁺ concentration outside the cell
　　　R, T, and F as above

In this case, the concentration gradient is outward and the electrical gradient inward. In the frog muscle cells, the calculated equilibrium potential for potassium (E_K) is − 101 mV. Since the resting membrane potential of −99 mV is almost identical, it is apparent that the distribution of K⁺ at rest can be explained primarily by passive forces. However, a small amount of K⁺ is actively transported into the cell as well (see below).

The situation for Na⁺ is quite different from that for K⁺ and Cl⁻. The direction of the chemical gradient for Na⁺ is inward, to the area where it is in lesser concentration, and the electrical gradient is in the same direction. Experiments with radioactive sodium have established the fact that the membrane has a relatively low but definite permeability to Na⁺ (Table 1–4). However, the intracellular Na⁺ remains low. Therefore, Na⁺ must be actively transported out of the cell against its electrical and chemical gradients.

The situation is apparently similar in some nerve fibers. In squid giant axon, for example, the resting membrane potential is −77 mV and the equilibrium potentials for K⁺, Cl⁻, and Na⁺ are −89, −48, and +49, respectively. The ion fluxes across the nerve cell membrane at rest are summarized in Fig 1–8. In red cells, on the other hand, the membrane potential is low (−9 mV) and near the Cl⁻ equilibrium potential, whereas both Na⁺ and K⁺ are actively transported across the cell membrane. Cl⁻ appears to be actively transported in some mammalian neurons and is actively transported in the kidney.

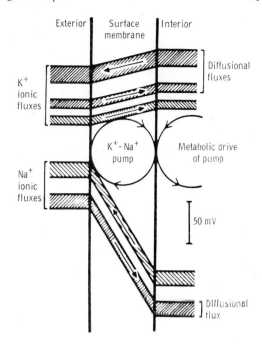

Figure 1–8. Na⁺ and K⁺ fluxes through the resting nerve cell membrane. The Na⁺ and K⁺ fluxes that are not labeled "diffusional fluxes" are due to active transport of these ions. The diffusional efflux of Na⁺, less than 1% of the influx, has been omitted. (Reproduced, with permission, from Eccles: *The Physiology of Nerve Cells.* Johns Hopkins Univ Press, 1957.)

The Sodium-Potassium Pump

The mechanism responsible for the active transport of sodium out of the cell and potassium into the cell is a **sodium-potassium pump** that is sometimes referred to simply as the **sodium pump**. The pump is located in the membrane. The energy for pumping is provided by ATP, and an adequate supply of ATP depends on the metabolic processes in the cell. Application of ATP by micropipet to the inside of the membrane increases transport, while application to the outside has no effect. The transport of Na⁺ is coupled to that of K⁺, but the coupling ratio of Na⁺ to K⁺ varies from 1 to 4 or more. The activity of the pump is also directly proportional to the intracellular concentration of Na⁺. The rate of Na⁺ extrusion from the cell is thus proportionate to the amount of Na⁺ in it, a feedback arrangement that tends to keep the internal ionic composition of the cell constant. When the coupling ratio of Na⁺ to K⁺ is 1, there is no net movement of charge by the pump, and the pump is said to be nonelectrogenic. However, when more than 1 Na⁺ is transported out for each K⁺ transported into the cell, there is a net flux of positive charge out of the cell with the production of hyperpolarization. Under these circumstances, the pump is **electrogenic**. The transport mechanism is inhibited by ouabain and related cardiac glycosides and by metabolic poisons which prevent the formation of ATP. It is markedly temperature dependent, as would be expected in view of its dependence on metabolic processes. When the temperature is reduced, Na^+ efflux and K^+ influx are reduced several times as much as the passive processes of Na^+ influx and K^+ efflux.

The details of the operation of the Na^+ and K^+ pump are currently the subject of intensive research. An enzyme that is intimately related to the pumping mechanism has been identified in red blood cells, brain cells, and the membranes of a great many other types of cells in a wide variety of species. This enzyme hydrolyzes ATP to adenosine diphosphate (ADP; see Chapter 17), and it is activated by Na^+ and K^+. It is therefore known as the **sodium-potassium-activated adenosine triphosphatase**, or **Na^+-K^+ ATPase**. Its concentration in cell membranes is proportionate to the rate of Na^+ and K^+ transport in the cells. It is a large lipoprotein with a molecular weight of 670,000 which requires Mg^{++} for activity and is inhibited by ouabain. There is evidence that it extends through the membrane and that it contains 2 polypeptide units which form a channel through the membrane. It is postulated to exist in 2 conformational states. In one, it has a binding site for Na^+ accessible only from the intracellular side of the membrane. Na^+ binding activates a change to the other conformation, which leaves Na^+ on the outside of the cell. In this second conformation, a K^+ binding site is accessible only from the outside of the cell. K^+ binding activates a change to the first configuration, and this leaves K^+ inside the cell. It appears that Na^+ binding is associated with phosphorylation of a component of the membrane and that K^+ binding is associated with dephosphorylation.

Genesis of the Membrane Potential

The distribution of ions across the cell membrane and the nature of this membrane provide the explanation for the membrane potential. K^+ diffuses out of the cell along its concentration gradient, while the nondiffusible anion component stays in the cell, creating a potential difference across the membrane. There is thus a slight excess of cations outside of the membrane and a slight excess of anions inside it. It should be emphasized, however, that the number of ions responsible for the membrane potential is a minute fraction of the total number present. Na^+ influx does not compensate for the K^+ efflux because the membrane at rest is much less permeable to Na^+ than K^+. Cl^- diffuses inward down its concentration gradient, but its movement is balanced by the electrical gradient. The sodium pump does not generate the membrane potential when the coupling ratio is 1, because it moves an equal number of cations in each direction. However, it maintains the concentration gradients on which the existence of the membrane potential depends. If the pump is shut off by the administration of metabolic inhibitors, Na^+ enters the cell, K^+ leaves it, and the membrane potential declines. The rate of this decline varies with the size of the cell. In large cells, it takes hours, but in nerve fibers with diameters of less than 1 μm, complete depolarization can occur in less than 4 minutes.

The magnitude of the membrane potential at any given time depends, of course, upon the distribution of Na^+, K^+, and Cl^-, and the permeability of the membrane to each of these ions. An equation that describes this relationship with considerable accuracy is the **Goldman constant-field equation**:

$$V = \frac{RT}{F} \ln \left(\frac{P_{K^+}[K_o^+] + P_{Na^+}[Na_o^+] + P_{Cl^-}[Cl_i^-]}{P_{K^+}[K_i^+] + P_{Na^+}[Na_i^+] + P_{Cl^-}[Cl_o^-]} \right)$$

where V is the membrane potential, R the gas content, T the absolute temperature, F the faraday, and P_{K^+}, P_{Na^+}, and P_{Cl^-} the permeability of the membrane to K^+, Na^+, and Cl^-, respectively. The brackets signify concentration, and i and o refer to the inside and outside of the cell. Since P_{Na^+} is low relative to P_{K^+} and P_{Cl^-} in the resting cells, Na^+ contributes little to the value of V. As would be predicted from the Goldman equation, changes in external Na^+ produce little change in the resting membrane potential whereas increases in external K^+ decrease it.

Variations in Membrane Potential

If the resting membrane potential is decreased by the passage of a current through the membrane, the electrical gradient which keeps K^+ inside the cell is decreased and there is an increase in K^+ diffusion out of the cell. This K^+ efflux and the simultaneous movement of Cl^- into the cell result in a net movement of positive charge out of the cell, with consequent restoration of the resting membrane potential. When the membrane potential increases, these ions move in the opposite direction. These processes occur in all polarized cells, and tend to keep the resting membrane potential of the cells constant within narrow limits. However, in nerve and muscle cells, reduction of the membrane potential triggers a sudden increase in Na^+ permeability. This unique feature permits these cells to generate self-propagating impulses which are transmitted along their membranes for great distances. These impulses are considered in detail in Chapter 2.

Effects of the Sodium-Potassium Pump on Metabolic Rate

Active transport of Na^+ and K^+ is one of the major energy-using processes in the body, and probably accounts for a large part of the basal metabolism. Furthermore, there is a direct link between Na^+ and K^+ transport and metabolism; the greater the rate of pumping, the more ADP is formed, and the available supply of ADP determines the rate at which ATP is formed by oxidative phosphorylation (see Chapter 17).

Effects of the Sodium-Potassium Pump on Cell Volume

In animals, the maintenance of normal cell volume and pressure depend on Na^+ and K^+ pumping. In the absence of such pumping, Cl^- and Na^+ would enter the cells down their concentration gradients, and water would follow along the osmotic gradient thus created, causing the cells to swell until the pressure inside them balanced the influx. This does not occur, and the osmolality and pressure of the cells remain the same as those of the interstitial fluid because Na^+ and K^+ are actively transported, the membrane potential is maintained, and $[Cl_i^-]$ remains low.

THE CAPILLARY WALL

The structure of the capillary wall, the barrier between the plasma and the interstitial fluid, varies from one vascular bed to another. However, in skeletal muscle and many other organs, water and relatively small solutes are the only substances that cross the wall with ease. The apertures in the wall (probably the junctions between the endothelial cells) are too small to permit plasma proteins and other colloids to pass through in significant quantities. The colloids have a high molecular weight but are present in large amounts. The capillary wall therefore behaves like a membrane impermeable to colloids, which exert an osmotic pressure of about 25 mm Hg. The colloid osmotic pressure due to the plasma colloids is called the **oncotic pressure**. Filtration across the capillary membrane due to the hydrostatic pressure head in the vascular system is opposed by the oncotic pressure. The balance between the hydrostatic and oncotic pressures controls exchanges across the capillary wall.

Moderate amounts of protein do cross the capillary walls and enter the lymph. The size and frequency of the pores necessary to explain this movement have been calculated. Studies with the electron microscope have failed to demonstrate pores of the necessary size, but there are numerous vesicles in the capillary endothelium. Tagged protein molecules have been found in these vesicles, suggesting that proteins are transported out of capillaries across endothelial cells by pinocytosis followed by exocytosis on the interstitial side of the cells. Transport by this putative mechanism has been called **vesicular transport** or **cytopempsis**.

SODIUM & POTASSIUM DISTRIBUTION & TOTAL BODY OSMOLALITY

The foregoing discussion of the various compartments of the body fluids and the barriers between them facilitates consideration of the total body stores of the principal cations, Na^+ and K^+.

Total Body Sodium

The total amount of exchangeable Na^+ in the body (Na_E)—as opposed to its concentration in any particular body fluid—can be determined by the same dilution principle used to measure the body fluid compartments. A radioactive isotope of sodium (usually

Table 1–6. Distribution of sodium in the body in mEq/kg body weight and percentage of total body sodium.*

	mEq/kg	% of Total
Total	58	100
Exchangeable body sodium (Na_E)	41	70.7
Total intracellular	5.2	9.0
Total extracellular	52.8	91.0
Plasma	6.5	11.2
Interstitial fluid	16.8	29.0
Dense connective tissue and cartilage	6.8	11.7
Bone sodium		
Exchangeable	6.4	11.0
Nonexchangeable	14.8	25.5
Transcellular	1.5	2.6

*Data courtesy of IS Edelman.

^{24}Na) is injected, and after equilibration the fraction of the sodium in the body which is radioactive is determined. The fraction of a substance that is radioactive—ie, the concentration of radioactive molecules divided by the concentration of radioactive plus nonradioactive molecules—is the **specific activity** (SA) of the substance. The SA of sodium in plasma after the injection of ^{24}Na, for example, is

$$\frac{^{24}Na \text{ (counts per minute/liter)}}{^{24}Na + \text{nonradioactive Na (mEq/liter)}}$$

The total exchangeable body sodium (Na_E) =

$$\frac{^{24}Na \text{ injected} - {}^{24}Na \text{ excreted}}{SA \text{ of plasma}}$$

The average normal value for Na_E in healthy adults is 41 mEq/kg, whereas the total amount of Na^+ in the body is about 58 mEq/kg. Therefore, approximately 17 mEq/kg are not available for exchange. The vast majority of this nonexchangeable Na^+ is in the hydroxyapatite crystal lattice of bone. The amount of Na^+ in the various body compartments is summarized in Table 1–6.

Total Body Potassium

The total exchangeable body K^+ can be determined by measuring the dilution of radioactive potassium (^{42}K). The average value in young adult men is about 45 mEq/kg body weight. It is somewhat less in women, and declines slightly with advancing age. About 10% of the total body K^+ is bound, mostly in red blood cells, brain, and bone, and the remaining 90% is exchangeable (Fig 1–9).

Interrelationships of Sodium & Potassium

Since the salts of sodium and potassium dissociate in the body to such a great extent, and since they are so plentiful, they determine in large part the osmolality of the body fluids. A change in the amount of electrolyte in one compartment is followed by predict-

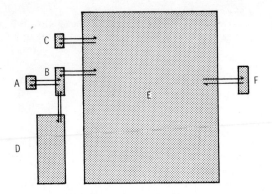

A: Plasma potassium, 0. 4% of total body potassium
B: Interstitial lymph potassium, 1%
C: Dense connective tissue and cartilage potassium, 0. 4%
D: Bone potassium, 7. 6%
E: Intracellular potassium, 89. 6%
F: Transcellular potassium, 1%

Figure 1–9. Body potassium distribution. Figures are percentages of total body potassium. (Data from Edelman & Liebman: Am J Med 27:256, 1959.)

able changes in the electrolyte concentration in the others. Fig 1–10 shows, for example, the changes in osmolal concentration and volume of the intracellular and extracellular fluid spaces that follow removal of 500 mOsm of extracellular electrolyte. Loss of electrolyte in excess of water from the ECF leads to hypotonicity of the ECF relative to the intracellular fluid. Consequently, water moves into the cells by osmosis until osmotic equilibrium between the ECF and the intracellular fluid is again attained.

Total Body Osmolality

Since Na^+ is the principal cation of the plasma, the plasma osmotic pressure correlates well with the plasma Na^+ level. However, plasma Na^+ does not necessarily correlate well with Na_E. Total body osmolality reflects the electrolyte concentration in the body, ie, the total exchangeable body sodium plus the total exchangeable body potassium divided by the total body water:

$$\frac{Na_E + K_E}{TBW}$$

Because this latter figure has been found to correlate well with plasma Na^+, plasma Na^+ is a relatively accurate measure of total body osmolality. It is worth noting that plasma Na^+ can be affected by changes in any

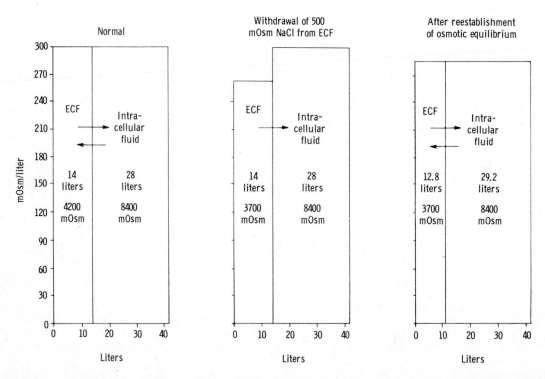

Figure 1–10. Response of body fluid to removal of 500 mOsm from ECF without change in total body water in a 70 kg man. The hypotonicity of the ECF causes water to enter cells until osmotic equilibrium is reestablished. Total mOsm in body after removal of 500 mOsm = (14 × 300) + (28 × 300)–500 = 12,100 mOsm. New osmotic equilibrium = 12,100/(28 + 14) = 288 mOsm/liter. This means that the new volume of the ECF will be (4200–500)/288 = 12.8 liters, and the new volume of the intracellular fluid will be 8400/288 = 29.2 liters. (After Darrow & Yannet. Modified and reproduced, with permission, from Gamble: *Chemical Anatomy, Physiology, and Pathology of Extracellular Fluid.* Harvard Univ Press, 1942.)

of 3 body components: Na_E itself, K_E, or TBW. A detailed discussion of the effects of disease on electrolyte and water balance is beyond the scope of this book, but the facts discussed above are basic to any consideration of pathologic water and electrolyte changes.

Plasma K^+ levels are not a good indicator of the total body K^+ since most of the K^+ is in the cells. There is a correlation between the K^+ and H^+ content of plasma, the 2 rising and falling together.

pH & BUFFERS

The maintenance of a stable pH in the body fluids is essential to life. The pH of a solution is the logarithm to the base 10 of the reciprocal of the H^+ concentration ($[H^+]$), ie, the negative logarithm of the $[H^+]$. The pH of water, in which H^+ and OH^- ions are present in equal numbers, is 7.0. For each pH unit less than 7.0, the $[H^+]$ is increased tenfold; and for each pH unit above 7.0, it is decreased tenfold.

Buffers

The pH of the ECF is maintained at 7.40. In health, this value usually varies less than ±0.05 pH unit. Body pH is stabilized by the **buffering capacity** of the body fluids. A buffer is a substance which has the ability to bind or release H^+ in solution, thus maintaining the pH of the solution relatively constant despite the addition of considerable quantities of acid or base. One buffer in the body is carbonic acid, which is normally only slightly dissociated into H^+ and bicarbon-

ate: $H_2CO_3 \rightleftarrows H^+ + HCO_3^-$. If H^+ is added to a solution of carbonic acid, the equilibrium shifts and most of the added H^+ is removed from solution. If OH^- is added, H^+ and OH^- combine and more H_2CO_3 dissociates. Other buffers include the blood proteins and the proteins in cells. The quantitative aspects of buffering and the respiratory and renal adjustments that operate with the buffers to maintain a stable ECF pH of 7.40 are discussed elsewhere.

HOMEOSTASIS

The actual environment of the cells of the body is the interstitial component of the ECF. Since normal cell function depends upon the constancy of this fluid, it is not surprising that in higher animals an immense number of regulatory mechanisms have evolved to maintain it. To describe "the various physiologic arrangements which serve to restore the normal state, once it has been disturbed," W.B. Cannon coined the term **homeostasis**. The buffering properties of the body fluids and the renal and respiratory adjustments to the presence of excess acid or alkali are examples of homeostatic mechanisms. There are countless other examples, and a large part of physiology is concerned with regulatory mechanisms which act to maintain the constancy of the internal environment. Many of these regulatory mechanisms operate on the principle of negative feedback; deviations from a given normal setpoint are detected by a sensor, and signals from the sensor trigger compensatory changes which continue until the setpoint is again reached.

● ● ●

References: Section I.
Introduction

Altman PL, Katz PD (editors): *Cell Biology*. Federation of American Societies of Experimental Biology, 1976.

Berlin RD & others: The cell surface. N Engl J Med 292:515, 1975.

Bloom W, Fawcett DW: *A Textbook of Histology*, 10th ed. Saunders, 1975.

Cannon WB: *The Wisdom of the Body*. Norton, 1932.

Cohen SS: Are/were mitochondria and chloroplasts microorganisms? Am Sci 58:281, 1970.

Edelman GM: Surface modulation in cell recognition and cell growth. Science 192:218, 1976.

Haggis GH & others: *Introduction to Molecular Biology*, 2nd ed. Wiley, 1973.

Hayflick L: The cell biology of human aging. N Engl J Med 295:1302, 1976.

Jackson RL, Gotto AM Jr: Phospholipids in biology and medicine. N Engl J Med 290:24, 1974.

Kolodny EH: Lysosomal storage diseases. N Engl J Med 294:1217, 1976.

Loeb JN: The hyperosmolar state. N Engl J Med 290:1184, 1974.

Palade G: Intracellular aspects of the process of protein synthesis. Science 189:347, 1975.

Schwartz A, Lindenmayer GE, Allen JC: The sodium-potassium adenosine triphosphatase: Pharmacological, physiological, and biochemical aspects. Pharmacol Rev 27:3, 1975.

Stephens RE, Edds KT: Microtubules: Structure, chemistry, and function. Physiol Rev 56:709, 1976.

Weissman G, Claiborne R (editors): *Cell Membranes: Biochemistry, Cell Biology and Pathology*. HP Publishing Co, 1975.

Welt L: *Clinical Disorders of Hydration and Acid-Base Equilibrium*, 3rd ed. Little, Brown, 1971.

Wessells NK: How living cells change shape. Sci Am 225:76, Oct 1971.

Whaley WG, Dauwalder M, Kephart JE: Golgi apparatus: Influence on cell surfaces. Science 175:596, 1972.

Symposium: Comparative aspects of transport of hypertonic, isotonic and hypotonic solutions by epithelial membranes. Fed Proc 30:3, 1971.

Symposium: The nature and function of peroxisomes (microbodies, glyoxysomes). Ann NY Acad Sci 168:209, 1969.

II. Physiology of Nerve & Muscle Cells

2...

Excitable Tissue: Nerve

The human nervous system contains more than 10 billion neurons. These basic building blocks of the nervous system have evolved from primitive neuro-effector cells which respond to various stimuli by contracting. In higher animals, contraction has become the specialized function of muscle cells, while transmission of nerve impulses has become the specialized function of neurons.

NERVE CELLS

Morphology

A typical spinal motor neuron such as that shown in Fig 2–1 has 5–7 processes called **dendrites** which extend out from the cell body and arborize extensively. It also has a long fibrous **axon** which originates from a somewhat thickened area of the cell body, the **axon hillock**. A short distance from its origin, the axon acquires a sheath of **myelin**, a protein-lipid complex made up of many layers of unit membrane (Fig 2–2). The myelin sheath envelops the axon except at its ending and at periodic constrictions about 1 mm apart called the **nodes of Ranvier**. The axon ends in a number of **synaptic knobs**, which are also called **terminal buttons** or **axon telodendria**. These knobs contain granules or vesicles in which the synaptic transmitter secreted by the nerve is stored (see Chapter 4). Some mammalian neurons and most neurons in invertebrates are unmyelinated; the axons are invested in Schwann cells, but there has been no rotation of the axon to produce multiple layers of membrane (Fig 2–2).

The conventional terminology used above for the parts of a neuron works well enough for spinal motor neurons and interneurons, but it has obvious shortcomings in terms of "dendrites" and "axons" when it is applied to other types of neurons found in the nervous system (Fig 2–3). A terminology for the parts of neurons which generally harmonizes morphologic and functional considerations is shown in Fig 2–4. According to this terminology, the **dendritic zone** of the neuron is the receptor membrane of the neuron (see below and Chapters 4 and 5). The axon is the single, elongated cytoplasmic extension with the specialized function of conducting impulses away from the dendritic zone. The cell body is often located at the dendritic zone end of the axon, but it can be within the axon (eg, auditory neurons) or attached to the side of the axon (eg, cutaneous neurons). Its location makes no difference as far as the receptor function of the dendritic zone and the transmission function of the axon are concerned. It is worth pointing out, however, that some dendrites appear to be able to

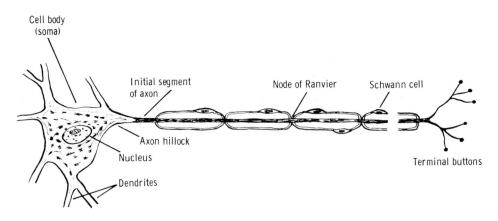

Figure 2–1. Motor neuron with myelinated axon.

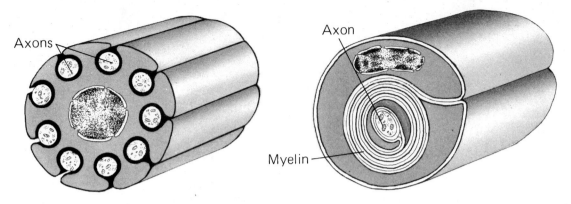

Figure 2—2. Diagrammatic representation of the relation of axons to Schwann cell in unmyelinated *(left)* and myelinated nerve *(right)*. In the former, the axons are simply buried in the cell. In the latter, the Schwann cell membrane is coiled many times around the axon, forming the multiple layers of membrane that make up myelin.

generate impulses as well as integrate activity. Indeed, transmission of impulses from one dendrite to another has been demonstrated in the CNS.

The size of the neurons and the length of their processes vary considerably in different parts of the nervous system. In some cases, the dimensions of the neurons are truly remarkable. In the case of spinal motor neurons supplying the muscles of the foot, for example, it has been calculated that if the cell body were the size of a tennis ball the dendrites of the cell would fill an average-sized living room and the axon

would be up to 1.6 km (almost a mile) long though only 13 mm (½ inch) in diameter.

Protein Synthesis & Axoplasmic Transport

Despite the extremely long axons of some neurons, it is the cell body that maintains the functional and anatomic integrity of the axon; if the axon is cut, the part distal to the cut degenerates (**Wallerian degeneration**). The materials responsible for maintaining the axon, probably mostly proteins, are formed in the cell body and transported down the axon

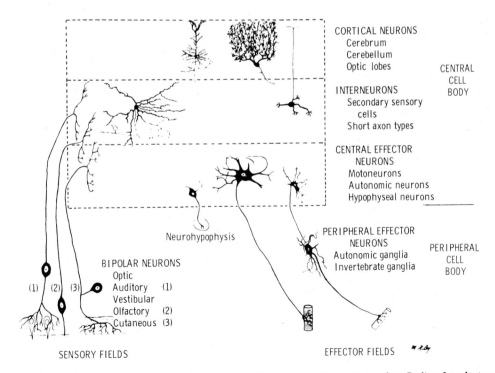

Figure 2—3. Types of neurons in the mammalian nervous system. (Reproduced, with permission, from Bodian: Introductory survey of neurons. Cold Spring Harbor Symposium on Quantitative Biology 17:1, 1952.)

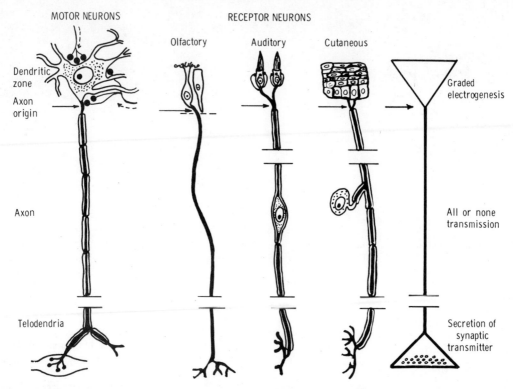

Figure 2—4. A variety of mammalian receptor and effector neurons. The neurons are arranged to illustrate the concept that impulse origin (indicated in each case by the arrow) rather than location of the cell body is the logical point of departure for analyzing neuronal structure in functional terms. Thus the dendritic zone, the area where the activity that generates the impulses occurs, may be dendrites or cell body. The axon conducts the impulses to the axon telodendria. The location of the cell body varies, and has no direct effect on impulse generation or transmission. (Modified after Grundfest and reproduced, with permission, from Bodian: The generalized vertebrate neuron. Science 137:323, 1962. Copyright 1962 by the American Association for the Advancement of Science.)

(axoplasmic transport). Proteins associated with synaptic transmitters are also synthesized in the endoplasmic reticulum of the cell body and transported to the axon terminals. There is both fast (400 mm/day) and slow (approximately 200 mm/day) transport. The fast transport mechanism depends on the oxidative metabolism of the neuron and probably on ATP. It appears to depend on the microtubules, and, since it has some similarities to the contraction of muscle, the hypothesis has been advanced that the transported material is attached to filaments formed in the cell body and slides along the microtubules in a manner analogous to the way actin slides along myosin in skeletal muscle.

Excitation

The nerve cell has a low threshold for excitation. The stimulus may be electrical, chemical, or mechanical. The physicochemical disturbance created by the stimulus, the **impulse**, is normally transmitted (or **conducted**) along the axon to its termination. Nerves are not "telephone wires" which transmit impulses passively; and conduction of nerve impulses, although rapid, is much slower than that of electricity. Nerve tissue is in fact a relatively poor passive conductor, and

it would take a potential of many volts to produce a signal of a fraction of 1 volt at the other end of a 1 meter axon in the absence of active processes in the nerve. Conduction is an active, self-propagating process which requires expenditure of energy by the nerve, and the impulse moves along the nerve at a constant amplitude and velocity. The process is often compared to what happens when a match is applied to one end of a train of gunpowder; by igniting the powder particles immediately in front of it, the flame moves steadily down the train to its end.

ELECTRICAL PHENOMENA IN NERVE CELLS

For over 100 years it has been known that there are electrical potential changes in a nerve when it conducts impulses, but it was not until suitable equipment was developed that these electrical events could be measured and studied in detail. Special instruments are necessary because the events are rapid, being measured in **milliseconds (msec)**; and the potential changes are

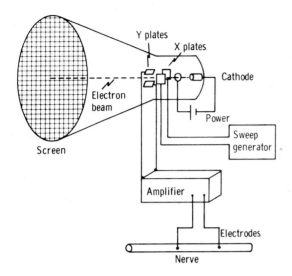

Figure 2—5. Cathode ray oscilloscope. Simplified diagram of principal connections when arranged to record potential changes in nerve. (Modified and reproduced, with permission, from Erlanger & Gasser: *Electrical Signs of Nervous Activity.* Univ of Pennsylvania Press, 1937.)

small, being measured in **millivolts (mV)**. The principal advances which made detailed study of the electrical activity in nerves possible were the development of electronic amplifiers and the cathode ray oscilloscope. Modern amplifiers magnify potential changes 1000 times or more, and the cathode ray oscilloscope provides an almost inertialess and almost instantaneously responding "lever" for recording electrical events.

The Cathode Ray Oscilloscope

The cathode ray oscilloscope (CRO) is used to measure the electrical events in living tissue. A cathode emits electrons when a high voltage is applied across it and a suitable anode in a vacuum. In the CRO the electrons are directed into a focused beam which strikes the face of the glass tube in which the cathode is located. The face is coated with one of a number of substances (phosphors) which emit light when struck by electrons. A vertical metal plate is placed on either side of the electron beam. When a voltage is applied across these plates, the negatively charged electrons are drawn toward the positively charged plate and repelled by the negatively charged plate. If the voltage applied to the vertical plates (X plates) is increased slowly and then reduced suddenly and increased again, the beam moves steadily toward the positive plate, snaps back to its former position, and moves toward the positive plate again. Application of a "saw-tooth voltage" of this type thus causes the beam to sweep across the face of the tube, and the speed of the sweep is proportionate to the rate of rise of the applied voltage.

In the CRO (Fig 2—5), another set of plates (Y plates) is arranged horizontally, with one plate above and one below the beam. Voltages applied to these plates move the beam up and down as it sweeps across

the face of the tube, the magnitude of the vertical deflection being proportionate to the potential difference between the horizontal plates at any given instant. In practice, electrodes placed on or in the nerve are connected through a suitable amplifier to the horizontal plates of the oscilloscope. Any changes in potential occurring in the nerve are thus recorded as vertical deflections of the beam as it moves across the tube. The tracing of the beam on the face of the oscilloscope may be photographed to make a permanent record.

Recording From Single Axons

With the CRO the electrical events occurring in a piece of peripheral nerve dissected from a laboratory animal can be demonstrated. However, such preparations contain many axons, and it is important to be able to study the properties of a single axon. Mammalian axons are relatively small (20 μm or less in diameter) and are difficult to separate from other axons, but giant unmyelinated nerve cells exist in a number of invertebrate species. Such giant cells are found, for example, in crabs (Carcinus) and cuttlefish (Sepia), but the largest known axons are found in the squid (Loligo). The neck region of the muscular mantle of the squid contains single axons up to 1 mm in diameter. It appears that their fundamental properties are similar to those of mammalian axons.

Another important technical advance in neurophysiology has been the development of microelectrodes which can be inserted into nerve cells. These electrodes are made by drawing out glass capillary pipets so that the diameter of the tip is very small. They are filled with a solution of electrolyte, usually potassium chloride. Electrodes with tip diameters of a few micrometers can be inserted into invertebrate giant axons, and ultramicroelectrodes with tip diameters of less than 1 μm can be inserted into mammalian nerve cells.

Resting Membrane Potential

When 2 electrodes are connected through a suitable amplifier to a CRO and placed on the surface of a single axon, no potential difference is observed. However, if one electrode is inserted into the interior of the cell, a constant potential difference is observed between the inside and the outside of the cell at rest. The magnitude of this **resting membrane potential** in most neurons is approximately 70 mV. It is expressed as a negative potential, −70 mV, because the inside of the cell is negatively charged relative to the exterior.

Latent Period

If the axon is stimulated and a conducted impulse occurs, a characteristic series of potential changes is observed as the impulse passes the exterior electrode. When the stimulus is applied there is a brief irregular deflection of the baseline, the **stimulus artifact**. This artifact is due to current leakage from the stimulating electrodes to the recording electrodes. It usually occurs despite careful shielding, but it is of value because it marks on the cathode ray screen the point at which the stimulus was applied.

The stimulus artifact is followed by an isopotential interval or **latent period** which ends with the next potential change and corresponds to the time it takes the impulse to travel along the axon from the site of stimulation to the recording electrodes. Its duration is proportionate to the distance between the stimulating and recording electrodes and the speed of conduction of the axon. If the duration of the latent period and the distance between the electrodes are known, the speed of conduction in the axon can be calculated. For example, assume that the distance between the cathodal stimulating electrode and the exterior electrode in Fig 2–6 is 4 cm. The cathode is normally the stimulating electrode, as described below. If the latent period is 2 msec long, the speed of conduction is 4 cm/2 msec, or 20 meters/sec.

Action Potential

The first manifestation of the approaching impulse is a beginning depolarization of the membrane. After an initial 15 mV of depolarization, the rate of depolarization increases. The point at which this change in rate occurs is called the **firing level**. Thereafter, the tracing on the oscilloscope rapidly reaches and **overshoots** the isopotential (zero potential) line to approximately +35 mV. It then reverses and falls rapidly toward the resting level. When repolarization is about 70% completed, the rate of repolarization decreases and the tracing approaches the resting level more slowly. The sharp rise and rapid fall are the **spike potential** of the axon, and the slower fall at the end of the process is the **after-depolarization**. After reaching

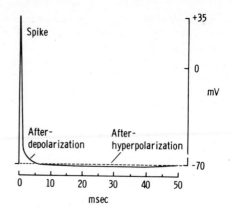

Figure 2–7. Diagram of complete action potential of large mammalian myelinated fiber, drawn without time or voltage distortion to show proportions of components. (Modified and redrawn from Gasser: The control of excitation in the nervous system. Harvey Lectures 32:169, 1957.)

the previous resting level, the tracing overshoots slightly in the hyperpolarizing direction to form the small but prolonged **after-hyperpolarization**. The after-depolarization is sometimes called the **negative after-potential** and the after-hyperpolarization the **positive after-potential**, but the terms are now rarely used. The whole sequence of potential changes is called the **action potential**.

The proportions of the tracing in Fig 2–6 are intentionally distorted to illustrate these various components of the action potential. A tracing with the components plotted on exact temporal and magnitude scales for a mammalian neuron is shown in Fig 2–7. Note that the rise of the action potential is so rapid that it fails to show clearly the change in depolarization rate at the firing level, and also that the after-hyperpolarization is only about 1–2 mV in amplitude although it lasts about 35–40 msec. The duration of the after-depolarization is about 4 msec in this instance. It is shorter and less prominent in many other neurons. Changes may occur in the after-polarization without changes in the rest of the action potential. For example, if the nerve has been conducting repetitively for a long time, the after-hyperpolarization is usually quite large. These potentials represent recovery processes in the neuron rather than the events responsible for the spike portion of the action potential.

"All or None" Law

If an axon is arranged for recording as shown in Fig 2–6 with the recording electrodes at an appreciable distance from the stimulating electrodes, it is possible to determine the minimal intensity of stimulating current (**threshold intensity**) which will just produce an impulse. This threshold varies with the experimental conditions and the type of axon, but once it is reached, a full-fledged action potential is produced. Further increases in the intensity of a stimulus produce no increment or other change in the action

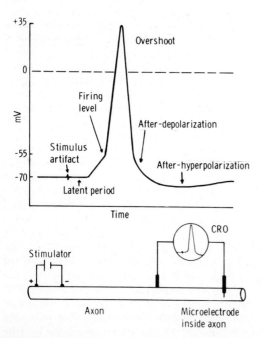

Figure 2–6. Action potential ("spike potential") recorded with one electrode inside cell.

potential as long as the other experimental conditions remain constant. The action potential fails to occur if the stimulus is subthreshold in magnitude, and it occurs with a constant amplitude and form regardless of the strength of the stimulus if the stimulus is at or above threshold intensity. The action potential is therefore "all or none" in character, and is said to obey the **"all or none law."**

Strength-Duration Curve

In a preparation such as that in Fig 2–6, it is possible to determine experimentally the relationship between the strength of the stimulating current and the length of time it must be applied to the nerve to produce a response. Stimuli of extremely short duration will not excite the axon no matter how intense they may be. With stimuli of longer duration, threshold intensity is related to the duration of stimulus as shown in Fig 2–8. With weak stimuli, a point is reached where no response occurs no matter how long the stimulus is applied. The relationship shown in Fig 2–8 applies only to currents that rise to peak intensity rapidly. Slowly rising currents sometimes fail to fire the nerve because the nerve in some way adapts to the applied stimulus, a process called **accommodation.**

Classically, the magnitude of the current just sufficient to excite a given nerve or muscle is called the **rheobase** and the time for which it must be applied the **utilization time.** Another common measurement is the **chronaxie,** ie, the length of time a current of twice rheobasic intensity must be applied to produce a response. Within limits, the chronaxie of any given excitable tissue is constant for that tissue, and chronaxie values have been used to compare excitability of various tissues.

Electrotonic Potentials, Local Response, & Firing Level

Although subthreshold stimuli do not produce an action potential, they do have an effect on the membrane potential. This can be demonstrated by placing

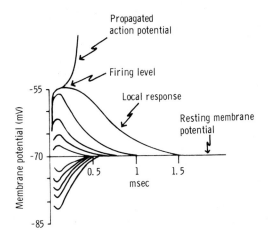

Figure 2–9. Electrotonic potentials and local response. The changes in the membrane potential of a neuron following application of stimuli of 0.2, 0.4, 0.6, 0.8, and 1.0 times threshold intensity are shown superimposed on the same time scale. The responses below the horizontal line are those recorded near the anode, and the responses above the line are those recorded near the cathode. The stimulus of threshold intensity was repeated twice. Once it caused a propagated action potential (top line), and once it did not. (Based on a diagram from Hodgkin: The subthreshold potentials in a crustacean nerve fiber. Proc Roy Soc London s.B 126:87, 1938.)

recording electrodes within a few millimeters of a stimulating electrode and applying subthreshold stimuli of fixed duration. Application of such currents with a cathode leads to a localized depolarizing potential change which rises sharply and decays exponentially with time. The magnitude of this response drops off rapidly as the distance between the stimulating and recording electrodes is increased. Conversely, an anodal current produces a hyperpolarizing potential change of similar duration. These potential changes are called **electrotonic potentials,** those produced at a cathode being **catelectrotonic** and those at an anode **anelectrotonic.** They are passive changes in membrane polarization caused by addition or subtraction of charge by the particular electrode. At low current intensities producing up to about 7 mV of depolarization or hyperpolarization, their size is proportionate to the magnitude of the stimulus. With stronger stimuli, this relationship remains constant for anelectrotonic responses but not for responses at the cathode. The cathodal responses are greater than would be expected from the magnitude of the applied current. Finally, when the cathodal stimulation is great enough to produce about 15 mV of depolarization, ie, at a membrane potential of −55 mV, the membrane potential suddenly begins to fall rapidly and a propagated action potential occurs. The disproportionately greater response at the cathode to stimuli of sufficient strength to produce 7–15 mV of depolarization indicates active participation by the membrane in the process and is called the **local response** (Fig 2–9). The point at which a runaway spike potential is initiated is the **firing level.** Thus, cathodal

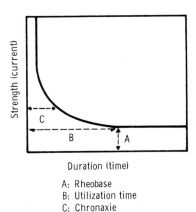

A: Rheobase
B: Utilization time
C: Chronaxie

Figure 2–8. Strength-duration curve. The curve relates the strength of a stimulus to the time for which it must be applied to an excitable tissue to produce a response.

currents which produce up to 7 mV of depolarization have a purely passive effect on the membrane caused by addition of negative charges. Those producing 7–15 mV of depolarization produce in addition a slight active change in the membrane, and this change contributes to the depolarizing process. However, the repolarizing forces are still stronger than the depolarizing forces, and the potential decays. At 15 mV of depolarization, the depolarizing forces are strong enough to overwhelm the repolarizing processes and an action potential results. These facts indicate that at 15 mV of depolarization some fundamental change which leads to runaway depolarization occurs in the membrane.

Stimulation normally occurs at the cathode because cathodal stimuli are depolarizing. Anodal currents, by taking the membrane potential farther away from the firing level, actually inhibit impulse formation. However, cessation of an anodal current may lead to an overshoot of the membrane potential in the depolarizing direction. This rebound is sometimes large enough to cause the nerve to fire at the end of an anodal stimulus.

Changes in Excitability During Electrotonic Potentials & the Action Potential

During the action potential as well as during catelectrotonic and anelectrotonic potentials and the local response, there are changes in the threshold of the neuron to stimulation. Hyperpolarizing anelectrotonic responses elevate the threshold and catelectrotonic potentials lower it as they move the membrane potential closer to the firing level. During the local response the threshold is also lowered, but during the

rising and much of the falling phases of the spike potential the neuron is refractory to stimulation. This **refractory period** is divided into an **absolute refractory period**, corresponding to the period from the time the firing level is reached until repolarization is about one-third complete; and a **relative refractory period**, lasting from this point to the start of after-depolarization. During the absolute refractory period no stimulus, no matter how strong, will excite the nerve, but during the relative refractory period stronger than normal stimuli can cause excitation. During after-depolarization the threshold is again decreased, and during after-hyperpolarization it is increased. These changes in threshold are correlated with the phases of the action potential in Fig 2–10.

Electrogenesis of the Action Potential

The descriptive data discussed above may be formulated into a picture of the electrical events underlying the action potential. The nerve cell membrane is polarized at rest, with positive charges lined up along the outside of the membrane and negative charges along the inside. During the action potential, this polarity is abolished and for a brief period is actually reversed (Fig 2–11). Positive charges from the membrane ahead of and behind the action potential flow into the area of negativity represented by the action potential ("current sink"). By drawing off positive charges, this flow decreases the polarity of the membrane ahead of the action potential. Such electrotonic depolarization initiates a local response, and when the firing level is reached a propagated response occurs which in turn electrotonically depolarizes the membrane in front of it. This sequence of events moves regularly along an unmyelinated axon to its end. Thus, the self-propagating nature of the nerve impulse is due to circular current flow and successive electrotonic depolarizations to the firing level of the membrane ahead of the action potential. Once initiated, a moving impulse does not depolarize the area behind it to the firing level because this area is refractory.

The action potentials produced at synaptic junctions also depend upon electrotonic depolarization of the nerve cell membrane to the firing level. The details of the process by which the nerve cell body and dendrites serve as a large current sink to draw off positive charges from the axon are described in Chapter 4.

Saltatory Conduction

Conduction in myelinated axons depends upon a similar pattern of circular current flow. However, myelin is a relatively effective insulator, and current flow through it is negligible. Instead, depolarization in myelinated axons jumps from one node of Ranvier to the next, with the current sink at the active node serving to electrotonically depolarize to the firing level the node ahead of the action potential (Fig 2–11). This jumping of depolarization from node to node is called **saltatory conduction**. It is a rapid process, and myelinated axons conduct up to 50 times faster than the fastest unmyelinated fibers.

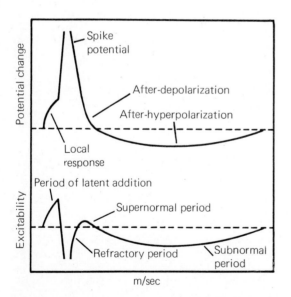

Figure 2–10. Relative changes in excitability of a nerve cell membrane during the passage of an impulse. Note that excitability is the reciprocal of threshold. (Modified and reproduced, with permission, from Morgan: *Physiological Psychology.* McGraw-Hill, 1943.)

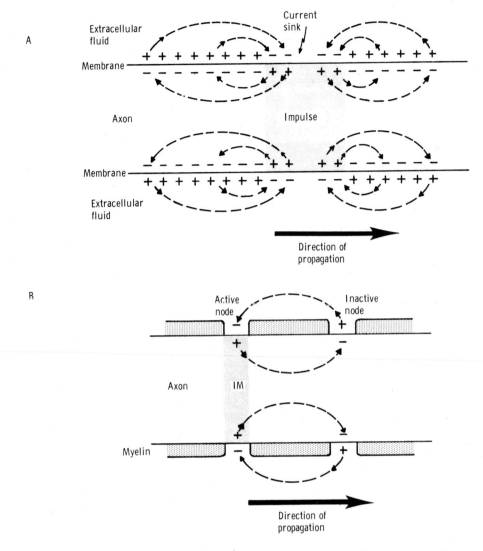

Figure 2—11. Local current flow around an impulse in an axon. Note that current flow is represented as movement of positive charges. *A* represents the situation in nonmyelinated nerves, *B* that in myelinated nerves (saltatory conduction). IM = impulse.

Orthodromic & Antidromic Conduction

An axon can conduct in either direction. When an action potential is initiated in the middle of it, 2 impulses traveling in opposite directions are set up by electrotonic depolarization on either side of the initial current sink.

In a living animal, impulses normally pass in one direction only, ie, from synaptic junctions or receptors along axons to their termination. Such conduction is called **orthodromic.** Conduction in the opposite direction is called **antidromic.** Since synapses, unlike axons, permit conduction in one direction only, any antidromic impulses that are set up fail to pass the first synapse they encounter (see Chapter 4) and die out at that point.

Biphasic & Monophasic Action Potentials

The descriptions of the resting membrane poten-

tial and action potential outlined above are based on recording with 2 electrodes, one on the surface of the axon and the other inside the axon. If both recording electrodes are placed on the surface of the axon, there is no potential difference between them at rest. When the nerve is stimulated and an impulse is conducted past the 2 electrodes, a characteristic sequence of potential changes results. As the wave of depolarization reaches the electrode nearest the stimulator, this electrode becomes negative to the other electrode (Fig 2—12). When the impulse passes to the portion of the nerve between the 2 electrodes, the potential returns to zero and then, as it passes the second electrode, the first electrode becomes positive to the second. It is conventional to connect the leads in such a way that when the first electrode becomes negative to the second an upward deflection is recorded. Therefore, the record shows an upward deflection followed by an

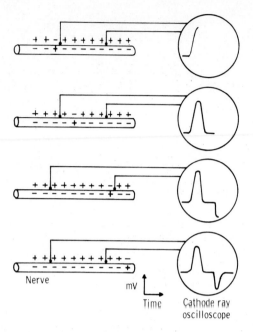

Figure 2–12. Biphasic action potential. Both recording electrodes are on the outside of the nerve membrane.

isoelectric interval and then a downward deflection. This sequence is called a **biphasic action potential** (Fig 2–12). The duration of the isoelectric interval is proportionate to the speed of conduction of the nerve and the distance between the 2 recording electrodes.

If the axon under one of the external electrodes is damaged (eg, by crushing), the damaged area becomes negative relative to the healthy portion at rest. The potential difference between the 2 electrodes is called the **demarcation potential**. Its magnitude is variable, depending upon the extent of the disruption of the membrane. The negativity of the damaged area is due to breakdown of the membrane. If such a preparation is stimulated, an upward deflection is recorded as the impulse passes under the electrode on healthy tissue. No downward deflection is observed because the impulse stops at the damaged area. The single deflection

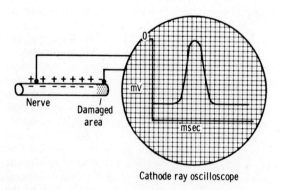

Figure 2–13. Monophasic action potential.

produced in this way is called a **monophasic action potential** (Fig 2–13).

Conduction in a Volume Conductor

Because the body fluids contain large quantities of electrolytes, the nerves in the body function in a conducting medium which is often called a **volume conductor**. The monophasic and biphasic action potentials described above are those seen when an axon is stimulated in a nonconducting medium outside the body. The potential changes observed during extracellular recording in a volume conductor are basically similar to these action potentials, but they are complicated by the effects of current flow in the volume conductor. These effects are complex, depending upon such factors as the orientation of the electrodes relative to the direction the action potential is moving and the distance between the recording electrode over active tissue and the indifferent electrode. In general, when an action potential is recorded in a volume conductor, there are positive deflections before and after the negative spike. A simplified diagram of the genesis of these deflections is shown in Fig 2–14.

IONIC BASIS OF EXCITATION & CONDUCTION

Ionic Basis of Resting Membrane Potential

The ionic basis of the resting membrane potential has been discussed in Chapter 1, using frog skeletal muscle cells as an example. In nerve, as in other tissues, Na^+ is actively transported out of the cell and a small amount of K^+ is actively transported in. K^+ diffuses back out of the cell down its concentration gradient, and Na^+ diffuses back in, but since the permeability of the membrane to K^+ is much greater than it is to Na^+ at rest, the passive K^+ efflux is much greater than the passive Na^+ influx. Since the membrane is impermeable to most of the anions in the cell, the K^+ efflux is not accompanied by an equal flux of anions and the membrane is maintained in a polarized state with the outside positive to the inside. The ion fluxes across the nerve cell membrane at rest are summarized in Fig 1–8.

Ionic Fluxes During the Action Potential

In nerve, as in other tissues, a slight decrease in resting membrane potential leads to increased movement of K^+ out of and Cl^- into the cell, restoring the resting membrane potential. In the case of nerve and muscle, however, there is a unique change in the cell membrane when depolarization exceeds 7 mV. This change is a voltage-dependent increase in membrane permeability to Na^+, so that the closer the membrane potential is to the firing level the greater the Na^+ permeability. The electrical and concentration gradients for Na^+ are both directed inward. During the local response, Na^+ permeability is slightly increased,

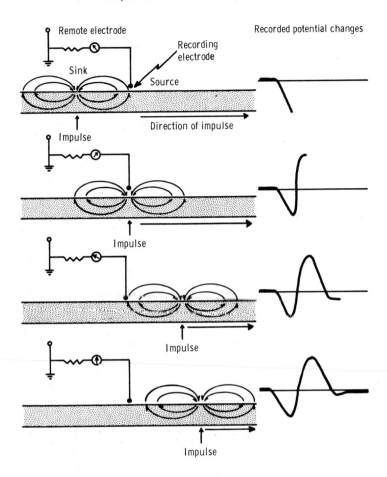

Figure 2–14. Potential changes recorded during passage of an impulse along an axon in a volume conductor. One electrode (recording electrode) is on the surface of the axon; the other (remote or indifferent electrode) is on inactive tissue at a distance in the conducting medium. (Reproduced, with permission, from Brazier: *The Electrical Activity of the Nervous System,* 3rd ed. Pitman, 1968.)

but K^+ efflux is able to restore the potential to the resting value. When the firing level is reached, permeability is great enough so that Na^+ influx further lowers the membrane potential and Na^+ permeability is further increased. The consequent Na^+ influx swamps the repolarizing processes, and runaway depolarization results, producing the spike potential.

The equilibrium potential for Na^+ in mammalian neurons calculated by using the Nernst equation is about +60 mV. With the great increase in Na^+ permeability at the start of the action potential, the membrane potential approaches this value. It does not reach it, however, primarily because the change in Na^+ permeability is short-lived. Na^+ permeability starts to return to the resting value during the rising phase of the spike potential, and Na^+ conductance is decreased during repolarization. In addition, the direction of the electrical gradient for Na^+ is reversed during the overshoot because the membrane potential is reversed. These factors limit Na^+ influx and help bring about repolarization.

Another important factor producing repolariza-

tion of the nerve membrane is the increase in K^+ permeability that accompanies the increase in Na^+ permeability. The change in K^+ permeability starts more slowly and reaches a peak during the falling phase of the action potential. The increase in permeability decreases the barrier to K^+ diffusion, and K^+ consequently leaves the cell. The resulting net transfer of positive charge out of the cell serves to complete repolarization.

The changes in membrane permeability during the action potential have been documented in a number of ways, perhaps most clearly by the voltage clamp technic. This research technic, the details of which are beyond the scope of this book, has made it possible to measure changes in the **conductance** of the membrane for various ions. The conductance of an ion is the reciprocal of its electrical resistance in a membrane and is a measure of membrane permeability to that ion. The changes in Na^+ and K^+ conductance during the action potential are shown in Fig 2–15. Additional evidence that this ionic hypothesis of the basis of the action potential is correct is provided by the observa-

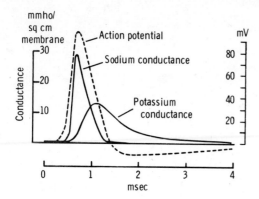

Figure 2–15. Changes in Na⁺ and K⁺ conductance during the action potential in giant squid axon. The dotted line represents the action potential superimposed on the same time coordinate. The unit of conductance, the mmho, is the reciprocal of the unit of resistance, the mOhm (milliOhm). (Redrawn and reproduced, with permission, from Hodgkin: Ionic movements and electrical activity in giant nerve fibers. Proc R Soc Lond [Biol] 148:1, 1958.)

tion that decreasing the external Na⁺ concentration decreases the size of the action potential but has little effect on the resting membrane potential. The lack of much effect on the resting membrane potential would be predicted from the Goldman equation (see Chapter 1) since the permeability of the membrane to Na⁺ at rest is relatively low. Conversely, increasing the external K⁺ concentration decreases the resting membrane potential. The way in which partial depolarization causes the change in membrane permeability to Na⁺ has not been determined. However, it is clear that separate "pores" or channels are involved in the transport of Na⁺ and K⁺. The Na⁺ channels can be blocked by a poison called tetrodotoxin (TTX) without affecting the K⁺ channels.

Although Na⁺ enters the nerve cell and K⁺ leaves it during the action potential, the number of ions involved is not large relative to the total numbers present. The fact that the nerve gains Na⁺ and loses K⁺ during activity has been demonstrated experimentally, but significant differences in ion concentrations can be measured only after prolonged, repeated stimulation.

As noted above, the after-depolarization (negative after-potential) and the after-hyperpolarization (positive after-potential) represent restorative processes in the cell that are separate from those causing the action potential. Relatively little is known about their origin. The after-depolarization is reduced by agents that inhibit metabolism. The after-hyperpolarization is also reduced and it now seems clear that it is due to the sodium pump acting in an electrogenic fashion. The net flux of Na⁺ to the exterior hyperpolarizes the membrane.

Energy Sources & Metabolism of Nerve

The major part of the energy requirement of nerve is the portion used to maintain polarization of the membrane. The energy for the sodium-potassium pump is derived from the hydrolysis of ATP. During maximal activity, the metabolic rate of the nerve doubles; by comparison, that of skeletal muscle increases as much as 100-fold. Inhibition of lactic acid production does not influence nerve function.

Like muscle, nerve has a resting heat while inactive, an initial heat during the action potential, and a recovery heat that follows activity. However, in nerve, the recovery heat after a single impulse is about 30 times the initial heat. There is some evidence that the initial heat is produced during the after-depolarization rather than the spike. The metabolism of muscle is discussed in detail in Chapter 3.

PROPERTIES OF MIXED NERVES

Peripheral nerves in mammals are made up of many axons bound together in a fibrous envelope called the **epineurium**. Potential changes recorded from such nerves therefore represent an algebraic summation of the all or none action potentials of many axons. The thresholds of the individual axons in the nerve and their distance from the stimulating electrodes vary. With subthreshold stimuli, none of the axons are stimulated and no response occurs. When the stimuli are of threshold intensity, axons with low thresholds fire and a small potential change is observed. As the intensity of the stimulating current is increased, the axons with higher thresholds are also discharged. The electrical response increases proportionately until the stimulus is strong enough to excite all of the axons in the nerve. The stimulus which produces excitation of all the axons is the **maximal stimulus**, and further application of greater, **supramaximal** stimuli produces no further increase in the size of the observed potential.

Compound Action Potentials

Another property of mixed nerves, as opposed to single axons, is the appearance of multiple peaks in the action potential. The multi-peaked action potential is called a **compound action potential**. Its shape is due to the fact that a mixed nerve is made up of families of fibers with varying speeds of conduction. Therefore, when all the fibers are stimulated, the activity in fast-conducting fibers arrives at the recording electrodes sooner than the activity in slower fibers; and the farther away from the stimulating electrodes the action potential is recorded, the greater is the separation between the fast and slow fiber peaks. The number and size of the peaks vary with the types of fibers in the particular nerve being studied. If less than maximal stimuli are used, the shape of the compound action potential also depends upon the number and type of fibers stimulated.

Erlanger and Gasser have divided mammalian nerve fibers into A, B, and C groups, further subdivid-

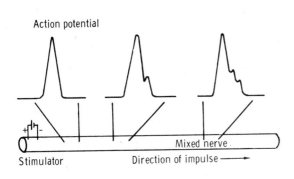

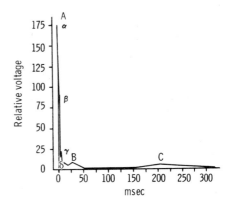

Figure 2—16. Compound action potential. *Left:* Record obtained with recording electrodes at various distances from the stimulating electrodes along a mixed nerve. *Right:* Reconstruction of a compound action potential to show relative sizes and time relationships of the components. (Redrawn and reproduced, with permission, from Erlanger & Gasser: *Electrical Signs of Nervous Activity.* Univ of Pennsylvania Press, 1937.)

ing the A group into α, β, γ, and δ fibers. The relative latencies of the electrical activity due to each of these components are shown in Fig 2–16. It should be emphasized that the drawing is not the compound action potential of any particular peripheral nerve; none of the peripheral nerves show all the components illustrated in this composite diagram because none contain all of the fiber types.

NERVE FIBER TYPES & FUNCTION

By comparing the neurologic deficits produced by careful dorsal root section and other nerve cutting experiments with the histologic changes in the nerves, the functions and histologic characteristics of each of the families of axons responsible for the various peaks of the compound action potential have been established. In general, the greater the diameter of a given nerve fiber, the greater its speed of conduction. The larger axons are concerned with proprioceptive sensation and somatic motor function, while the smaller axons subserve pain sensation and autonomic function. In Table 2–1, the various fiber types are listed with their diameters, electrical characteristics, and functions. There is evidence that the dorsal root C fibers conduct impulses generated by touch and other cutaneous receptors in addition to pain receptors, but only the latter are relayed to consciousness. The other fibers presumably are concerned with reflex responses integrated in the spinal cord and brain stem.

Further research has shown that not all the classically described lettered components are homogeneous, and a numerical system (Ia, Ib, II, III, IV) has been used by some physiologists to classify sensory fibers. Unfortunately, this has led to some confusion. A comparison of the number system and the letter system is shown in Table 2–2.

In addition to variations in speed of conduction and fiber diameter, the various classes of fibers in peripheral nerves differ in their sensitivity to hypoxia and anesthetics (Table 2–3). This fact has clinical as well as physiologic significance. Local anesthetics depress transmission in the group C fibers before they affect the touch fibers in the A group. Conversely, pressure on a nerve can cause loss of conduction in

Table 2—1. Nerve fiber types in mammalian nerve.

Fiber Type		Function	Fiber Diameter (μm)	Conduction Velocity (m/sec)	Spike Duration (msec)	Absolute Refractory Period (msec)
A	α	Proprioception; somatic motor	12–20	70–120	0.4–0.5	0.4–1
	β	Touch, pressure	5–12	30–70		
	γ	Motor to muscle spindles	3–6	15–30		
	δ	Pain, temperature, touch	2–5	12–30		
B		Preganglionic autonomic	<3	3–15	1.2	1.2
C dorsal root		Pain, reflex responses	0.4–1.2	0.5–2	2	2
	sympathetic	Postganglionic sympathetics	0.3–1.3	0.7–2.3	2	2

Table 2–2. Numerical classification sometimes used for sensory neurons.

Number		Origin	Fiber Type
I	a	Muscle spindle, annulospiral ending	A α
	b	Golgi tendon organ	A α
II		Muscle spindle, flower-spray ending; touch, pressure	A β
III		Pain and temperature receptors; some touch receptors	A δ
IV		Pain and other receptors	Dorsal root C

Table 2–3. Relative susceptibility of mammalian A, B, and C nerve fibers to conduction block produced by various agents.

	Most Susceptible	Inter-mediate	Least Susceptible
Sensitivity to hypoxia	B	A	C
Sensitivity to pressure	A	B	C
Sensitivity to cocaine and local anesthetics	C	B	A

Table 2–4. Types of fibers in peripheral and cranial nerves.

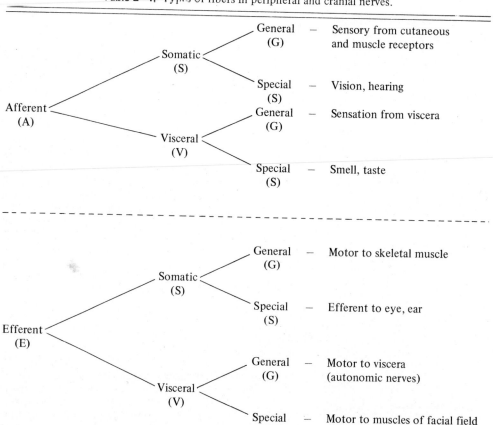

Thus, GVA = general visceral afferent; SVE = special visceral efferent; etc.

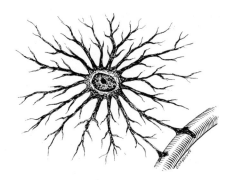

Protoplasmic astrocyte

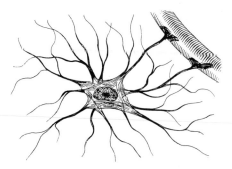

Fibrous astrocyte

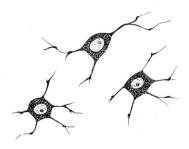

Oligodendrocytes

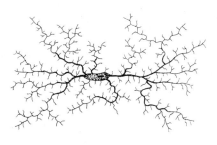

Microglia

Figure 2—17. Glial cells. (Reproduced, with permission, from Junqueira, Carneiro, & Contopoulos: *Basic Histology*, 2nd ed. Lange, 1977.)

motor, touch, and pressure fibers while pain sensation remains relatively intact. Patterns of this type are sometimes seen in individuals who sleep with their arms under their heads for long periods of time, causing compression of the nerves in the arms. Because of the association of deep sleep with alcoholic intoxication, the syndrome is common on weekends, and has acquired the interesting name Saturday night or Sunday morning paralysis.

Peripheral nerve fibers in man are also classified on a physio-anatomic basis. This classification (Table 2—4) divides nerves into afferent and efferent categories, and further subdivides them according to whether they have somatic or visceral and general or special functions. The term special is applied to nerves which supply the organs of the special senses and the musculature which is branchiomeric in origin, ie, musculature arising from the branchial arches during embryonic development.

NERVE GROWTH FACTOR

The salivary glands of certain species of laboratory mammals contain **nerve growth factor** (NGF). This protein, which is made up of 5 subunits, stimulates the growth of neurons, particularly in the autonomic nervous system. Antiserum against it has been prepared, and injection of this antiserum in newborn animals leads to near total destruction of the sympathetic ganglia; it thus produces an **immunosympathectomy**. The structure of NGF somewhat resembles that of insulin, and it appears to be one of a number of different hormone-like protein factors that stimulate the growth of various tissues in the body. It is found in the circulation, but it also appears to be transported along neurons from their endings to their cell bodies.

GLIA

In addition to neurons, the nervous system contains glial cells, or neuroglia (Fig 2—17). Glial cells are very numerous; indeed, there are approximately 10 times as many glial cells as neurons. The Schwann cells which invest axons in peripheral nerves are classified as glia. In the CNS, there are 3 types of glia. **Microglia** are scavenger cells that enter the nervous system from the blood vessels. The **oligodendroglia** are involved in myelin formation. The **astrocytes** are found throughout the brain and many send end feet to blood vessels (see Chapter 17). They have a membrane potential which varies with the external K^+ concentration, but do not generate propagated potentials. Despite many theories, their function remains uncertain.

3...

Excitable Tissue: Muscle

Muscle cells, like neurons, can be excited chemically, electrically, and mechanically to produce an action potential which is transmitted along their cell membrane. They contain contractile proteins and, unlike neurons, they have a contractile mechanism which is activated by the action potential.

Muscle is generally divided into 3 types, **skeletal**, **cardiac**, and **smooth**, although smooth muscle is not a homogeneous single category. Skeletal muscle comprises the great mass of the somatic musculature. It has well developed cross-striations, does not normally contract in the absence of nervous stimulation, lacks anatomic and functional connections between individual muscle fibers, and is generally under voluntary control. Cardiac muscle also has cross-striations, but it is functionally syncytial in character and contracts rhythmically in the absence of external innervation due to the presence in the myocardium of pacemaker cells that discharge spontaneously. Smooth muscle lacks cross-striations. The type found in most hollow viscera is

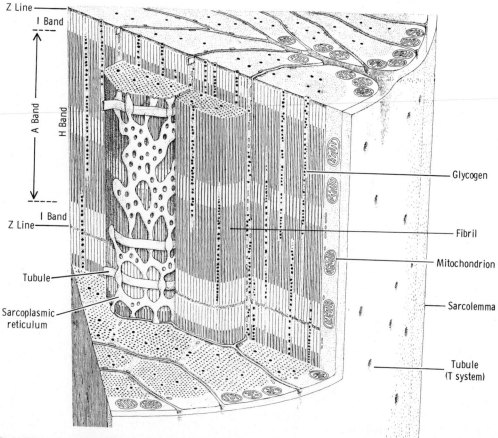

Figure 3–1. Structure of skeletal muscle fiber. The fiber is made up of a number of fibrils and surrounded by a membrane, the sarcolemma. Each fibril is surrounded by sarcoplasmic reticulum and by the T system of tubules, which opens to the exterior of the fiber. (Reproduced, with permission, from: How is muscle turned on and off? by Hoyle. Scientific American 222:84 [April], 1970. Copyright © 1970 by Scientific American, Inc. All rights reserved.)

functionally syncytial in character and contains pace-makers that discharge irregularly. The type found in the eye and in some other locations is not spontaneously active and resembles skeletal muscle. There are contractile proteins similar to those in muscle in many other cells and it appears that these proteins are responsible for cell motility, mitosis, and the movement of various components within cells (see Chapter 1).

SKELETAL MUSCLE

MORPHOLOGY

Organization

Skeletal muscle is made up of individual muscle fibers which are the "building blocks" of the muscular system in the same sense that the neurons are the building blocks of the nervous system. Most skeletal muscles begin and end in tendons, and the muscle fibers are arranged in parallel between the tendinous ends so that the force of contraction of the units is additive (Fig 3–1). Each muscle fiber is a single cell, multinucleated, long, and cylindrical in shape. There are no syncytial bridges between cells.

The muscle fibers are made up of fibrils, as shown in Fig 3–1, and the fibrils are divisible into individual filaments. The filaments are made up of the contractile proteins.

Muscle contains the proteins **myosin** (molecular weight about 500,000), **actin** (molecular weight about 45,000), **tropomyosin** (molecular weight about 70,000), and **troponin**. Troponin is made up of 3 subunits, **troponin I, troponin T,** and **troponin C.** The 3 subunits have molecular weights ranging from 18,000–35,000.

Striations

The cross-striations characteristic of skeletal muscle are due to differences in the refractive indexes of the various parts of the muscle fiber. The parts of the cross-striations are identified by letters (Fig 3–2). The light I band is divided by the dark Z line, and the dark A band has the lighter H band in its center. A transverse M line is seen in the middle of the H band, and this line plus the narrow light areas on either side of it are sometimes called the pseudo-H zone. The area between 2 adjacent Z lines is called a **sarcomere.** The arrangement of thick and thin filaments that is responsible for the striations is diagrammed in Fig 3–3. The thick filaments, which are about twice the diameter of the thin filaments, are made up of myosin; the thin filaments are made up of actin, tropomyosin, and troponin. The thick myosin filaments are lined up to form the A bands, whereas the array of thin actin filaments forms the less dense I bands. The lighter H bands in the center of the A bands are the regions

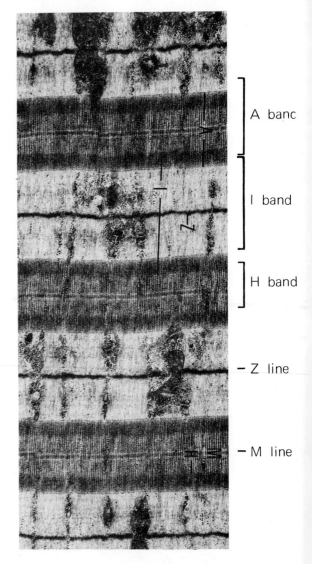

Figure 3–2. Electron micrograph of human gastrocnemius muscle. The various bands and lines are identified on the right. (× 13,500.) (Courtesy of SM Walker and GR Schrodt.)

where, when the muscle is relaxed, the actin filaments do not overlap the myosin filaments. The Z lines transect the fibrils and connect to the actin filaments. If a transverse section through the A band is examined under the electron microscope, each myosin filament is found to be surrounded by 6 actin filaments in a regular hexagonal pattern.

Observations with x-ray diffraction technics and the electron microscope indicate that the individual myosin molecules have enlarged heads and that they are arranged as shown in Fig 3–3. Cross-linkages form between the heads of the myosin molecules and the actin molecules. The myosin molecules are arranged symmetrically on either side of the center of the sarcomere, and it is this arrangement that creates the light

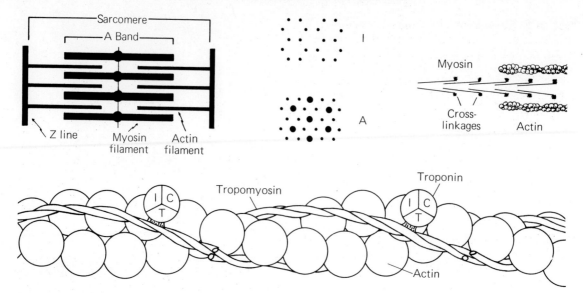

Figure 3–3. ***Top left:*** Arrangement of actin and myosin filaments in skeletal muscle. I and A represent a cross-section through the I band and the lateral portion of the A band, respectively. ***Top right:*** Detail of structure of myosin and actin. ***Bottom:*** Diagrammatic representation of the arrangement of actin, tropomyosin, and the 3 subunits of troponin (see text).

areas in the pseudo-H zone. The M line is due to a central bulge in each of the thick filaments. At these points, there are slender cross-connections which hold the myosin filaments in proper array. There are several hundred myosin molecules in each thick segment.

The actin filaments are made up of 2 chains of globular units which form a long double helix. Tropomyosin molecules are long filaments located in the groove between the 2 chains in the actin (Fig 3–3). Each thin filament contains 300–400 actin molecules and 40–60 tropomyosin molecules. Troponin molecules are small globular units located at intervals along the tropomyosin molecules. Troponin T binds the other troponin components to tropomyosin, troponin I inhibits the interaction of myosin with actin (see below), and troponin C contains the binding sites for the Ca^{++} that initiates contraction.

Sarcotubular System

The muscle fibrils are surrounded by structures made up of membrane which appear in electron photomicrographs as vesicles and tubules. These structures form the **sarcotubular system,** which is made up of a **T system** and a **sarcoplasmic reticulum.** The T system of transverse tubules, which is continuous with the membrane of the muscle fiber, forms a grid perforated by the individual muscle fibrils (Fig 3–1). The space between the 2 layers of the T system is an extension of the extracellular space. The sarcoplasmic reticulum forms an irregular curtain around each of the fibrils between its contacts with the T system, which in mammalian skeletal muscle is at the junction of the A and I bands. At these junctions, the arrangement of the central T system with sarcoplasmic reticulum on either

side has led to the use of the term **triads** to describe the system. The function of the T system is the rapid transmission of the action potential from the cell membrane to all the fibrils in the muscle. The sarcoplasmic reticulum is concerned with calcium movement and muscle metabolism (see below).

ELECTRICAL PHENOMENA & IONIC FLUXES

Electrical Characteristics of Skeletal Muscle

The electrical events in skeletal muscle and the ionic fluxes underlying them are similar to those in nerve, although there are quantitative differences in timing and magnitude. The resting membrane potential of skeletal muscle is about −90 mV. The action potential lasts 2–4 msec; and is conducted along the muscle fiber at about 5 meters/sec. The absolute refractory period is 1–3 msec long and the after-polarizations, with their related changes in threshold to electrical stimulation, are relatively prolonged. The chronaxie of skeletal muscle is generally somewhat longer than that of nerve. The initiation of impulses at the myoneural junction is discussed in Chapter 4.

Although the electrical properties of the individual fibers in a muscle do not differ sufficiently to produce anything resembling a compound action potential, there are slight differences in the thresholds of the various fibers. Furthermore, in any stimulation experiment some fibers are farther from the stimulating electrodes than others. Therefore, the size of the

Table 3–1. Steady-state distribution of ions in the intracellular and extracellular compartments of mammalian skeletal muscle, and the equilibrium potentials for these ions.* A⁻ represents organic anions. The value for intracellular Cl⁻ is calculated from the membrane potential, using the Nernst equation.

Ion	Concentration, mmol/liter		Equilibrium Potential (mV)
	Intracellular Fluid	Extracellular Fluid	
Na⁺	12	145	+65
K⁺	155	4	−95
H⁺	13×10^{-5}	3.8×10^{-5}	−32
Cl⁻	3.8	120	−90
HCO₃⁻	8	27	−32
A⁻	155	0	...
Membrane Potential = −90 mV			

*Data from Ruch TC, Patton HD (editors): *Physiology and Biophysics,* 19th ed. Saunders, 1965.

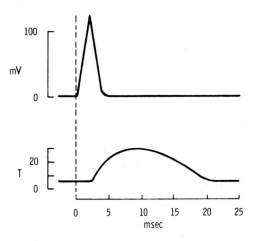

Figure 3–4. The electrical and mechanical responses of a mammalian skeletal muscle fiber to a single maximal stimulus. The mechanical response (tension) and the electrical response (mV potential change) are plotted on the same abscissa (time). T = tension in arbitrary units.

action potential recorded from a whole muscle preparation is proportionate to the intensity of the stimulating current between threshold and maximal current intensities.

Ion Distribution & Fluxes

The distribution of ions across the muscle fiber membrane is similar to that across the nerve cell membrane. The values for the various ions and their equilibrium potentials are shown in Tables 1–3 and 3–1. Depolarization is a manifestation of Na⁺ influx; repolarization, of K⁺ efflux (as described in Chapter 2 for nerve).

CONTRACTILE RESPONSES

It is important to distinguish between the electrical and mechanical events in muscle. Although one response does not normally occur without the other, their physiologic basis and characteristics are different. Muscle fiber membrane depolarization normally starts at the motor end-plate, the specialized structure under the motor nerve ending (see Chapter 4); the action potential is transmitted along the muscle fiber and initiates the contractile response.

The Muscle Twitch

A single action potential causes a brief contraction followed by relaxation. This response is called a **muscle twitch**. In Fig 3–4, the action potential and the twitch are plotted on the same time scale. The twitch starts about 2 msec after the start of depolarization of the membrane, before repolarization is complete. The duration of the twitch varies with the type of muscle being tested. "Fast" muscle fibers, primarily those concerned with fine, rapid, precise movement, have twitch durations as short as 7.5 msec. "Slow" muscle fibers,

principally those involved in strong, gross, sustained movements, have twitch durations up to 100 msec.

Molecular Basis of Contraction

The process by which the shortening of the contractile elements in muscle is brought about is a sliding of the actin filaments over the myosin filaments. The width of the A bands is constant, whereas the Z lines move closer together when the muscle contracts and farther apart when it is stretched (Fig 3–5). As the muscle shortens, the actin filaments from the opposite ends of the sarcomere approach each other; when the shortening is marked, these filaments apparently overlap.

The sliding during muscle contraction is produced by breaking and reforming of the cross-linkages between actin and myosin. The heads of the myosin molecules link to actin at an angle, produce movement of myosin on actin by swiveling, and then disconnect and reconnect at the next linking site, repeating the process in serial fashion (Fig 3–6). Each single cycle of attaching, swiveling, and detaching shortens the muscle 1%.

The immediate source of energy for muscle contraction is ATP. Hydrolysis of the bonds between the phosphate residues of this compound is associated with the release of a large amount of energy, and the bonds are therefore referred to as high-energy phosphate bonds. In muscle, the hydrolysis of ATP to adenosine diphosphate (ADP) is catalyzed by the contractile protein, myosin; and this **adenosine triphosphatase** activity is found in the heads of the myosin molecules, where they are in contact with actin.

The process by which depolarization of the muscle fiber initiates contraction is called **excitation-contraction coupling**. The action potential is transmitted

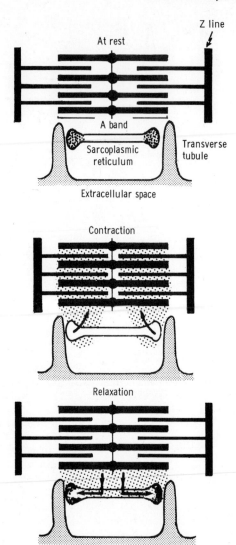

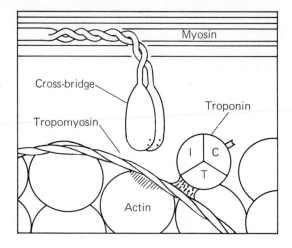

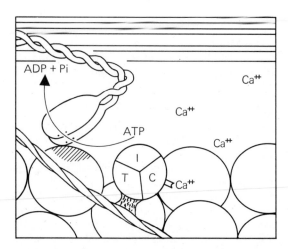

Figure 3–6. Initiation of muscle contraction by Ca⁺⁺. The cross-bridges (heads of myosin molecules) attach to binding sites on actin (striped areas) and swivel when tropomyosin is displaced laterally by binding of Ca⁺⁺ to troponin C. (Modified from Katz: Congestive heart failure. N Engl J Med 293:1184, 1975.)

Figure 3–5. Muscle contraction. Calcium ions (represented by black dots) are normally stored in the cisterns of the sarcoplasmic reticulum. The action potential spreads via the transverse tubules and releases Ca⁺⁺. The actin filaments (thin lines) slide on the myosin filaments, and the Z lines move closer together. Ca⁺⁺ is then pumped into the sarcoplasmic reticulum and the muscle relaxes. (Modified from Layzer & Rowland: Cramps. N Engl J Med 285:31, 1971.)

to all the fibrils in the fiber via the T system. It triggers the release of calcium ions from the **terminal cisterns,** the lateral sacs of the sarcoplasmic reticulum next to the T system (Fig 3–5). The Ca⁺⁺ initiates contraction.

Ca⁺⁺ initiates contraction by binding to troponin C. In resting muscle, troponin I is tightly bound to actin, and tropomyosin covers the sites where myosin heads bind to actin. Thus, the troponin-tropomyosin complex constitutes a "relaxing protein" which inhibits the interaction between actin and myosin. When the Ca⁺⁺ released by the action potential binds to troponin C, the binding of troponin I to actin is presum-

ably weakened, and this permits the tropomyosin to move laterally (Fig 3–6). This movement uncovers binding sites for the myosin heads, so that ATP is split and contraction occurs. Seven myosin binding sites are uncovered for each molecule of troponin that binds a calcium ion.

Shortly after releasing Ca⁺⁺, the sarcoplasmic reticulum begins to reaccumulate Ca⁺⁺. The Ca⁺⁺ is actively pumped into longitudinal portions of the reticulum and diffuses from there to the cisterns, where it is stored (Fig 3–5). Once the Ca⁺⁺ concentration outside of the reticulum has been lowered sufficiently, chemical interaction between myosin and actin ceases and the muscle relaxes. If the active transport of Ca⁺⁺ is inhibited, relaxation does not occur even though there are no more action potentials; the resulting sustained contraction is called a **contracture.** It should be noted that ATP provides the energy for the active transport

Table 3—2. Sequence of events in contraction and relaxation of skeletal muscle. (Steps 1—4 in contraction are discussed in Chapter 4.)

Steps in contraction
(1) Discharge of motor neuron.
(2) Release of transmitter (acetylcholine) at motor end plate.
(3) Generation of end-plate potential.
(4) Generation of action potential in muscle fibers.
(5) Inward spread of depolarization along T tubules.
(6) Release of Ca^{++} from lateral sacs of sarcoplasmic reticulum and diffusion to thick and thin filaments.
(7) Binding of Ca^{++} to troponin C, uncovering myosin binding sites on actin.
(8) Formation of cross-linkages between actin and myosin and sliding of thin on thick filaments, producing shortening.

Steps in relaxation
(1) Ca^{++} pumped back into sarcoplasmic reticulum.
(2) Release of Ca^{++} from troponin.
(3) Cessation of interaction between actin and myosin.

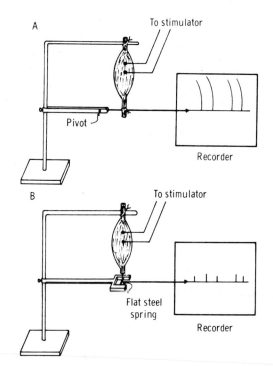

Figure 3—7. *A:* Muscle preparation arranged for recording isotonic contractions. *B:* Preparation arranged for recording isometric contractions. In A, the muscle is fastened to a writing lever which swings on a pivot. In B, it is attached to a steel spring to which is fastened a writing lever. Contraction deforms the spring and the slight motion is indicated by deflection of the writing lever.

of Ca^{++} into the sarcoplasmic reticulum. Thus, both contraction and relaxation of muscle require ATP.

The events involved in muscle contraction and relaxation are summarized in Table 3—2.

Types of Contraction

Muscular contraction involves shortening of the contractile elements, but because muscles have elastic and viscous elements in series with the contractile mechanism it is possible for contraction to occur without an appreciable decrease in the length of the whole muscle. Such a contraction is called **isometric** ("same measure" or length). Contraction against a constant load, with approximation of the ends of the muscle, is **isotonic** ("same tension").

A whole muscle preparation arranged for recording isotonic contractions is shown in Fig 3—7A. The muscle lifts the lever, and the distance the lever moves indicates the degree of shortening. In this situation, the muscle does external work, since the lever is being moved a certain distance. The muscle preparation in Fig 3—7B is arranged for recording isometric contractions. It is attached to a strong metal spring, and contraction deforms the spring. The slight motion produced is proportionate to the tension developed. Since the product of force times distance in this situation is very small, little external work is done by the muscle. In other situations, it is possible for muscles to do external work (Fig 3—8) or even negative work while contracting. This happens, for example, when a heavy weight is lowered onto a table. In this case the biceps muscle actively resists the descent of the object, but the net effect of the effort is to lengthen the biceps muscle while it is contracting.

Summation of Contractions

The electrical response of a muscle fiber to repeated stimulation is like that of nerve. The fiber is electrically refractory only during the rising and part

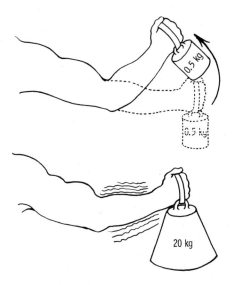

Figure 3—8. *Above:* Isotonic (free) contraction. Biceps shortens freely, weight is lifted. *Below:* Isometric contraction. Biceps generates force but cannot shorten and raise weight.

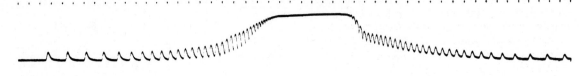

Figure 3—9. Tetanus. Isometric tension of a single muscle fiber during continuously increasing and decreasing stimulation frequency. Dots at top are at 0.2 sec intervals. (Reproduced, with permission, from Buchtal: Dan Biol Med 17:1, 1942.)

of the falling phase of the spike potential. At this time, the contraction initiated by the first stimulus is just beginning. However, because the contractile mechanism does not have a refractory period, repeated stimulation before relaxation has occurred produces additional activation of the contractile elements and a response which is added to the contraction already present. This phenomenon is known as **summation of contractions.** The tension developed during summation is considerably greater than that during the single muscle twitch. With rapidly repeated stimulation, activation of the contractile mechanism occurs repeatedly before any relaxation has occurred and the individual responses fuse into one continuous contraction. Such a response is called a **tetanus,** or **tetanic contraction.** It is a **complete tetanus** when there is no relaxation between stimuli, and an **incomplete tetanus** when there are periods of incomplete relaxation between the summated stimuli. During a complete tetanus, the tension developed is about 4 times that developed by the individual twitch contractions. The development of an incomplete and a complete tetanus in response to stimuli of increasing frequency is shown in Fig 3–9.

The stimulation frequency at which summation of contractions will occur is determined by the twitch duration of the particular muscle being studied. For example, if the twitch duration is 10 msec, frequencies less than 1 per 10 msec (100/sec) will cause discrete responses interrupted by complete relaxation, and frequencies greater than 100/sec will cause summation.

Treppe

When a series of maximal stimuli are delivered to skeletal muscle at a frequency just below the tetanizing frequency, there is an increase in the tension developed during each twitch until, after several contractions, a uniform tension per contraction is reached. This phenomenon is known as **treppe,** or the "staircase" phenomenon (German *Treppe* = "staircase"). It also occurs in cardiac muscle. Treppe is believed to be due to increased availability of Ca^{++} for binding to troponin C. It should not be confused with summation of contractions and tetanus.

Relation Between Muscle Length, Tension, & Velocity of Contraction

Both the tension that a muscle develops when stimulated to contract isometrically (the **total tension**), and the **passive tension** exerted by the unstimulated muscle vary with the length of the muscle fiber. This relationship can be studied in a whole skeletal muscle

preparation such as that shown in Fig 3–7B. The length of the muscle can be varied by changing the distance between the 2 rods to which it is attached. At each length, the passive tension is measured and the muscle is then stimulated electrically and the total tension measured. The difference between the 2 values at any length is the amount of tension actually generated by the contractile process, the **active tension.** The records obtained by plotting passive tension and total tension against muscle length are shown in Fig 3–10. Similar curves are obtained when single muscle fibers are studied. Passive tension rises slowly at first, and then rapidly as the muscle is stretched. Rupture of the muscle occurs when it is stretched to about 3 times its **equilibrium length,** ie, the length of the relaxed muscle cut free from its bony attachments.

The total tension curve rises to a maximum and then declines until it reaches the passive tension curve, ie, until no additional tension is developed upon further stimulation. The length of the muscle at which the active tension is maximal is usually called its rest-

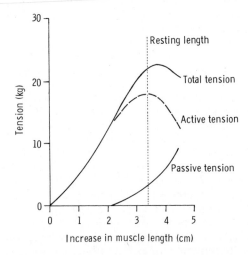

Figure 3—10. Length-tension diagram for skeletal muscle. The passive tension curve measures the tension exerted by the muscle at each length when it is not stimulated. The total tension curve represents the tension developed when the muscle contracts isometrically in response to a maximal stimulus. The active tension is the difference between the 2. (Drawn from data on human triceps muscle, with permission, from: *Report to the NRC, Committee on Artificial Limbs, on Fundamental Studies of Human Locomotion and other Information Relating to Design of Artificial Limbs.* Univ of California [Berkeley], 1947, Vol 2.)

ing length. The term comes originally from experiments demonstrating that the length of many of the muscles in the body at rest is the length at which they develop maximal tension. Other definitions of resting length are sometimes used, but that given here is the most widely accepted and has the greatest physiologic validity.

The observed length-tension relation in skeletal muscle is explained by the sliding filament mechanism of muscle contraction. When the muscle fiber contracts isometrically, the tension developed is proportionate to the number of cross-linkages between the actin and the myosin molecules. When muscle is stretched, the overlap between actin and myosin is reduced and the number of cross-linkages is reduced. Conversely, when the muscle is shorter than resting length, the actin filaments overlap, and this also reduces the number of cross-linkages.

The velocity of muscle contraction varies inversely with the load on the muscle. At a given load, the velocity is maximal at the resting length and declines if the muscle is shorter or longer than this length.

ENERGY SOURCES & METABOLISM

Muscle contraction requires energy, and muscle has been called "a machine for converting chemical into mechanical energy." The immediate source of this energy is the energy-rich organic phosphate derivatives in muscle; the ultimate source is the intermediary metabolism of carbohydrate and lipids. The hydrolysis of ATP to provide the energy for contraction has been discussed above.

Phosphocreatine

ATP is resynthesized from ADP by the addition of a phosphate group. Under normal conditions the energy for this endothermic reaction is supplied by the breakdown of glucose to CO_2 and H_2O, but there also exists in muscle another energy-rich phosphate compound which can supply this energy. This compound is **phosphocreatine**, which is hydrolyzed to creatine and phosphate groups with the release of considerable energy. At rest, some ATP transfers its phosphate to creatine, so that a phosphocreatine store is built up. During exercise the phosphocreatine is hydrolyzed, forming ATP from ADP and thus permitting contraction to continue.

Carbohydrate Breakdown

Much of the energy for phosphocreatine and ATP resynthesis comes from the breakdown of glucose to CO_2 and H_2O. The major metabolic pathways involved are discussed in detail elsewhere. For the purposes of the present discussion, it is sufficient to point out that glucose in the blood stream enters cells, where it is degraded through a series of chemical reactions to pyruvic acid. Another source of intracellular

$$ATP + H_2O \rightarrow ADP + H_3PO_4 + 12{,}000 \text{ calories}$$

$$\text{Phosphocreatine} + ADP \rightleftarrows \text{Creatine} + ATP$$

$$\text{Glucose} + 2\,ATP\ (\text{or glycogen} + 1\,ATP) \xrightarrow[\text{Anaerobic}]{} 2\ \text{Lactic acid} + 4\,ATP$$

$$\text{Glucose} + 2\,ATP\ (\text{or glycogen} + 1\,ATP) \xrightarrow[\text{Oxygen}]{} 6\,CO_2 + 6\,H_2O + 40\,ATP$$

$$FFA \xrightarrow[\text{Oxygen}]{} CO_2 + H_2O + ATP$$

Figure 3–11. Energy sources for muscle contraction. The amount of ATP formed per mol of free fatty acid (FFA) oxidized is large, but varies with the size of the FFA. For example, complete oxidation of 1 mol of palmitic acid generates 140 mols of ATP.

glucose, and consequently of pyruvic acid, is glycogen, the carbohydrate polymer which is especially abundant in liver and skeletal muscle. When adequate O_2 is present, pyruvic acid enters the citric acid cycle and is metabolized—through this cycle and the so-called respiratory enzyme pathway—to CO_2 and H_2O. This process is called **aerobic glycolysis.** The metabolism of glucose or glycogen to CO_2 and H_2O liberates sufficient energy to form large quantities of ATP from ADP. If O_2 supplies are insufficient, the pyruvic acid formed from glucose does not enter the tricarboxylic acid cycle but is reduced to lactic acid. This process of **anaerobic glycolysis** is associated with the net production of much smaller quantities of energy-rich phosphate bonds, but it does not require the presence of O_2. Skeletal muscle also takes up free fatty acids (FFA) from the blood and oxidizes them to CO_2 and H_2O. Indeed, FFA are probably the major substrates for muscle at rest and during recovery after contraction. The various reactions involved in supplying energy to skeletal muscle are summarized in Fig 3–11.

The Oxygen Debt Mechanism

During muscular exercise, the muscle blood vessels dilate and blood flow is increased so that the available O_2 supply is increased. Up to a point, the increase in O_2 consumption is proportionate to the energy expended, and all the energy needs are met by aerobic processes. However, when muscular exertion is very great, aerobic resynthesis of energy stores cannot keep pace with their utilization. Under these conditions, phosphocreatine is used to resynthesize ATP. Phosphocreatine resynthesis is accomplished by using the energy released by the anaerobic breakdown of glucose to lactic acid. This use of the anaerobic pathway is self-limiting, because in spite of rapid diffusion of lactic acid into the blood stream, enough accumulates in the muscles to eventually exceed the capacity of the tissue buffers and produce an enzyme-inhibiting decline in pH. However, for short periods, the presence of an anaerobic pathway for glucose breakdown permits muscular exertion of a far greater magnitude than would be possible without it. Without this pathway, for example, walking or running at a slow jog would be possible but sprinting and all other forms of short-term, violent exertion would not.

After a period of exertion is over, extra O_2 is consumed to remove the excess lactic acid and replenish the ATP and phosphocreatine stores. The amount of extra O_2 consumed is proportionate to the extent to which the energy demands during exertion exceeded the capacity for the aerobic synthesis of energy stores, ie, the extent to which an **oxygen debt** was incurred. The O_2 debt is measured experimentally by determining O_2 consumption after exercise until a constant, basal consumption is reached, and subtracting the basal consumption from the total. The amount of this debt may be 6 times the basal O_2 consumption, which indicates that the subject is capable of 6 times the exertion that would have been possible without it. Obviously, the maximal debt can be incurred rapidly or slowly; violent exertion is possible for only short periods of time, whereas less strenuous exercise can be carried on for longer periods of time.

Trained athletes are able to increase the O_2 consumption of their muscles to a greater degree than untrained individuals. Consequently, they are capable of greater exertion without increasing their lactic acid production, and they contract smaller oxygen debts for a given amount of exertion.

Heat Production in Muscle

Thermodynamically, the energy supplied to a muscle must equal its energy output. The energy output appears in work done by the muscle, in energy-rich phosphate bonds formed for later use, and in heat. The overall mechanical efficiency of skeletal muscle (work done/total energy expenditure) ranges up to 50% while lifting a weight during isotonic contraction and is essentially 0% during isometric contraction. Energy storage in phosphate bonds is a small factor. Consequently, heat production is considerable. The heat produced in muscle can be measured accurately with suitable thermocouples.

Resting heat, the heat given off at rest, is the external manifestation of basal metabolic processes. The heat produced in excess of resting heat during contraction is called the **initial heat.** This is made up of **activation heat,** the heat that muscle produces whenever it is contracting; and **shortening heat,** which is proportionate in amount to the distance the muscle shortens. Shortening heat is apparently due to some change in the structure of the muscle during shortening.

Following contraction, heat production in excess of resting heat continues for as long as 30 minutes. This **recovery heat** is the heat liberated by the metabolic processes which restore the muscle to its precontraction state. The recovery heat of muscle is approximately equal to the initial heat, ie, the heat produced during recovery is equal to the heat produced during contraction.

If a muscle which has contracted isotonically is restored to its previous length, extra heat in addition to recovery heat is produced (**relaxation heat**). External work must be done on the muscle to return it to its previous length, and relaxation heat is mainly a manifestation of this work.

PROPERTIES OF MUSCLES IN THE INTACT ORGANISM

Effects of Denervation

In the intact animal or human, healthy skeletal muscle does not contract except in response to stimulation of its motor nerve supply. Destruction of this nerve supply causes muscle atrophy. It also leads to abnormal excitability of the muscle and increases its sensitivity to circulating acetylcholine (denervation hypersensitivity; see Chapter 4). Fine, irregular contractions of individual fibers (**fibrillations**) appear. If the motor nerve regenerates, these disappear. Such contractions usually are not visible grossly and should not be confused with **fasciculations**, which are jerky, visible contractions of groups of muscle fibers due to pathologic discharge of spinal motor neurons.

The Motor Unit

Since the axons of the spinal motor neurons supplying skeletal muscle each branch to innervate several muscle fibers, the smallest possible amount of muscle which can contract in response to the excitation of a single motor neuron is not one muscle fiber but all the fibers supplied by the neuron. Each single motor neuron and the muscle fibers it innervates constitute a **motor unit.** The number of muscle fibers in a motor unit varies. In muscles such as those of the hand and those concerned with motion of the eye—ie, muscles concerned with fine, graded, precise movement—there are 3–6 muscle fibers per motor unit. On the other hand, values of 120–165 fibers per unit have been reported in cat leg muscles, and some of the large muscles of the back in humans probably contain even more.

Electromyography

Activation of motor units can be studied by **electromyography,** the process of recording the electrical activity of muscle on a cathode ray oscilloscope. This may be done in unanesthetized humans by using small metal disks on the skin overlying the muscle as the pick-up electrodes, or by using hypodermic needle electrodes. The record obtained with such electrodes is the **electromyogram (EMG).** With needle electrodes, it is usually possible to pick up the activity of single muscle fibers. A typical EMG is shown in Fig 3–12.

Factors Responsible for Grading of Muscular Activity

It has been shown by electromyography that

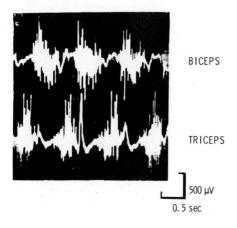

BICEPS

TRICEPS

500 μV

0.5 sec

Figure 3–12. Electromyographic tracings from human biceps and triceps muscles during alternate flexion and extension of the elbow. (Courtesy of BC Garoutte.)

there is little if any spontaneous activity in the skeletal muscles of normal individuals at rest. With minimal voluntary activity, a few motor units discharge, and with increasing voluntary effort more and more are brought into play. This process is sometimes called **recruitment of motor units**. Gradation of muscle response is therefore in part a function of the number of motor units activated. In addition, the frequency of discharge in the individual nerve fibers plays a role, the tension developed during a tetanic contraction being greater than that during individual twitches. The length of the muscle is also a factor. Finally, the motor units fire asynchronously, ie, out of phase with each other. This asynchronous firing causes the individual muscle fiber responses to merge into a smooth contraction of the whole muscle.

Muscle Types

The properties of the various muscles in humans vary with the character of the muscle fibers they contain. There are 3 types of skeletal muscle fibers: A fibers, which are large and pale and contain relatively little mitochondrial ATPase; C fibers, which are small and dark and contain large quantities of ATPase; and B fibers, which are intermediate in size and ATPase content. Most muscles contain a mixture of all 3 types of fibers and are pale or **white**. However, certain muscles are made up solely of B fibers, and these muscles are called **red** muscles because they are darker than the other muscles. The red muscles, which are also called **slow** muscles, respond slowly and have a longer latency than the white muscles. They are adapted for long, slow, posture-maintaining contractions. The long muscles of the back are red muscles. White muscles generally have short twitch durations and are called **fast** muscles. They are specialized for fine, skilled movements. The extraocular muscles and some of the hand muscles contain large numbers of A fibers. Each spinal motor neuron innervates only one

kind of muscle fiber, so that all the muscle fibers in a motor unit are of the same type.

The differences between these types of muscles are not inherent but are determined in part by their innervation. The nerves to fast and slow muscles have been crossed and allowed to regenerate. When regrowth was complete and the nerve which previously supplied the slow muscle innervated the fast one, the fast muscle became slow. The reverse change occurred in the previously slow muscle. There were also appropriate changes in ATPase content. There is evidence that substances can flow down neurons and enter muscle. However, the effect of the nerve on the chemistry of the muscle appears to be due to the pattern of discharge in the nerve rather than a trophic factor per se.

Denervation of skeletal muscle leads to atrophy and flaccid paralysis, with the appearance of fibrillations. These effects are the classical consequences of a **lower motor neuron lesion**. The muscle also becomes hypersensitive to acetylcholine (denervation hypersensitivity; see Chapter 4).

The Strength of Skeletal Muscles

Human skeletal muscle can exert 3–4 kg of tension per sq cm of cross-sectional area. This figure is about the same as that obtained in a variety of experimental animals, and seems to be constant for all mammalian species. Since many of the muscles in humans have a relatively large cross-sectional area, the tension they can develop is quite large. The gastrocnemius, for example, not only supports the weight of the whole body during climbing but resists a force several times this great when the foot hits the ground during running or jumping. An even more striking example is the gluteus maximus, which can exert a tension of 1200 kg. The total tension that could be developed by all muscles in the body of an adult man is approximately 22,000 kg (nearly 25 tons).

Body Mechanics

Body movements are generally organized in such a way that they take maximal advantage of the physiologic principles outlined above. For example, the attachments of the muscles in the body are such that many of them are normally at or near their resting length when they start to contract. In the case of muscles that extend over more than one joint, movement at one joint may compensate for movement at another in such a way that relatively little shortening of the muscle occurs during contraction. Nearly isometric contractions of this type permit development of maximal tension per contraction. The hamstring muscles extend from the pelvis over the hip joint and the knee joint to the tibia and fibula. Hamstring contraction produces flexion of the leg on the thigh. If the thigh is flexed on the pelvis at the same time, the lengthening of the hamstrings across the hip joint tends to compensate for the shortening across the knee joint. In the course of walking and other activities, the body moves in a way which takes advantage of this.

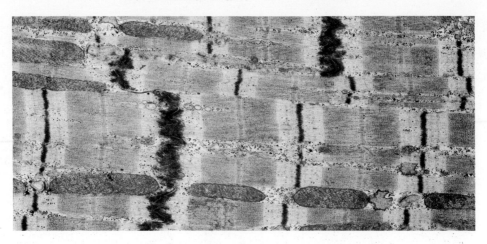

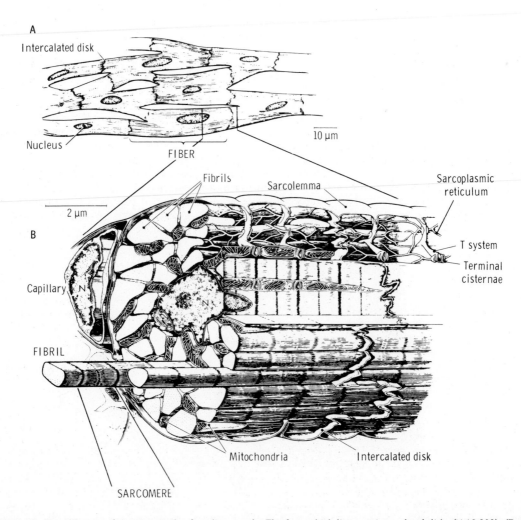

Figure 3–13. *Top:* Electron photomicrograph of cardiac muscle. The fuzzy thick lines are intercalated disks (✕ 12,000). (Reproduced, with permission, from Bloom & Fawcett: *A Textbook of Histology,* 10th ed. Saunders, 1975.) *Bottom:* Diagram of cardiac muscle as seen under the light microscope *(A)* and the electron microscope *(B).* N, nucleus. (Reproduced, with permission, from Braunwald & others: Mechanisms of contraction of the normal and failing heart. N Engl J Med 277:794, 1967. Courtesy of Little, Brown, Inc.)

Such factors as momentum and balance are integrated into body movement in ways which make possible maximal motion with minimal muscular exertion. In walking, for example, there is a brief burst of activity in the leg flexors at the start of each step, and then the leg is swung forward with little more active muscular contraction. Therefore, the muscles are active for only a fraction of each step, and walking for long periods of time causes relatively little fatigue.

CARDIAC MUSCLE

MORPHOLOGY

The striations in cardiac muscle are similar to those in skeletal muscle, and Z lines are present. The muscle fibers branch and interdigitate, but each is a complete unit surrounded by a cell membrane. Where the end of one muscle fiber abuts on another, the membranes of both fibers parallel each other through an extensive series of folds. These areas, which always occur at Z lines, are called **intercalated disks** (Fig 3–13). They provide a strong union between fibers, maintaining cell to cell cohesion, so that the pull of one contractile unit can be transmitted along its axis to the next. Along the sides of the muscle fibers next to the disks, the cell membranes of adjacent fibers fuse for considerable distances. These gap junctions provide low resistance bridges for the spread of excitation from one fiber to another (see Chapter 1). They permit cardiac muscle to function as if it were a syncytium, even though there are no protoplasmic bridges between cells. The T system in cardiac muscle is located at the Z lines rather than at the A–I junction (as it is in mammalian skeletal muscle). Cardiac muscle contains large numbers of elongated mitochondria in close contact with the fibrils.

ELECTRICAL PROPERTIES

Resting Membrane & Action Potentials

The resting membrane potential of individual mammalian cardiac muscle cells is about −80 mV (interior negative to exterior). Stimulation produces a propagated action potential which is responsible for initiating contraction. Depolarization proceeds rapidly and an overshoot is present, as in skeletal muscle and nerve, but repolarization is a slow process (Fig 3–14). In mammalian hearts, depolarization lasts about 2 msec, but repolarization lasts 200 msec or more. Repolarization is therefore not complete until the contraction is half over. With extracellular recording, the

electrical events include a spike and a later wave that bear a resemblance to the QRS complex and T wave of the electrocardiogram. Intracellular records indicate that repolarization is a 3-phase process. After the spike, repolarization starts rapidly but then becomes prolonged, with a final more rapid return to the resting membrane potential.

As in other excitable tissues, changes in the external K^+ concentration affect the resting membrane potential of cardiac muscle, whereas changes in the external Na^+ concentration affect the magnitude of the action potential (Fig 3–15). Depolarization and the first rapid phase of repolarization are apparently due to a rapid change in Na^+ permeability similar to that occurring in nerve and skeletal muscle, whereas the second plateau phase is due to a slower starting, less intense, and more prolonged increase in Ca^{++} permeability. The third phase is the manifestation of a delayed increase in K^+ permeability. This increase produces the K^+ efflux which completes the repolarization process.

In cardiac muscle, the repolarization time decreases as the cardiac rate increases. At a cardiac rate of 75 beats per minute, the duration of the action potential (0.25 sec) is almost 70% longer than it is at a cardiac rate of 200 (0.15 sec).

MECHANICAL PROPERTIES

Refractory Period

The contractile response of cardiac muscle begins just after the start of depolarization and lasts about 1½ times as long as the action potential (Fig 3–14). The

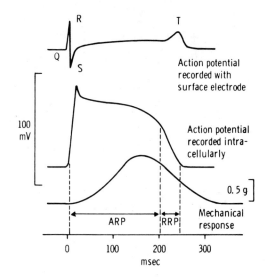

Figure 3–14. Action potentials and contractile response of mammalian cardiac muscle fiber plotted on the same time axis. ARP, absolute refractory period; RRP, relative refractory period.

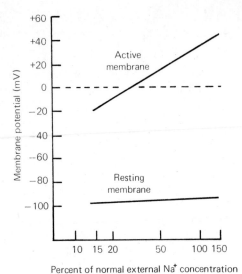

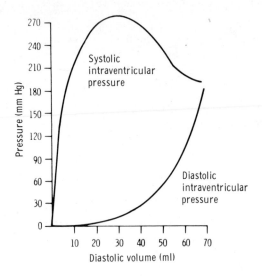

Percent of normal external Na⁺ concentration

Diastolic volume (ml)

Figure 3—15. Effect of changes in the external concentration of Na⁺ on the peak amplitude of the action potential (top curve) and the resting membrane potential (bottom curve) in cardiac muscle. (Modified from Weidmann: *Elektrophysiologie der Herzmuskelfaser.* Verlag Hans Huber, 1956).

Figure 3—16. "Length-tension" relationship for cardiac muscle. The values are for dog heart. (Modified from Patterson & others: The regulation of the heart beat. J Physiol 48:465, 1914.)

role of Ca^{++} in excitation-contraction coupling is similar to its role in skeletal muscle (see above). Responses of the muscle are all or none in character, ie, the muscle fibers contract fully if they respond at all. Since cardiac muscle is absolutely refractory during most of the action potential, the contractile response is more than half over by the time a second response can be initiated. Therefore, tetanus of the type seen in skeletal muscle cannot occur. Of course, tetanization of cardiac muscle for any length of time would have lethal consequences, and in this sense the fact that cardiac muscle cannot be tetanized is a safety feature. Ventricular muscle is said to be in the "vulnerable period" just at the end of the action potential, because stimulation at this time will sometimes initiate ventricular fibrillation.

Correlation Between Muscle Fiber Length & Tension

The relation between initial fiber length and total tension in cardiac muscle is similar to that in skeletal muscle; there is a resting length at which the tension developed upon stimulation is maximal. In the body, the initial length of the fibers is determined by the degree of diastolic filling of the heart and the pressure developed in the ventricle is proportionate to the total tension developed. As the diastolic filling increases, the force of contraction of the ventricles is increased (Fig 3—16). The homeostatic value of this response is apparent.

The force of contraction of cardiac muscle is also increased by catecholamines (see Chapter 13), and this increase occurs without a change in muscle length. The increase, which is called the positively ino-

tropic effect of catecholamines, is mediated via β-adrenergic receptors and cyclic AMP. Cyclic AMP in turn increases Ca^{++} influx from the ECF, making more Ca^{++} available to bind to troponin C. Cyclic AMP via a protein kinase also increases the active transport of Ca^{++} to the sarcoplasmic reticulum, thus accelerating relaxation and consequently shortening systole. This is important when the cardiac rate is increased because it permits adequate diastolic filling. Digitalis glycosides increase cardiac contractions by decreasing Ca^{++} efflux.

METABOLISM

Although the general pattern of cardiac muscle metabolism resembles that of skeletal muscle, there are differences. Mammalian hearts have an abundant blood supply, numerous mitochondria, and a high content of myoglobin, a muscle pigment that may function as an O_2 storage mechanism. Normally, less than 1% of the total energy liberated is provided by anaerobic metabolism. During hypoxia, this figure may increase to nearly 10%; but under totally anaerobic conditions the energy liberated is inadequate to sustain ventricular contractions. Under basal conditions, 35% of the caloric needs of the human heart are provided by carbohydrate, 5% by ketones and amino acids, and 60% by fat. However, the proportions of substrates utilized vary greatly with the nutritional state. After feeding large amounts of glucose, more lactic acid and pyruvic acid are used; during prolonged starvation, more fat is used. Circulating free fatty acids normally account for almost 50% of the lipid utilized. In untreated diabetics, the carbohydrate utilization of cardiac muscle is reduced and that of fat increased.

PACEMAKER TISSUE

The heart continues to beat after all nerves to it are sectioned; indeed, if the heart is cut into pieces, the pieces continue to beat. This is because of the presence in the heart of specialized pacemaker tissue that can initiate repetitive action potentials. The pacemaker tissue makes up the conduction system that normally spreads impulses throughout the heart.

Pacemaker tissue is characterized by an unstable membrane potential. Instead of a steady value between impulses, the membrane potential declines steadily after each action potential until the firing level is reached and another action potential is triggered. This slow depolarization between action potentials is called a **pacemaker potential** or **prepotential** (Fig 3–17). The steeper its slope, the faster the rate at which the pacemaker fires. Some agents that modify the firing rate of pacemakers do so by changing the slope of the prepotential, although others act by altering the membrane potential and thus changing the amount of time required to reach the firing level. The prepotential has been shown to be due to a slow decrease in K^+ permeability. This causes a progressive decline in K^+ efflux and a resultant reduction in membrane potential. Prepotentials are not seen in atrial and ventricular muscle cells; and in these cells, K^+ permeability is constant during diastole.

SMOOTH MUSCLE

MORPHOLOGY

Smooth muscle is distinguished anatomically from skeletal and cardiac muscle because it lacks visible cross-striations. There is a sarcoplasmic reticulum, but it is poorly developed. The muscle contains actin and myosin, and there is debate about the arrangement of the filaments. In intestinal smooth muscle, there is evidence that the contractile units are made up of small bundles of interdigitating thick and thin filaments that are irregularly shaped and randomly arranged. When the muscle contracts, the thick and thin filaments are thought to slide on each other.

Types

There are various types of smooth muscle in the body. In general, smooth muscle can be divided into **visceral smooth muscle** and **multi-unit smooth muscle**. Visceral smooth muscle occurs in large sheets, has low resistance bridges between individual muscle cells, and functions in a syncytial fashion. The bridges, like those in cardiac muscle, are junctions where the membranes of the 2 adjacent cells fuse to form a single membrane. Visceral smooth muscle is found primarily in the walls of hollow viscera. The musculature of the intestine, the uterus, and the ureters are examples. Multi-unit smooth muscle is made up of individual units without interconnecting bridges. It is found in structures such as the iris of the eye in which fine, graded contractions occur. It is usually not under voluntary control, but it has many functional similarities to skeletal muscle.

VISCERAL SMOOTH MUSCLE

Electrical & Mechanical Activity

Visceral smooth muscle is characterized by the instability of its membrane potential and by the fact that it shows continuous, irregular contractions that are independent of its nerve supply. This maintained state of partial contraction is called **tonus**, or **tone**. The membrane potential has no true "resting" value, being relatively low when the tissue is active and higher when it is inhibited; but in periods of relative quiescence it averages about -50 mV. Superimposed on the membrane potential are waves of various types (Fig 3–18). There are slow sine wave-like fluctuations a few millivolts in magnitude and spikes that sometimes overshoot the zero potential line and sometimes do not. In many tissues the spikes have a duration of about 50 msec. However, in some tissues the action potentials have a prolonged plateau during repolarization, like the action potentials in cardiac muscle. The spikes may occur on the rising or falling phases of the sine wave

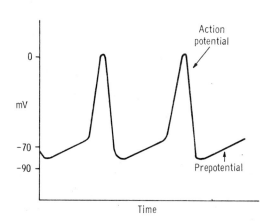

Figure 3–17. Diagram of the membrane potential of pacemaker tissue.

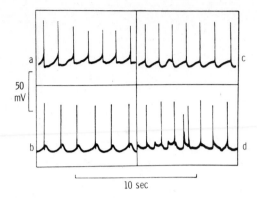

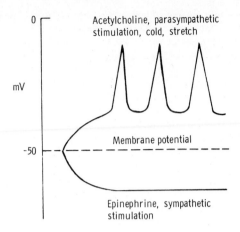

INTESTINAL SMOOTH MUSCLE

Figure 3–18. Spontaneous electrical activity in individual smooth muscle cells of teniae coli of guinea pig colon. *a:* Pacemaker type; *b:* sinusoidal waves with action potentials on the rising phases; *c:* sinusoidal waves with action potentials on the falling phases; *d:* mixture of pacemaker, oscillatory, and conducted action potentials. (Reproduced, with permission, from Bulbring: Physiology and pharmacology of intestinal smooth muscle. Lectures on the Scientific Basis of Medicine 7:374, 1957.)

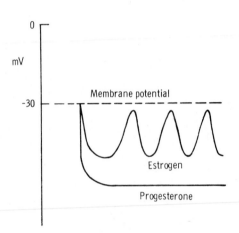

UTERINE SMOOTH MUSCLE

Figure 3–19. *Above:* Effects of various agents on the membrane potential of intestinal smooth muscle. *Below:* Effects of estrogens and of progesterone on the membrane potential of the uterus of the ovariectomized rabbit or rat. (Modified and reproduced, with permission, from Burnstock & others: Electrophysiology of smooth muscle. Physiol Rev 43:482, 1963.)

oscillations. There are, in addition, pacemaker potentials similar to those found in the cardiac pacemakers. However, in visceral smooth muscle, these potentials are generated in multiple foci which shift from place to place. Spikes generated in the pacemaker foci are conducted for some distance in the muscle. Because of the continuous activity, it is difficult to study the relation between the electrical and mechanical events in visceral smooth muscle; but in some relatively inactive preparations, a single spike can be generated. The muscle starts to contract about 200 msec after the start of the spike and 150 msec after the spike is over. The peak contraction is reached as long as 500 msec after the spike. Thus, the excitation-contraction coupling in visceral smooth muscle is a very slow process compared to skeletal and cardiac muscle, in which the time from initial depolarization to initiation of contraction is less than 10 msec. Ca^{++} is involved in the initiation of contraction of smooth muscle, but the details of its function remain unknown.

Visceral smooth muscle is unique in that, unlike other types of muscle, it contracts when stretched in the absence of any extrinsic innervation. Stretch is followed by a decline in membrane potential, an increase in the frequency of spikes, and a general increase in tone.

If epinephrine is added to a preparation of intestinal smooth muscle arranged for recording of intracellular potentials in vitro, the membrane potential usually becomes larger, the spikes decrease in frequency, and the muscle relaxes (Fig 3–19). Norepinephrine is the chemical mediator released at adrenergic nerve endings (see Chapter 13), and stimulation of the adrenergic nerves to the preparation has a similar effect. Stimulation of the adrenergic nerves to the intestine inhibits contractions in vivo. Norepinephrine

exerts both a and β actions (see Chapter 13) on the muscle. The β action, reduced muscle tension in response to excitation, is probably due to increased intracellular binding of Ca^{++}. The a action, which is also inhibition of contraction, is associated with increased Ca^{++} efflux from the muscle cells.

Acetylcholine has an effect opposite to that of norepinephrine on the membrane potential and contractile activity of intestinal smooth muscle. If acetylcholine is added to the fluid bathing a smooth muscle preparation in vitro, the membrane potential decreases and the spikes become more frequent (Fig 3–19). The muscle becomes more active, with an increase in tonic tension and the number of rhythmic contractions. The depolarization is apparently due to an increase in Na^+

permeability. In the intact animal, stimulation of cholinergic nerves causes release of acetylcholine and increased intestinal contractions. In vitro, similar effects are produced by cold and stretch.

Function of the Nerve Supply to Smooth Muscle

The effects of acetylcholine and norepinephrine on visceral smooth muscle serve to emphasize 2 of its important properties: (1) its spontaneous activity in the absence of nervous stimulation, and (2) its sensitivity to chemical agents released from nerves locally or brought to it in the circulation. In mammals, visceral muscle usually has a dual nerve supply from the 2 divisions of the autonomic nervous system. The structure and function of the contacts between these nerves and smooth muscle are discussed in Chapter 4. The function of the nerve supply is not to initiate activity in the muscle but rather to modify it. Stimulation of one division of the autonomic nervous system usually increases smooth muscle activity, whereas stimulation of the other decreases it. However, in some organs, adrenergic stimulation increases and cholinergic stimulation decreases smooth muscle activity; in others, the reverse is true.

Other chemical agents also affect smooth muscle. An interesting example is the uterus. Uterine smooth muscle is relatively inexcitable during diestrus and in the ovariectomized animal. During estrus or in the estrogen-treated ovariectomized animal, excitability is enhanced and tonus and spontaneous contractions occur. However, estrogen increases rather than decreases the membrane potential (Fig 3–19). Progesterone increases the membrane potential even further and inhibits the electrical and contractile activity of uterine muscle.

Relation of Length to Tension; Plasticity

Another special characteristic of smooth muscle is the variability of the tension it exerts at any given length. If a piece of visceral smooth muscle is stretched, it first exerts increased tension (see above). However, if the muscle is held at the greater length after stretching, the tension gradually decreases. Sometimes the tension falls to or below the level exerted before the muscle was stretched. It is consequently impossible to correlate length and developed tension accurately, and no resting length can be assigned. In some ways, therefore, smooth muscle behaves more like a viscous mass than a rigidly structured tissue, and it is this property which is referred to as the **plasticity** of smooth muscle.

The consequences of plasticity can be demonstrated in the intact animal. For example, the tension exerted by the smooth muscle walls of the bladder can be measured at varying degrees of distention. To obtain the data shown in Fig 3–20, a catheter was inserted into the empty bladder of an intact human and fluid introduced in 50 ml increments. After each addition of fluid, the tension was measured for a period of time. Immediately after each increment of fluid, the tension was higher; but after a short period of

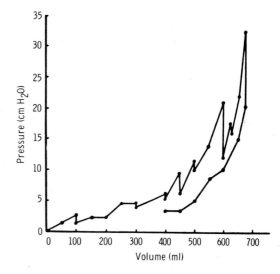

Figure 3–20. Change in pressure in the human bladder during filling and emptying. Water was instilled into the bladder by catheter 50 ml at a time, the inflow being stopped and the pressure measured after each increment (upper left curve). After 700 ml had been instilled, the bladder was allowed to empty 50 ml at a time (lower right curve). (Reproduced, with permission, from Denny-Brown & Robertson: Physiology of micturition. Brain 56:149, 1933.)

time it decreased. Therefore, the filling curve in Fig 3–20 is not a smooth curve but a jagged line. After 700 ml had been infused into the bladder, the subject voided in 50 ml increments and the tension was recorded after each increment. Plotting these tensions produced an emptying curve which was different from the filling curve, again due to the absence of any constant relationship between fiber length and tension.

MULTI-UNIT SMOOTH MUSCLE

Unlike visceral smooth muscle, multi-unit smooth muscle is nonsyncytial and contractions do not spread widely through it. Because of this, the contractions of multi-unit smooth muscle are more discrete, fine, and localized than those of visceral smooth muscle. Like visceral smooth muscle, multi-unit smooth muscle is very sensitive to circulating chemical substances and is normally activated by chemical mediators (acetylcholine and norepinephrine) released at the endings of its motor nerves. Especially in the case of norepinephrine, the mediator tends to persist and to cause repeated firing of the muscle after a single stimulus rather than a single action potential. Therefore, the contractile response produced is usually an irregular tetanus rather than a single twitch. When a single twitch response is obtained, it resembles the twitch contraction of skeletal muscle except that its duration is 10 times as long.

4 . . .

Synaptic & Junctional Transmission

The all or none type of conduction seen in axons and skeletal muscle has been discussed in Chapters 2 and 3. Impulses are transmitted from one nerve cell to another at **synapses** (Fig 4–1). These are the junctions where the axon or some other portion of one cell (the **presynaptic cell**) terminates on the soma, the dendrites, or some other portion of another neuron (the **postsynaptic cell**). It is worth noting that dendrites as well as axons can be presynaptic or postsynaptic. Transmission at most of the junctions is chemical; the impulse in the presynaptic axon liberates a **chemical mediator**. The chemical mediator binds to receptors on the surface of the postsynaptic cell, and this triggers intracellular events which alter the permeability of the membrane of the postsynaptic neuron. At some of the junctions, however, transmission is **electrical**, and at a few **conjoint synapses** it is both electrical and chemical (Fig 4–2). In any case, impulses in the presynaptic fibers usually contribute to the initiation of conducted responses in the postsynaptic cell, but transmission is not a simple jumping of one action potential from the presynaptic to the postsynaptic neuron. It is a complex process which permits the grading and modulation of neural activity necessary for normal function.

In the case of electrical synapses, the membranes of the presynaptic and postsynaptic neurons come close together, forming a gap junction (see Chapter 1). Like the intercellular junctions in other tissues (see Chapter 1), these junctions form low-resistance bridges through which ions pass with relative ease. Electrical and conjoint synapses are being found with increasing frequency in mammals, and there is electrical coupling, for example, between some of the neurons in the lateral vestibular nucleus. However, most synaptic transmission is chemical. Consideration in this chapter is limited, unless otherwise specified, to chemical transmission.

Transmission from nerve to muscle resembles chemical synaptic transmission. The **myoneural junction**, the specialized area where a motor nerve terminates on a skeletal muscle fiber, is the site of a stereotyped transmission process. The contacts between autonomic neurons and smooth and cardiac muscle are less specialized, and transmission is a more diffuse process.

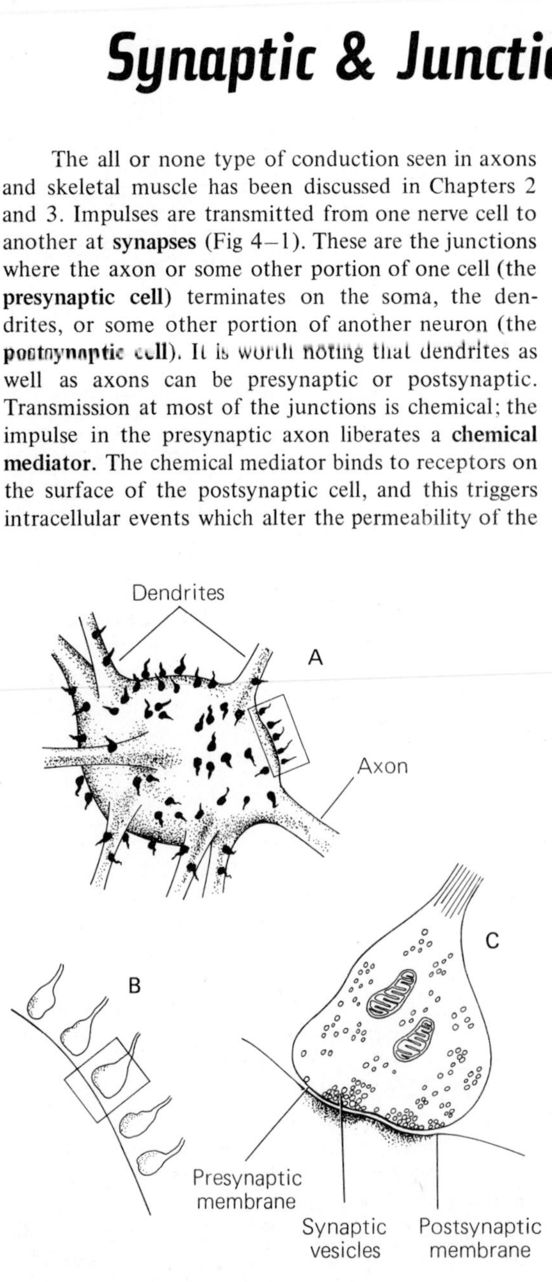

SYNAPTIC TRANSMISSION

SYNAPTIC ANATOMY

There is considerable variation in the anatomic structure of synapses in various parts of the mammalian nervous system. The ends of the presynaptic fibers are generally enlarged to form **terminal buttons**, or **synaptic knobs** (Figs 4–1, 4–2). Endings are com-

Figure 4–1. Synapses on a spinal motor neuron. *A:* Cell body of spinal motor neuron. The dark objects are synaptic knobs at the ends of the axons of presynaptic neurons. The area in the rectangle in *A* is enlarged in *B*, and the area in the rectangle in *B* is enlarged in *C*. (Modified from Junqueira, Carneiro, & Contopoulos: *Basic Histology,* 2nd ed. Lange, 1977.)

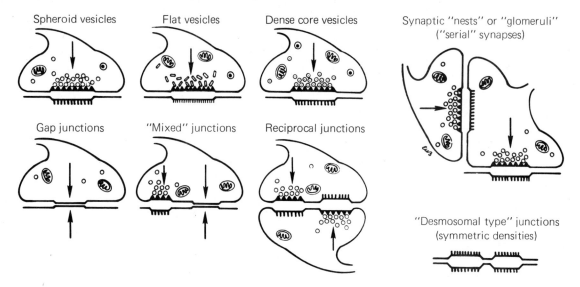

Figure 4—2. Major types of synaptic junctions. At synapses where there are vesicles, conduction is chemical, whereas conduction at gap junctions is electrical. Flattened vesicles appear to contain inhibitory mediator, whereas dense core vesicles contain catecholamines. The "desmosomal type" junctions occur in sympathetic ganglia, but their function is unknown. (Reproduced, with permission, from Bodian: Neuron junctions: A revolutionary decade. Anat Rec 174:73, 1973.)

monly located on **dendritic spines**, which are small knobs projecting from dendrites. In some instances the terminal branches of the axon of the presynaptic neuron form a basket or net around the soma of the postsynaptic cell ("basket cells" of the cerebellum and autonomic ganglia). In other locations, they intertwine with the dendrites of the postsynaptic cell (climbing fibers of the cerebellum) or end on the dendrites directly (apical dendrites of cortical pyramids) or on the axons (axo-axonal endings). In the spinal cord, the presynaptic endings are closely applied to the soma and the proximal portions of the dendrites of the postsynaptic neuron. The number of synaptic knobs varies from one per postsynaptic cell (in the midbrain) to a very large number. The number of synaptic knobs applied to a single spinal motor neuron has been calculated to be about 5500; there are so many knobs that the neuron appears to be encrusted with them. The portion of the soma membrane covered by any single synaptic knob is small, but the synaptic knobs are so numerous that, in aggregate, the area covered by them all is often 40% of the total membrane area (Fig 4–1). There are even more endings on the dendrites.

Synaptic Knobs

Under the electron microscope, the synaptic knobs at synapses where transmission is chemical are found to be separated from the soma of the postsynaptic cell by a definite **synaptic cleft** about 20 nm wide. The synaptic knob and the soma each have an intact membrane. Inside the knob, there are many mitochondria and small vesicles or granules, the latter being especially numerous in the part of the knob closest to the synaptic cleft. The vesicles or granules contain small "packets" of the chemical transmitter responsi-

ble for synaptic transmission (see below). They vary in morphology depending on the particular transmitter they contain.

The transmitter is released from the synaptic knobs when action potentials pass along the axon to the endings. The membranes of the vesicles or granules fuse to the nerve cell membrane and the area of fusion breaks down, releasing the contents by the process of exocytosis (see Chapter 1). Ca^{++} triggers this process, and the action potential increases the permeability of the nerve cell membrane to Ca^{++} The amount of transmitter released is proportionate to the Ca^{++} influx.

Convergence & Divergence

Only a few of the synaptic knobs on a postsynaptic neuron are endings of any single presynaptic neuron. The inputs to the cell are multiple. In the case of spinal motor neurons, for example, some inputs come directly from the dorsal root, some from the long descending spinal tracts, and many from **interneurons**, the short interconnecting neurons of the spinal cord. Thus, many presynaptic neurons **converge** on any single postsynaptic neuron. Conversely, the axons of most presynaptic neurons divide into many branches which **diverge** to end on many postsynaptic neurons. Convergence and divergence are the anatomic substrates for facilitation, occlusion, and reverberation (see below). It has been calculated that there are approximately 10^{14} synapses in the human brain and that, on the average, each of the more than 10 billion neurons in the nervous system has 100 inputs converging on it while it in turn diverges to 100 other neurons. The number of possible paths an impulse can take through a neuron net of this complexity is astronomically large.

ELECTRICAL EVENTS AT SYNAPSES

Synaptic activity in the spinal cord has been studied in detail by inserting a microelectrode into the soma of a motor neuron in the cat and recording the electrical events that follow stimulation of the excitatory and inhibitory inputs to these cells. Activity at other synapses has not been so well studied in mammals, but the events occurring at these synapses are apparently similar to those occurring at spinal synapses.

Penetration of an anterior horn cell is achieved by advancing a microelectrode through the ventral portion of the spinal cord. Puncture of a cell membrane is signalled by the appearance of a steady 70 mV potential difference between the microelectrode and an electrode outside the cell. The cell can be identified as a spinal motor neuron by stimulating the appropriate ventral root and observing the electrical activity of the cell. Such stimulation initiates an antidromic impulse (see Chapter 2) which is conducted to the soma and stops at this point. Therefore, the presence of an action potential in the cell after antidromic stimulation indicates that the cell that has been penetrated is a motor neuron rather than an interneuron. Activity in some of the presynaptic terminals impinging on the impaled spinal motor neuron (Fig 4–3) can be initiated by stimulating the dorsal roots.

Excitatory Postsynaptic Potentials

Single stimuli applied to the sensory nerves in the experimental situation described above characteristically do not lead to the formation of a propagated action potential in the postsynaptic neuron. Instead, the stimulation produces either a transient, partial depolarization or a transient hyperpolarization.

The depolarizing response produced by a single stimulus to the proper input begins about 0.5 msec after the afferent impulse enters the spinal cord. It reaches its peak 1–1.5 msec later, and then declines exponentially, with a **time constant** (time required for the response to decay to 1/e, or 1/2.718 of its maximum) of about 4 msec. During this potential, the excitability of the neuron to other stimuli is increased, and consequently the potential is called an **excitatory postsynaptic potential (EPSP)**.

The EPSP is due to depolarization of the postsynaptic cell membrane immediately under the active synaptic knob. The area of inward current flow thus created is so small that it will not drain off enough positive charges to depolarize the whole membrane. Instead, an EPSP is inscribed. The EPSP due to activity in one synaptic knob is small, but the depolarizations produced by each of the active knobs summate.

Summation may be **spatial** or **temporal**. When activity is present in more than one synaptic knob at the same time, spatial summation occurs and activity in one synaptic knob is said to **facilitate** activity in another to approach the firing level. Temporal summation occurs if repeated afferent stimuli cause new EPSPs before previous EPSPs have decayed. Spatial and temporal facilitation are illustrated in Fig 4–4. The EPSP is therefore not an all or none response but is proportionate in size to the strength of the afferent stimulus. If the EPSP is large enough to reach the firing level of the cell, a full-fledged action potential is produced.

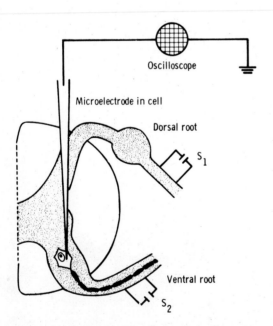

Figure 4–3. Arrangement of recording electrodes and stimulators for studying synaptic activity in spinal motor neurons in mammals. One stimulator (S_2) is used to produce antidromic impulses for identifying the cell; the other (S_1) is used to produce orthodromic stimulation via reflex pathways.

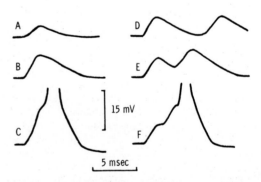

Figure 4–4. Spatial summation (A–C) and temporal summation (D–F) of EPSPs. Records are potential changes recorded with one electrode inside the postsynaptic cell. In A–C, afferent volleys of increasing strength were delivered. In C, the firing level was reached and an action potential generated. In D–F, 2 different volleys of the same strength were delivered but the time interval between them was shortened. In F, the firing level was reached and an action potential generated. (Based on Eccles: *The Physiology of Nerve Cells.* Johns Hopkins Univ Press, 1957.)

Synaptic Delay

When an impulse reaches the presynaptic terminals, there is an interval of at least 0.5 msec, the **synaptic delay**, before a response is obtained in the postsynaptic neuron. The delay following maximal stimulation of the presynaptic neuron corresponds to the latency of the EPSP, and is due to the time it takes for the synaptic mediator to be released and to act on the membrane of the postsynaptic cell. Because of it, conduction along a chain of neurons is slower if there are many synapses in the chain than if there are only a few. This fact is important in comparing, for example, transmission in the lemniscal sensory pathways to the cerebral cortex and transmission in the reticular activating system (see Chapter 11). Since the minimum time for transmission across one synapse is 0.5 msec, it is also possible to determine whether a given reflex pathway is monosynaptic or polysynaptic (contains more than one synapse) by measuring the delay in transmission from the dorsal to the ventral root across the spinal cord.

Ionic Basis of EPSPs

The ionic events underlying excitatory synaptic activity have been worked out in considerable detail. Depolarization of the synaptic knob of an excitatory input is followed by an increase in the permeability of the soma membrane underlying it to Na^+. Consequently, Na^+ moves along its concentration and electrical gradients into the cell (see Chapter 2) and a depolarizing potential is produced. However, the area in which this influx occurs is so small that the repolarizing forces are able to overcome its influence, and runaway depolarization of the whole membrane does not result. If more excitatory synaptic knobs are active, more Na^+ enters and the depolarizing potential is greater. If Na^+ influx is great enough, the firing level is reached and a propagated action potential results.

Inhibitory Postsynaptic Potentials

An EPSP is usually produced by afferent stimulation, but stimulation of certain presynaptic fibers regularly initiates a hyperpolarizing response in spinal motor neurons. This response begins 1–1.25 msec after the afferent stimulus enters the cord, reaches its peak in 1.5–2 msec, and declines exponentially with a time constant of 3 msec. During this potential, the excitability of the neuron to other stimuli is decreased; consequently, it is called an **inhibitory postsynaptic potential (IPSP)**. Spatial summation of IPSPs occurs, as shown by the increasing size of the response as the strength of an inhibitory afferent volley is increased (Fig 4–5). Temporal summation also occurs. This type of inhibition is called **postsynaptic** or **direct inhibition**.

Ionic Basis of IPSPs

At least in some neurons, the IPSP is apparently due to a localized increase in membrane permeability to Cl^- but not to Na^+. When an inhibitory synaptic knob becomes active, the area of the postsynaptic cell membrane under the knob permits increased Cl^- influx

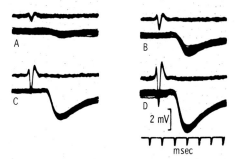

Figure 4–5. Inhibitory postsynaptic potentials. The lower tracing in each case is the intracellular response of a biceps semitendinosus motor neuron to stimulation of the nerve from the quadriceps. The upper tracing is the externally recorded response from the dorsal root. Note that the IPSPs increase in size as the stimulus strength is increased from A to D. All records were obtained by superimposing about 40 traces. (Reproduced, with permission, from Eccles, in: *Handbook of Physiology.* Field J, Magoun HW [editors]. Washington: American Physiological Society, 1959. Section 1, pp 59–74.)

as the ions flow down their concentration gradients. The net effect is the transfer of negative charge into the cell, so that the membrane potential increases. However, the permeability change is short-lived, and resting conditions are rapidly restored. There is evidence that this restoration is due to active transport of Cl^- out of the cell.

The decreased excitability of the nerve cell during the IPSP is due in part to moving the membrane potential away from the firing level. Consequently, more

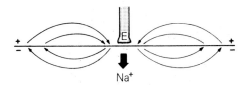

Excitatory transmitter ⟶
increased permeability of
postsynaptic cell membrane
to Na^+

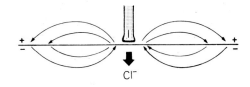

Inhibitory transmitter ⟶
increased permeability of
postsynaptic cell membrane
to Cl^-, not to Na^+

Figure 4–6. Summary of events occurring at synapses in mammals.

excitatory (depolarizing) activity is necessary to reach the firing level. However, additional factors are involved; when the membrane potential is held at −80 mV, inhibitory stimulation still decreases excitability even though the membrane potential does not change. The actions of excitatory and inhibitory synaptic activity on the membrane of the postsynaptic cell are summarized in Fig 4–6.

Neurons Responsible for Postsynaptic Inhibition

Stimulation of certain sensory nerve fibers known to pass directly to motor neurons in the spinal cord produces EPSPs in these neurons and IPSPs in other neurons. If these afferent fibers also passed directly to the neurons in which IPSPs are produced, it would be necessary to postulate that a single presynaptic neuron has 2 kinds of endings, some excitatory and some inhibitory, or, alternatively, that the soma membrane of the postsynaptic cell is a patchwork of 2 kinds of membrane. However, evidence has accumulated that a single interneuron is inserted between afferent dorsal root fibers and inhibitory endings. This special interneuron, called a Golgi bottle neuron, is short and plump and has a thick axon. Discharge of the chemical mediator from the synaptic knobs of this neuron causes formation of an IPSP due to an increase in the permeability of the postsynaptic cell membrane to Cl⁻ but not to Na⁺. In this way, excitatory input is "converted" into inhibitory input by interposing a single Golgi bottle neuron between the excitatory ending and the spinal motor neuron.

Generation of the Action Potential in the Postsynaptic Neuron

The constant interplay of excitatory and inhibitory activity on the postsynaptic neuron produces a fluctuating membrane potential that is the algebraic sum of the hyperpolarizing and depolarizing activity. The soma of the neuron thus acts as a sort of integrator. When the 10–15 mV of depolarization sufficient to reach the firing level is attained, a propagated spike results. However, the discharge of the neuron is slightly more complicated than this. In motor neurons, the portion of the cell with the lowest threshold for the production of a full-fledged action potential is the **initial segment,** the portion of the axon at and just beyond the axon hillock. This unmyelinated segment is depolarized or hyperpolarized electronically by the current sinks and sources under the excitatory and inhibitory synaptic knobs. It is the first part of the neuron to fire, and its discharge is propagated in 2 directions: down the axon and back into the soma. Retrograde firing of the soma in this fashion probably has value in "wiping the slate clean" for subsequent renewal of the interplay of excitatory and inhibitory activity on the cell.

Function of the Dendrites

Dendrites usually do not conduct like the axons. Action potentials are generated in some of the dendrites, but they are usually part of the "receptor membrane" of the neuron (see Chapter 2), the site of current sources or sinks which electrotonically change the membrane potential of the axon hillock region or other locus from which the action potentials are generated. In the CNS, there are in addition neurons with dendrites but no axons. These cells transmit action potentials or spread EPSPs and IPSPs from one neuron to another without a propagated action potential. When the dendritic tree of a neuron is extensive and has multiple presynaptic knobs ending on it, there is room for a great interplay of inhibitory and excitatory activity. Current flow to and from the dendrites in these situations waxes and wanes. The role of the dendrites in the genesis of the electroencephalogram is discussed in Chapter 11.

Electrical Transmission

At synaptic junctions where transmission is electrical, the impulse reaching the presynaptic terminal generates an EPSP in the postsynaptic cell which, because of the low-resistance bridge between the 2, has a much shorter latency than the EPSP at a synapse where transmission is chemical. In conjoint synapses, there is both a short latency response and a longer latency, chemically mediated, postsynaptic response.

CHEMICAL TRANSMISSION OF SYNAPTIC ACTIVITY

The nature of the chemical mediators at many of the synapses is not known. However, acetylcholine is the mediator at all synapses between preganglionic and postganglionic fibers of the autonomic nervous system, at the myoneural junction, and at all postganglionic parasympathetic and some postganglionic sympathetic endings. It is also a mediator in the CNS. The chemical and biophysical events occurring at synapses where it is a mediator are relatively well understood, and the mediator function of acetylcholine provides a good example of chemical mediation of synaptic activity. It should be emphasized, however, that acetylcholine is only one of the mediators in the nervous system.

Acetylcholine

The relatively simple structure of acetylcholine, which is the acetyl ester of choline, is shown in Fig 4–7. It exists, largely enclosed in clear synaptic vesicles, in high concentration in the terminal buttons of cholinergic neurons. Neurons which release acetylcholine are known as **cholinergic** neurons. The arrival of an impulse at a synaptic knob increases the Ca⁺⁺ permeability of the membrane, and the resultant Ca⁺⁺ influx causes liberation of acetylcholine into the synaptic cleft by the process of exocytosis. The transmitter crosses the cleft, and, at those synaptic junctions where acetylcholine is an excitatory mediator, it acts on receptors on the membrane of the postsynaptic cell to increase the permeability of the membrane to Na⁺.

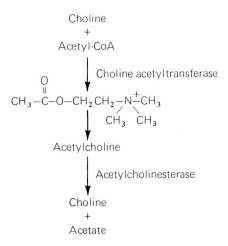

Choline
+
Acetyl-CoA

Choline acetyltransferase

$$CH_3-\overset{\overset{O}{\|}}{C}-O-CH_2CH_2-\overset{+}{N}\overset{CH_3}{\underset{CH_3\quad CH_3}{\diagdown}}$$

Acetylcholine

Acetylcholinesterase

Choline
+
Acetate

Figure 4–7. Biosynthesis and catabolism of acetylcholine.

Cholinesterases

Acetylcholine must be rapidly removed from the synapse if repolarization is to occur. Some is taken up again by the presynaptic terminals, but most is hydrolyzed by a process catalyzed by the enzyme **acetylcholinesterase**. This enzyme is also called **true** or **specific cholinesterase**. It is present in high concentrations in the cell membranes at nerve terminals which are cholinergic, but it is also found in some other membranes, in red blood cells, and in the placenta. Its greatest affinity is for acetylcholine, but it also hydrolyzes other choline esters. There are a variety of esterases in the body. One found in plasma is capable of hydrolyzing acetylcholine but has different properties from acetylcholinesterase. It is therefore called **pseudocholinesterase** or **nonspecific cholinesterase**. The plasma moiety is partly under endocrine control and is affected by variations in liver function. On the other hand, the specific cholinesterase at nerve endings is highly localized. Hydrolysis of acetylcholine by this enzyme is rapid enough to explain the observed changes in Na^+ permeability and electrical activity during synaptic transmission.

Acetylcholine Synthesis

Synthesis of acetylcholine involves the reaction of choline with acetate. There is an active uptake of choline into cholinergic neurons (Fig 13–4). The acetate is activated by the combination of acetate groups with reduced coenzyme A. The reaction between active acetate (acetyl-coenzyme A) and choline is catalyzed by the enzyme **choline acetyltransferase**. This enzyme is found in high concentration in the cytoplasm of cholinergic nerve endings; indeed, its localization is so specific that the presence of a high concentration in any given neural area has been taken as evidence that the synapses in that area are cholinergic.

Inhibitory Mediator

The chemical mediator released at the endings of the inhibitory interneurons in the spinal cord produces IPSPs in the postsynaptic neurons. The chemical nature of this **inhibitory mediator** has not been conclusively determined, although it appears to be the amino acid **glycine**. The action of the mediator is inhibited, possibly competitively, by strychnine and tetanus toxin. Thus, the action of these 2 poisons is to inhibit inhibition, with consequent unopposed play of excitatory impulses. The clinical picture of convulsions and muscular hyperactivity produced by tetanus toxin and strychnine emphasizes the importance of postsynaptic inhibition in normal neural function.

Other Chemical Mediators

Norepinephrine is the mediator of activity at most postganglionic sympathetic endings in the autonomic nervous system. Its synthesis and metabolism are discussed in Chapter 13. Neurons which liberate norepinephrine are called **adrenergic neurons**. Dopamine-secreting neurons which modulate the activity of the adrenergic neurons are found in sympathetic ganglia. Norepinephrine, dopamine, epinephrine, and 5-hydroxytryptamine (serotonin) are mediators in the CNS. Unlike acetylcholine, these amines are found in vesicles containing a dense core (granulated vesicles). Histamine, polypeptides such as "substance P" and somatostatin, and other agents may also be mediators in the brain (see Chapter 15).

One-Way Conduction

Synapses generally permit conduction of impulses in one direction only, from the presynaptic to the postsynaptic neurons. An impulse conducted antidromically up the axons of the ventral root dies out after depolarizing the cell bodies of the spinal motor neurons. Since axons will conduct in either direction with equal facility, the one-way gate at the synapses is necessary for orderly neural function. Chemical mediation at synaptic junctions explains one-way conduction. The mediator is located in the synaptic knobs of the presynaptic fibers, and very little if any is present in the postsynaptic membrane. Therefore, an impulse arriving at the postsynaptic membrane cannot liberate synaptic mediator. Progression of impulse traffic occurs only when the action potential arrives in the presynaptic terminals and causes liberation of stored chemical transmitter.

Pharmacologic Implications

The fact that transmission at most if not all synapses is chemical is of great pharmacologic importance. Transmission is also chemical at the endings of motor neurons on skeletal muscles, and at the points of contact between autonomic nerve fibers and smooth muscle (see below and Chapter 13). The biochemical events occurring at the synapse are much more sensitive than the events in the nerve fibers themselves to hypoxia and to drugs. For instance, polysynaptic pathways are more affected by anesthesia than those with few synapses, a factor which probably helps to explain the mechanism by which general anesthesia is produced (see Chapter 11). During deep anesthesia, synaptic transmission is blocked but long fibers still conduct impulses.

Nerve endings have been called biologic transducers that convert electrical energy into chemical energy. In broad terms, this conversion process involves the synthesis of the transmitter agents, their storage in the synaptic knobs, their release by the nerve impulses into the synaptic cleft, their action on the membrane of the postsynaptic cell, and their removal or their destruction, which is catalyzed by enzymes concentrated in the area around the endings. In theory, at least, all these processes can be inhibited or facilitated by drugs, with resultant changes in synaptic transmission. The synapses are thus a logical point for pharmacologic manipulation of neural function. Since transmission is chemical not only in the autonomic nervous system and at the myoneural junction but in the CNS as well, the pharmacologist can look forward to eventually regulating not only somatic and visceral motor activity but also emotions, behavior, and the other complex functions of the brain.

INHIBITION & FACILITATION AT SYNAPSES

Direct & Indirect Inhibition

Postsynaptic inhibition during the course of an IPSP is also called **direct inhibition** because it is not a consequence of previous discharges of the postsynaptic neuron. Various forms of **indirect inhibition,** inhibition due to the effects of previous postsynaptic neuron discharge, also occur. For example, the postsynaptic cell can be refractory to excitation because it has just fired and is in its refractory period. During after-hyperpolarization it is also less excitable; and in spinal neurons, especially after repeated firing, this after-hyperpolarization may be large and prolonged. In addition, there is evidence that with repeated stimulation of a given pathway the amount of transmitter released or the sensitivity of postsynaptic membrane to the transmitter decreases.

Postsynaptic Inhibition in the Spinal Cord

The various pathways in the nervous system which are known to mediate postsynaptic inhibition are discussed in Chapter 6, but one illustrative example will be presented here. Afferent fibers from the muscle spindles (stretch receptors) in skeletal muscle are known to pass directly to the spinal motor neurons of the motor units supplying the same muscle. Impulses in this afferent supply cause EPSPs and, with summation, propagated responses in the postsynaptic motor neurons. At the same time, IPSPs are produced in motor neurons supplying the antagonistic muscles. This latter response is probably mediated by collaterals of the afferent fibers which end on Golgi bottle neurons. These interneurons, in turn, end on the motor neurons which supply the antagonist (Fig 4–8). Therefore, activity in the afferent fibers from the muscle spindles excites the motor neurons supplying the

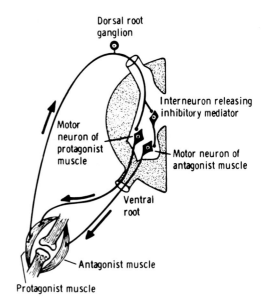

Figure 4–8. Diagram illustrating the probable anatomic connections responsible for inhibiting the antagonists to a muscle contracting in response to stretch. Activity is initiated in the spindle in the protagonist muscle. Impulses pass directly to the motor neurons supplying the same muscle and, via collaterals, to Golgi bottle neurons which end on the motor neurons of the antagonist muscle.

muscle from which the impulses come and inhibits those supplying its antagonists.

Presynaptic Inhibition

Another type of inhibition occurring in the CNS is **presynaptic inhibition,** a process which reduces the amount of synaptic mediator liberated by action potentials arriving at excitatory synaptic knobs. It has been demonstrated that the amount of mediator liberated at a nerve ending is markedly reduced if the magnitude of the action potential reaching the ending is reduced. The neurons producing presynaptic inhibition end on the excitatory endings (Fig 4–9). When they discharge, they produce a partial depolarization of the excitatory endings. Reducing the membrane potential of the excitatory endings to a level closer to the firing level makes the endings more excitable, but it also reduces the size of the action potentials reaching the ending by an amount equal to the amount of depolarization. Consequently, less mediator is released and there is less excitation of the postsynaptic cell. The neurons producing presynaptic inhibition often fire repetitively, and the partial depolarization may last 100 msec or more.

The chemical mediator released by the neurons responsible for presynaptic inhibition is antagonized by the convulsant drug picrotoxin, and there is reason to believe that it is γ-aminobutyric acid (GABA).

Organization of Inhibitory Systems

Presynaptic and postsynaptic inhibition are usu-

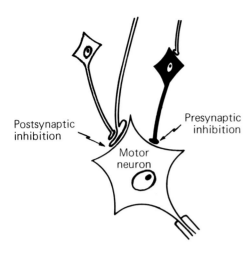

Figure 4—9. Arrangement of neurons producing presynaptic and postsynaptic inhibition. The neuron producing presynaptic inhibition is shown ending on an excitatory synaptic knob. Many of these neurons actually end higher up along the axon of the excitatory cell.

ally produced by stimulation of certain systems converging on a given postsynaptic neuron ("afferent inhibition"). Neurons may also inhibit themselves in a negative feedback fashion ("negative feedback inhibition"). For instance, spinal motor neurons regularly give off a recurrent collateral which synapses with an inhibitory interneuron that terminates on the cell body of the spinal neuron and other spinal motor neurons (Fig 4—10). This particular inhibitory neuron is sometimes called the Renshaw cell after its discoverer. Impulses generated in the motor neuron activate the inhibitory interneuron to liberate inhibitory mediator, and this slows or stops the discharge of the motor

neuron. Similar inhibition via recurrent collaterals is seen in the cerebral cortex and limbic system. Presynaptic inhibition appears to be in most cases a negative feedback inhibition in which cutaneous and other sensory neurons make connections which bring about presynaptic inhibition of their own terminals and surrounding terminals. In addition, fibers descending from the medulla in the pyramidal tract end on the excitatory endings of the afferent fibers from the muscle spindles. The muscle spindles are the receptors for the stretch reflex (see Chapter 6), and so impulses in the descending fibers presumably decrease stretch reflex activity.

Another type of inhibition is seen in the cerebellum. In this part of the brain, stimulation of basket cells produces IPSPs in the Purkinje cells. However, the basket cells and the Purkinje cells are excited by the same excitatory input. This arrangement, which has been called "feed-forward inhibition," presumably limits the duration of the excitation produced by any given afferent volley.

Summation & Occlusion

The interplay between excitatory and inhibitory influences at synaptic junctions in a nerve net illustrates the integrating and modulating activity of the nervous system.

In the hypothetical nerve net shown in Fig 4—11, neurons A and B converge on X, and neuron B diverges on X and Y. A stimulus applied to A or to B will set up an EPSP in X. If A and B are stimulated at the same time, 2 areas of depolarization will be produced in X and their actions will sum. The resultant EPSP in X will be twice as large as that produced by stimulation of A or B alone, and the membrane potential may well reach the firing level of X. The effect of the depolarization caused by the impulse in A is facilitated by that due to activity in B, and vice versa; spatial facilitation

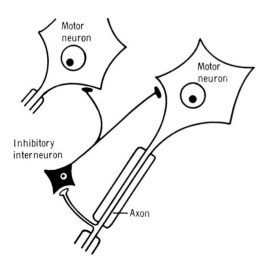

Figure 4—10. Negative feedback inhibition of a spinal motor neuron via an inhibitory interneuron (Renshaw cell).

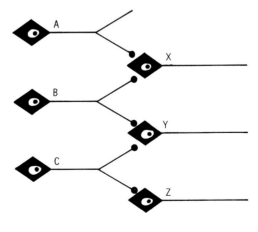

Figure 4—11. Simple nerve net. Neurons A, B, and C have excitatory endings on neurons X, Y, and Z.

has taken place. In this case, Y has not fired, but its excitability has been increased, and it is easier for activity in neuron C to fire it during the duration of the EPSP. Y is therefore said to be in the **subliminal fringe** of X. More generally stated, neurons are in the subliminal fringe if they are not discharged by an afferent volley (not in the **discharge zone**) but do have their excitability increased. The neurons that have few active knobs ending on them are in the subliminal fringe and those with many are in the discharge zone. However, this does not mean that with increasing strength of afferent stimulus the discharge zone becomes the same size as the subliminal fringe. In the case of stimulation of a dorsal root, the number of neurons discharged increases to a maximum with increasing strength of stimulation of the root, but so does the size of the subliminal fringe (Fig 4–12). Inhibitory impulses show similar temporal and spatial facilitation and subliminal fringe effects.

If neuron B in Fig 4–11 is stimulated repetitively, X and Y will discharge as a result of temporal summation of the EPSPs produced. If C is stimulated repetitively, Y and Z will discharge. If B and C are fired repetitively at the same time, X, Y, and Z will discharge. Thus, the response to stimulation of B and C together is not as great as the sum of responses to stimulation of B and C separately, because B and C both end on neuron Y. This decrease in expected response, due to presynaptic fibers sharing postsynaptic neurons, is called **occlusion**.

Excitatory and inhibitory subliminal effects and occlusive phenomena can have pronounced effects on transmission in any given pathway. Because of these effects, temporal patterns in peripheral nerves are usually altered as they pass through synapses on the way to the brain. These effects may also explain such important phenomena as referred pain (see Chapter 7).

POST-TETANIC POTENTIATION

The shifting patterns of facilitation and inhibition described above produce effects on neuronal excitability that are of relatively short duration. Another form of synaptic activity which has much more prolonged effects on excitability is the process of **post-tetanic potentiation**. This term refers to the decreased threshold for afferent stimulation of neurons in the CNS after their input has been subjected to prolonged repeated stimulation. It also occurs at autonomic ganglia and myoneural junctions. The potentiation may last several hours, and is localized to the afferent input that is stimulated. It does not spread to other afferent inputs. Inhibitory inputs also show post-tetanic potentiation, and the potentiation extends not only to the neurons directly fired but also to the subliminal fringe zone. This facilitation of transmission with repeated use of a pathway is in a sense an elementary form of learning. There is considerable evidence that the potentiation is due to an increase in transmitter release.

NEUROMUSCULAR TRANSMISSION

THE MYONEURAL JUNCTION

Anatomy

As the axon supplying a skeletal muscle fiber approaches its termination, it loses its myelin sheath and divides into a number of terminal buttons or end feet (Fig 4–13). The end feet contain many small clear vesicles which contain acetylcholine, the transmitter at these junctions. The endings fit into depressions in the **motor end-plate**, the thickened portion of the muscle membrane of the junction. Underneath the nerve ending, the muscle membrane of the end-plate is thrown into folds, the **palisades**. The space between the nerve and the thickened muscle membrane is comparable to the synaptic cleft at synapses. The whole structure is known as the **myoneural junction**. Only one nerve fiber ends on each end-plate, with no convergence of multiple inputs.

Sequence of Events During Transmission

The events occurring during transmission of impulses from the motor nerve to the muscle are some-

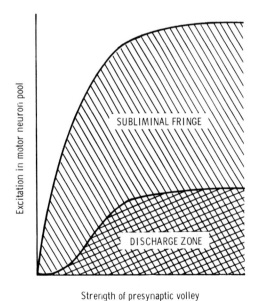

Figure 4–12. Relation of the size of the discharge zone and subliminal fringe to the strength of the presynaptic volley. (Redrawn and reproduced, with permission, from Lloyd: Reflex action in relation to pattern and peripheral source of afferent stimulation. J Neurophysiol 6:111, 1943.)

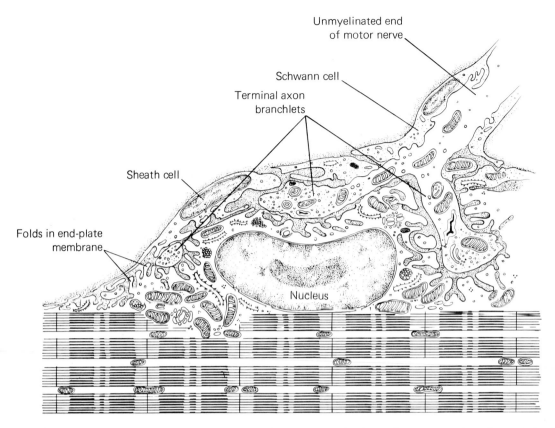

Figure 4–13. Myoneural junction. The drawing is based on electron micrographs of tissue from mice, and shows the terminal ends of a motor neuron axon buried in the end-plate cytoplasm, with the much folded end-plate membrane around them. (Modified and redrawn, with permission, from Anderson-Cedergren: Ultrastructure of motor end plate and sarcoplasmic components of skeletal muscle fiber. J Ultrastruct Res, Suppl 1, 1959.)

what similar to those occurring at synapses. The impulse arriving in the end of the motor neuron evokes liberation of acetylcholine from the vesicles in the nerve terminals. The acetylcholine increases the permeability of the underlying membrane, and Na⁺ influx produces a depolarizing potential, the **end-plate potential**. The current sink created by this local potential depolarizes the adjacent muscle membrane to its firing level. Action potentials are generated on either side of the end-plate and are conducted away from the end-plate in both directions along the muscle fiber. The muscle action potential, in turn, initiates muscle contraction, as described in Chapter 3.

End-Plate Potential

The end-plate potential is normally obscured by the propagated response initiated from the muscle fiber, but it can be seen if its magnitude is reduced to a size that is insufficient to fire the adjacent muscle membrane. Curare competes with acetylcholine for receptors on the end-plate membrane and forms a strong complex with the receptors. With small doses of curare, not all of the receptors are blocked, and acetylcholine acting at the unblocked receptors produces a small end-plate potential. The response is recorded

only at the end-plate region, and decrements exponentially away from it. Under these conditions, end-plate potentials can be shown to undergo temporal summation. Normally, however, the magnitude of the end-plate potential is sufficient to discharge the muscle membrane, and each impulse in the nerve ending produces a response in the muscle. Consequently, summation is not a usual phenomenon at the end-plate.

At the motor end-plate, it appears to be the complex formed by acetylcholine and the membrane receptor that induces the change in membrane permeability. There is a simultaneous increase in Na⁺ and K⁺ permeability, and the potential of the end-plate moves toward an equilibrium value of about −10 mV rather than the positive value reached during the action potential in nerve and muscle in which the peak increase in K⁺ permeability follows the increase in Na⁺ permeability. After triggering depolarization of the end-plate, the acetylcholine is probably bound to acetylcholinesterase, which hydrolyzes it. The end-plate membrane is depolarized if acetylcholine is dropped on it from a micropipet; but if the pipet is inserted through the muscle and the acetylcholine is applied to the underside of the end-plate membrane, no depolarization results.

Quantal Release of Transmitter

Small quanta, or "packets" of acetylcholine are released randomly from the nerve cell membrane at rest, each producing a minute depolarizing spike called a **minature end-plate potential,** which is about 0.5 mV in amplitude. The number of quanta of acetylcholine released in this way varies directly with the Ca^{++} concentration and inversely with the Mg^{++} concentration at the end-plate. When a nerve impulse reaches the ending, the number of quanta released increases by several orders of magnitude, and the result is the large end-plate potential that exceeds the firing level of the muscle fiber. The nerve impulse increases the permeability of the ending to Ca^{++} and the Ca^{++} is responsible for the increased quantal release.

Quantal release of acetylcholine similar to that seen at the myoneural junction has been observed at other cholinergic synapses, and similar processes are presumably operating at adrenergic and other synaptic junctions.

NERVE ENDINGS IN SMOOTH & CARDIAC MUSCLE

Anatomy

The postganglionic neurons in the various smooth muscles that have been studied in detail branch extensively and come in close contact with the muscle cells. Some of these nerve fibers contain vesicles and are cholinergic, whereas others contain the characteristic dense-core granules that are known to contain norepinephrine (see Chapter 13). There are no recognizable end-plates, and no discrete endings have been found; but the nerve fibers run along the membranes of the muscles cells and sometimes groove their surfaces. The adrenergic neurons have many branches and are beaded with enlargements or **varicosities** which contain adrenergic granules (Fig 4–14). The cholinergic neurons are probably similar. It has been suggested that transmitter is liberated at each varicosity, ie, at many locations along each axon. This arrangement permits one neuron to innervate many effector cells. The type of contact in which a neuron grooves the surface of a smooth muscle cell and then passes on to make similar contacts with other cells has been called a **synapse en passant.**

In the heart, cholinergic and adrenergic nerve fibers end on the sinoatrial node, the atrioventricular node, and the bundle of His. Adrenergic fibers also innervate the ventricular muscle. The exact nature of the endings on nodal tissue is not known. In the ventricle, the contacts between the adrenergic fibers and the cardiac muscle fibers resemble those found in smooth muscle.

Electrical Responses

In smooth muscles in which adrenergic discharge is excitatory, stimulation of the adrenergic nerves pro-

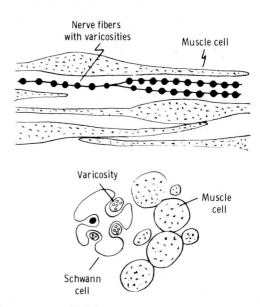

Figure 4–14. Relation of smooth muscle to autonomic nerve fibers. Longitudinal section *(top)* and transverse section *(bottom).* The Schwann cells which envelop the nerve fibers have been omitted from the top diagram. Note the areas of membrane fusion between muscle cells. (Modified from Bennett & Burnstock, in: *Handbook of Physiology.* Code CF [editor]. Washington: The American Physiological Society, 1968. Section 6, pp 1709–1732.)

duces discrete partial depolarizations that look like small end-plate potentials and are called **excitatory junction potentials (EJPs).** These potentials summate with repeated stimuli. Similar EJPs are seen in tissues excited by cholinergic discharges. In tissues inhibited by adrenergic stimuli, hyperpolarizing **inhibitory junction potentials (IJPs)** have been produced by stimulation of the adrenergic nerves.

These electrical responses are observed in many smooth muscle cells when a single nerve is stimulated, but their latency varies. This finding is consistent with the synapse en passant arrangement described above, but it could also be explained by transmission of the junction responses from cell to cell across low-resistance junctions or by diffusion of transmitter from its site of release to many smooth muscle cells. Miniature excitatory junction potentials similar to the miniature end-plate potentials in the skeletal muscle have been observed in some smooth muscle preparations, but they show considerable variation in size and duration. They may represent responses to single packets of transmitter, with the variation due to diffusion of the transmitter for variable distances.

DENERVATION HYPERSENSITIVITY

When the motor nerve to skeletal muscle is cut and allowed to degenerate, the muscle gradually becomes extremely sensitive to acetylcholine. This **denervation hypersensitivity** is also seen in smooth muscle. Smooth muscle, unlike skeletal muscle, does not atrophy when denervated, but it becomes hyperresponsive to the chemical mediator that normally activates it. Denervated glands, except for sweat glands, also become hypersensitive. A good example of denervation hypersensitivity is the response of the denervated iris. If the postganglionic sympathetic nerves to one pupil are cut in an experimental animal and, after several weeks, norepinephrine is injected intravenously, the denervated pupil dilates widely. A much smaller, less prolonged response is observed on the intact side. There is considerable evidence that other neural structures show a similar reaction to loss of their nerve supply. When higher centers in the nervous system are destroyed, the activity of the lower centers they control is generally increased ("release phenomenon"). The increased activity may be due in part to denervation hypersensitivity of the lower centers. Indeed, one theory holds that many of the signs and symptoms of neurologic disease are due to denervation hypersensitivity of various groups of neurons in the brain.

Hypersensitivity is limited to the structures immediately innervated by the destroyed neurons, and fails to develop in neurons and muscle farther "downstream." Suprasegmental spinal cord lesions do not lead to hypersensitivity of the paralyzed skeletal muscles to acetylcholine, and destruction of the preganglionic autonomic nerves to visceral structures does not cause hypersensitivity of the denervated viscera. This fact has practical implications in the treatment of diseases due to spasm of the blood vessels in the extremities. For example, if the upper extremity is sympathectomized by removing the upper part of the ganglion chain and the stellate ganglion, the hypersensitive smooth muscle in the vessel walls is stimulated by circulating norepinephrine, and episodic vasospasm continues to occur. However, if preganglionic sympathectomy of the arm is performed by cutting the ganglion chain below the third ganglion (to interrupt ascending preganglionic fibers) and the white rami of the first 3 thoracic nerves, no hypersensitivity results.

The cause of denervation hypersensitivity is still obscure. In skeletal muscle it is associated with an increase in the area of the muscle membrane sensitive to acetylcholine. Normally, only the end-plate region is depolarized by this mediator; after denervation, the sensitivity of the end-plate is no greater, but large portions of the muscle membrane respond. The sensitivity returns to normal if the nerve regrows. A similar spread of acetylcholine sensitivity has been demonstrated in denervated postganglionic cholinergic neurons. The hypersensitivity in smooth muscle may be due in part to loss of monoamine oxidase activity. Another factor is lack of re-uptake of liberated catecholamines; the nerve endings in normal tissue take up large amounts of norepinephrine, and after they have degenerated more norepinephrine is available to act on the receptors in the tissue (see Chapter 13).

5...
Initiation of Impulses in Sense Organs

SENSE ORGANS & RECEPTORS

Information about the internal and external environment reaches the CNS via a variety of **sensory receptors**. These receptors are transducers which convert various forms of energy in the environment into action potentials in neurons. The sensory receptor may be part of a neuron or, as in the case of the eye, a specialized cell that generates action potentials in neurons. The receptor is often associated with nonneural cells that surround it, forming a **sense organ**. The forms of energy converted by the receptors include, for example, mechanical (touch-pressure), thermal (degrees of warmth), electromagnetic (light), and chemical energy (odor, taste, and O_2 content of blood). The receptors in each of the sense organs are adapted to respond to one particular form of energy at a much lower threshold than other receptors respond to this form of energy. The particular form of energy to which a receptor is most sensitive is called its **adequate stimulus**. The adequate stimulus for the rods and cones in the eye, for example, is light. Receptors do respond to forms of energy other than their adequate stimulus, but the threshold for these nonspecific responses is much higher. Pressure on the eyeball will stimulate the rods and cones, for example, but the threshold of these receptors to pressure is much higher than the threshold of the pressure receptors in the skin.

THE SENSES

Sensory Modalities

Because the sensory receptors are specialized to respond to one particular form of energy and because many variables in the environment are perceived, it follows that there must be many different types of receptors. We learn in elementary school that there are "5 senses," but the inadequacy of this dictum is apparent if we list the major sensory modalities and their receptors in man. The list (Table 5–1) includes at least 11 conscious senses. There are, in addition, a large number of sensory receptors which relay information that does not reach consciousness. For example, the

muscle spindles provide information about muscle length, and other receptors provide information about such variables as arterial blood pressure, the temperature of the blood in the head, and the pH of the cerebrospinal fluid. The existence of other receptors of this type is suspected, and future research will undoubtedly add to the list of "unconscious senses." Furthermore, any listing of the senses is bound to be arbitrary. The rods and cones, for example, respond maximally to light of different wavelengths, and there probably are different cones for each of the 3 primary colors. There are 4 different modalities of taste—sweet, salt, sour, and bitter—and each is subserved by a more or less distinct type of taste bud. Sounds of different pitches are heard primarily because different groups of hair cells in the organ of Corti are activated maximally by sound waves of different frequencies. Whether these various responses to light, taste, and sound should be considered separate senses is a semantic question that in the present context is largely academic.

Classifications of Sense Organs

Numerous attempts have been made to classify the senses into groups, but none have been entirely successful. Traditionally, the special senses are smell, vision, hearing, rotational and linear acceleration, and taste; the cutaneous senses are those with receptors in the skin; and the visceral senses are those concerned with perception of the internal environment. Pain from visceral structures is usually classified as a visceral sensation. Another classification of the various receptors divides them into (1) teleceptors ("distance receivers"), the receptors concerned with events at a distance; (2) exteroceptors, those concerned with the external environment near at hand; (3) interoceptors, those concerned with the internal environment; and (4) proprioceptors, those which provide information about the position of the body in space at any given instant. However, the conscious component of proprioception, or "body image," is actually synthesized from information coming not only from receptors in and around joints but from cutaneous touch and pressure receptors as well. Certain other special terms are sometimes used. Because pain fibers have connections which mediate strong and prepotent withdrawal reflexes (see Chapter 6), and because pain is initiated by potentially noxious or damaging stimuli, pain receptors are some-

Table 5—1. Principal sensory modalities. (The first 11 are conscious sensations.)

Sensory Modality	Receptor	Sense Organ
Vision	Rods and cones	Eye
Hearing	Hair cells	Ear (organ of Corti)
Smell	Olfactory neurons	Olfactory mucous membrane
Taste	Taste receptor cells	Taste bud
Rotational acceleration	Hair cells	Ear (semicircular canals)
Linear acceleration	Hair cells	Ear (utricle and saccule)
Touch-pressure	Nerve endings	Various*
Warmth	Nerve endings	Various*
Cold	Nerve endings	Various*
Pain	Naked nerve endings	. . .
Joint position and movement	Nerve endings	Various*
Muscle length	Nerve endings	Muscle spindle
Muscle tension	Nerve endings	Golgi tendon organ
Arterial blood pressure	Nerve endings	Stretch receptors in carotid sinus and aortic arch
Central venous pressure	Nerve endings	Stretch receptors in walls of great veins, atria
Inflation of lung	Nerve endings	Stretch receptors in lung parenchyma
Temperature of blood in head	Neurons in hypothalamus	. . .
Arterial P_{O_2}	Nerve endings?	Carotid and aortic bodies
pH of CSF	Receptors on ventral surface of medulla oblongata	. . .
Osmotic pressure of plasma	Cells in anterior hypothalamus	. . .
Arteriovenous blood glucose difference	Cells in hypothalamus (glucostats)	. . .

*See text.

times called **nociceptors.** The term **chemoreceptor** is used to refer to those receptors which are stimulated by a change in the chemical composition of the environment in which they are located. These include receptors for taste and smell as well as visceral receptors such as those sensitive to changes in the plasma level of O_2, pH, and osmolality.

Cutaneous Sense Organs

There are 4 cutaneous senses: touch-pressure (pressure is sustained touch), cold, warmth, and pain. The skin contains various types of sensory endings. These include naked nerve endings, expanded tips on sensory nerve terminals, and encapsulated endings. The expanded endings include Merkel's disks and Ruffini endings (Fig 5–1), whereas the encapsulated endings include pacinian corpuscles, Meissner's corpuscles, and Krause's end bulbs. Ruffini endings and pacinian corpuscles are also found in deep fibrous tissues. In addition, sensory nerves end around hair follicles. However, none of the expanded or encapsulated endings appear to be necessary for cutaneous sensation. Their distribution varies in different regions of the body, and it has been repeatedly demonstrated that all 4 sensory modalities can be elicited from areas which on histologic examination contain only naked nerve endings. Where they are present, the expanded or encapsulated endings appear to function as mechanoreceptors that respond to tactile stimuli. The nerve endings around hair follicles mediate touch, and movements of hairs initiate tactile sensations. It should be emphasized that al-

though cutaneous sensory receptors lack histologic specificity, they are physiologically specific. Thus, any given ending signals one and only one kind of cutaneous sensation.

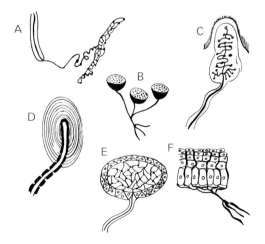

Figure 5—1. Sensory receptors in the skin. Ruffini endings (A) and Merkel's disks (B) are expanded ends of sensory nerve fibers. Meissner's corpuscle (C), pacinian corpuscles (D), and Krause's end bulbs (E) are encapsulated endings. F = naked nerve endings.

ELECTRICAL & IONIC EVENTS
IN RECEPTORS

Anatomic Relationships

The problem of how receptors convert energy into action potentials in the sensory nerves has been the subject of intensive study. In the complex sense organs such as those concerned with vision, hearing, equilibrium, and taste, there are separate receptor cells and synaptic junctions between receptors and afferent nerves. However, in most of the cutaneous sense organs, the receptors are specialized, histologically modified ends of sensory nerve fibers.

Pacinian corpuscles, which are touch receptors, have been studied in detail. Because of their relatively large size and accessibility in the mesentery of experimental animals, they can be isolated, studied with microelectrodes, and subjected to microdissection. Each capsule consists of the straight, unmyelinated ending of a sensory nerve fiber, 2 µm in diameter, surrounded by concentric lamellas of connective tissue which give the organ the appearance of a minute cocktail onion. The myelin sheath of the sensory nerve begins inside the corpuscle. The first node of Ranvier is also located inside, whereas the second is usually near the point at which the nerve fiber leaves the corpuscle (Fig 5–2).

Generator Potentials

Recording electrodes can be placed on the sensory nerve as it leaves a pacinian corpuscle and graded pressure applied to the corpuscle. When a small amount of pressure is applied, a nonpropagated depolarizing potential resembling an EPSP is recorded. This is called the **generator potential**, or **receptor potential**. As the pressure is increased, the magnitude of the receptor potential increases. When the magnitude of the generator potential is about 10 mV, an action potential is generated in the sensory nerve. As the pressure is further increased, the generator potential becomes even larger and the sensory nerve fires repetitively. Eventually, in the case of the pacinian corpuscle, the size of the generator potential reaches a maximum, but its rate of rise continues to increase as the magnitude of the applied pressure is increased.

Source of the Generator Potential

By microdissection technics it has been shown that removal of the connective tissue lamellas from the unmyelinated nerve ending in a pacinian corpuscle does not abolish the generator potential. When the first node of Ranvier is blocked by pressure or narcotics, the generator potential is unaffected but conducted impulses are abolished (Fig 5–2). When the sensory nerve is sectioned and the nonmyelinated terminal is allowed to degenerate, no generator potential is formed. These and other experiments have established the fact that the generator potential is produced in the unmyelinated nerve terminal. This potential electrotonically depolarizes the first node of Ranvier. The receptor therefore converts mechanical energy into an electrical response, the magnitude of which is proportionate to the intensity of the stimulus. The generator potential in turn depolarizes the sensory nerve at the first node of Ranvier. Once the firing level is reached,

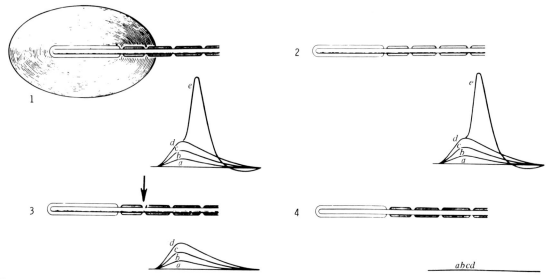

Figure 5–2. Demonstration that the generator potential in a pacinian corpuscle originates in the nonmyelinated nerve terminal. In 1, the electrical responses to a pressure of x (record a), 2 x (b), 3 x (c), and 4 x (d) were recorded. The strongest stimulus produced an action potential in the sensory nerve (e). In 2, the same responses persisted after removal of the connective tissue capsule. In 3, the generator responses persisted but the action potential was absent when the first node of Ranvier was blocked with pressure or narcotics (arrow). In 4, all responses disappeared when the sensory nerve was cut and allowed to degenerate before the experiment. (Reproduced, with permission, from Lowenstein: Biological transducers. Scientific American 203:98, Aug 1960. Copyright © 1960 by Scientific American, Inc. All rights reserved.)

an action potential is produced and the membrane repolarizes. If the generator potential is great enough, the neuron fires again as soon as it repolarizes, and it continues to fire as long as the generator potential is large enough to bring the membrane potential of the node to the firing level. Thus, the node converts the graded response of the receptor into action potentials, the frequency of which is proportionate to the magnitude of the applied stimuli.

Similar generator potentials have been studied in the muscle spindle. The relationship between the stimulus intensity and the size of the generator potential and between the stimulus intensity and the frequency of the action potentials in the afferent nerve fiber from a spindle is shown in Fig 5–3. The frequency of the action potentials is generally related to the intensity of the stimulus by a power function (see below). Generator potentials have also been observed in the organ of Corti, the olfactory and taste organs, and other sense organs. Presumably, they are in most

cases the mechanism by which sensory nerve fibers are activated.

Ionic Basis of Excitation

The biophysical events underlying the generator potential have not been completely clarified, but it is known that Na^+ depletion diminishes and eventually abolishes the generator potential in pacinian corpuscles. Presumably, the stimulus initiates an increase in the permeability of the membrane of the unmyelinated terminal to Na^+, the resultant influx of Na^+ produces the generator potential, and the magnitude of the permeability change is proportionate to the intensity of the stimulus. How the mechanical stimulus is converted into a change in membrane permeability is not known. It is possible that the change is due to stretching or distortion of the membrane, or it could be due to the release of some chemical mediator.

Adaptation

When a maintained stimulus of constant strength is applied to a receptor, the frequency of the action potentials in its sensory nerve declines over a period of time. This phenomenon is known as **adaptation**. The degree to which adaptation occurs varies with the type of sense organ (Fig 5–4). Touch adapts rapidly, and its receptors are called **phasic receptors**. Application of a maintained pressure to a pacinian corpuscle produces a generator potential that decays rapidly. On the other hand, the carotid sinus, the muscle spindles, and the organs for cold, pain, and lung inflation adapt very slowly and incompletely; the receptors involved are termed **tonic receptors**. This correlates with the fact that the generator potential of the muscle spindle is prolonged and decays very slowly when a steady stimu-

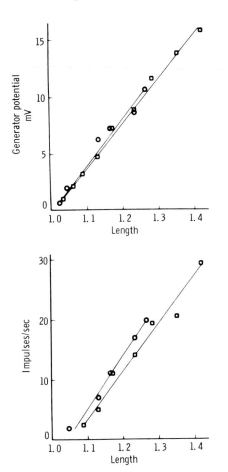

Figure 5–3. Relation between muscle length and size of generator potential *(above)* and impulse frequency *(below)* in crayfish stretch receptor. Squares and circles indicate values in 2 different preparations. (Reproduced, with permission, from Terzuolo & Washizu: Relation between stimulus strength, generator potential, and impulse frequency in stretch receptor of crustacea. J Neurophysiol 25:56, 1962.)

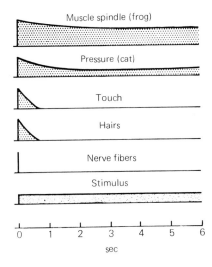

Figure 5–4. Adaptation. The height of the curve in each case indicates the frequency of the discharge in afferent nerve fibers at various times after beginning sustained stimulation. (Reproduced, with permission, from Adrian: *Basis of Sensation.* Christophers, 1928.)

lus is applied to it. Maintained pressure applied to the outside of a pacinian corpuscle causes steady displacement in the outer lamellas, but the lamellas near the nerve fiber slip back to their original position, ending the distortion of the nerve ending and causing the generator potential to decline. However, this is not the only factor producing adaptation; there is still a slow decline in the number of action potentials generated over a period of time by a steady stimulus after removal of the outer lamellas from the pacinian corpuscle. This decline is due to accommodation of the sensory nerve fiber to the generator potential.

The slow, incomplete adaptation of the carotid sinus and the organs for muscle stretch, pain, and cold is of some value to the animal. Muscle stretch plays a role in prolonged postural adjustments. The sensations of pain and cold are initiated by potentially noxious stimuli, and they would lose some of their warning value if their receptors showed marked adaptation. Carotid and aortic receptors operate continuously in the regulation of blood pressure, and adaptation of these receptors would limit the precision with which the regulatory system operates.

"CODING" OF SENSORY INFORMATION

There are minor variations in the speed of conduction and other characteristics of sensory nerve fibers (see Chapter 2), but in general action potentials are similar in all nerves. The action potentials in the nerve from a touch receptor, for example, are essentially identical to those in the nerve from a warmth receptor. This raises the question of why stimulation of a touch receptor causes a sensation of touch and not of warmth and how it is possible to tell whether the touch is light or heavy.

Doctrine of Specific Nerve Energies

The sensation evoked by impulses generated in a receptor depends upon the specific part of the brain they ultimately activate. The specific sensory pathways are discrete from sense organ to cortex. Therefore, when the nerve pathways from a particular sense organ are stimulated, the sensation evoked is that for which the receptor is specialized no matter how or where along the pathway the activity is initiated. This principle, first enunciated by Müller, has been given the rather cumbersome name of the **doctrine of specific nerve energies.** For example, if the sensory nerve from a pacinian corpuscle in the hand is stimulated by pressure at the elbow or by irritation from a tumor in the brachial plexus, the sensation evoked is one of touch. Similarly, if a fine enough electrode could be inserted into the appropriate fibers of the dorsal columns of the spinal cord, the thalamus, or the postcentral gyrus of the cerebral cortex, the sensation produced by stimulation would be touch. This doctrine has been questioned from time to time, especially by those who

claim that pain is produced by overstimulation of a variety of receptors. However, the overstimulation hypothesis has been largely discredited and the principle of specific nerve energies remains one of the cornerstones of sensory physiology.

Projection

No matter where a particular sensory pathway is stimulated along its course to the cortex, the conscious sensation produced is referred to the location of the receptor. This principle is called the **law of projection.** Cortical stimulation experiments during neurosurgical procedures on conscious patients illustrate this phenomenon. For example, when the cortical receiving area for impulses from the left hand is stimulated, the patient reports sensation in his left hand, not in his head. Another dramatic example is seen in amputees. These patients may complain, often bitterly, of pain and proprioceptive sensations in the absent limb ("phantom limb"). These sensations are due in part to pressure on the stump of the amputated limb. This pressure initiates impulses in nerve fibers which previously came from sense organs in the amputated limb, and the sensations evoked are projected to where the receptors used to be.

Intensity Discrimination

There are 2 ways in which information about intensity of stimuli is transmitted to the brain: by variation in the frequency of the action potentials generated by the activity in a given receptor, and by variation in the number of receptors activated. It has long been taught that the magnitude of the sensation felt is proportionate to the log of the intensity of the stimulus (**Weber-Fechner law**). It now appears, however, that a power function more accurately describes this relation. In other words, $R = KS^A$, where R is the sensation felt, S is the intensity of the stimulus, and, for any specific sensory modality, K and A are constants. The frequency of the action potentials a stimulus generates in a sensory nerve fiber is also related to the intensity of the initiating stimulus by a power function. An example of this relation is shown in Fig 5–3, in which the exponent is approximately 1.0. Another example is shown in Fig 5–5, in which the calculated exponent is 0.52. Current evidence indicates that in the CNS the relation between stimulus and sensation is linear; consequently, it appears that for any given sensory modality the relation between sensation and stimulus intensity is determined primarily by the properties of the peripheral receptors themselves.

Sensory Units

The term sensory unit is applied to a single sensory axon and all its peripheral branches. The number of these branches varies, but they may be numerous, especially in the case of the cutaneous senses. In the cornea and adjacent sclera of the eye, the surface area supplied by a single sensory unit is 50–200 sq mm. Generally, the areas supplied by one unit overlap and interdigitate with the areas supplied by others.

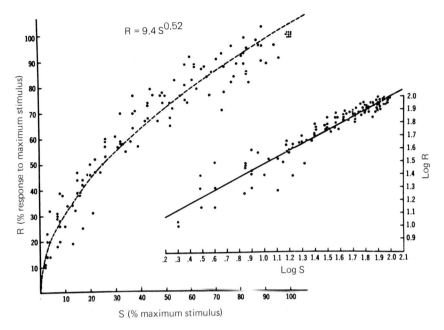

Figure 5–5. Relation between magnitude of touch stimulus (S) and frequency of action potentials in sensory nerve fibers (R). Dots are individual values from cats plotted on linear coordinates *(left)* and log-log coordinates *(right)*. The equation shows the calculated power function relationship between R and S. (Reproduced, with permission, from Werner & Mountcastle: Neural activity in mechanoreceptive cutaneous afferents, stimulus-response relations, Weber functions, and information transmission. J Neurophysiol 28:359, 1965.)

Recruitment of Sensory Units

As the strength of a stimulus is increased, it tends to spread over a large area and generally activates not only the sense organs immediately in contact with it but "recruits" those in the surrounding area as well. Furthermore, weak stimuli activate the receptors with the lowest thresholds, whereas stronger stimuli also activate those with higher thresholds. Some of the receptors activated are part of the same sensory unit, and impulse frequency in the unit therefore increases. Because of overlap and interdigitation of one unit with another, however, receptors of other units are also stimulated and consequently more units fire. In this way more afferent pathways are activated, and this is interpreted in the brain as an increase in intensity of the sensation.

• • •

References: Section II.
Physiology of Nerve & Muscle Cells

Basmajian JV: Electromyography comes of age. Science 176: 603, 1972.

Braunwald E, Ross J, Sonnenblick EH: *Mechanisms of Contraction of the Normal and Failing Heart,* 2nd ed. Little, Brown, 1976.

Bulbring E, Shuba MF (editors): *Physiology of Smooth Muscle.* Raven, 1975.

Cohen C: The protein switch of muscle contraction. Sci Am 233:36, Nov 1975.

Cowan WM, Cuénod M (editors): *Use of Axonal Transport for Studies of Neuronal Connectivity.* Elsevier, 1975.

Davson H: *A Textbook of General Physiology,* 4th ed. Williams & Wilkins, 1970.

Fleming WW, McPhillips JJ, Westfall DP: Postjunctional supersensitivity and subsensitivity of excitable tissues to drugs. Ergeb Physiol 68:55, 1973.

Geffen LB, Livett BG: Synaptic vesicles in sympathetic neurons. Physiol Rev 51:98, 1971.

Hodgkin AL: The ionic basis of nervous conduction. Science 145:1148, 1964.

Hubbard JI Microphysiology of vertebrate neuromuscular transmission. Physiol Rev 53:874, 1973.

Huxley AF: Excitation and conduction in nerve: Quantitative analysis. Science 145:1154, 1964.

Huxley AF: Muscular contraction. J Physiol 243:1, 1974.

Katz B: Quantal mechanism of neural transmitter release. Science 173:123, 1971.

Lester HA: The response to acetylcholine. Sci Am 236:106, Feb 1977.

Llinás R: Electrical synaptic transmission in the mammalian central nervous system. In: *Golgi Centennial Symposium Proceedings.* Santini M (editor). Raven, 1975.

Ochs S: Fast transport of materials in mammalian nerve fibers. Science 176:252, 1972.

Pappas GD, Purpura DP (editors): *Structure and Function of Synapses.* Raven, 1972.

Sharpless SK: Supersensitivity-like phenomena in the central nervous system. Fed Proc 34:1990, 1975.

Watson WE: Physiology of neuroglia. Physiol Rev 54:245, 1974.

Symposium: Membranes, ions and impulses. Fed Proc 34:1317, 1975.

Symposium: The synapse. Cold Spring Harbor Symp Quant Biol 40:1, 1976.

III. Functions of the Nervous System
6...
Reflexes

THE REFLEX ARC

The basic unit of integrated neural activity is the reflex arc. This arc consists of a sense organ, an afferent neuron, one or more synapses in a central integrating station, an efferent neuron, and an effector. In mammals, the connection between afferent and efferent somatic neurons is in the brain or spinal cord. The afferent neurons enter via the dorsal roots or cranial nerves, and have their cell bodies in the dorsal root ganglia or in the homologous ganglia on the cranial nerves. The efferent fibers leave via the ventral roots or corresponding motor cranial nerves. The principle that in the spinal cord the dorsal roots are sensory and the ventral roots are motor is known as the **Bell-Magendie law**.

In previous chapters the function of each of the components of the reflex arc has been considered in detail. As noted in Chapters 2 and 3, impulses generated in the axons of the afferent and efferent neurons and in muscle are "all or none" in character. On the other hand, there are 3 junctions or junction-like areas in the reflex arc where responses are graded (Fig 6–1). These are the receptor-afferent neuron region, the synapse between the afferent and efferent neurons, and the myoneural junction. At each of these points, a nonpropagated potential proportionate in size to the magnitude of the incoming stimulus is generated. The graded potentials serve to electrotonically depolarize the adjacent nerve or muscle membrane and set up all or none responses. The number of action potentials in the afferent nerve is proportionate to the magnitude of the applied stimulus at the sense organ. There is also a rough correlation between the magnitude of the stimulus and the frequency of action potentials in the efferent nerve; however, since the connection between the afferent and efferent neurons is in the CNS, activity in the reflex arc is modified by the multiple inputs converging on the efferent neurons.

The simplest reflex arc is one with a single synapse between the afferent and efferent neurons. Such arcs are **monosynaptic**, and reflexes occurring in them are **monosynaptic reflexes**. Reflex arcs in which one or more interneurons are interposed between the afferent and efferent neurons are **polysynaptic**, the number of synapses in the arcs varying from 2 to many hundreds. In both types, but especially in polysynaptic reflex arcs, activity is modified by spatial and temporal facilitation, occlusion, and subliminal fringe effects.

MONOSYNAPTIC REFLEXES: THE STRETCH REFLEX

When a skeletal muscle with an intact nerve supply is stretched, it contracts. This response is called the

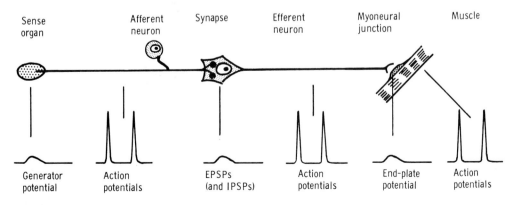

Figure 6–1. The reflex arc. Note that at the receptor and at each of the junctions in the arc there is a nonpropagated graded response which is proportionate to the magnitude of the stimulus, whereas in the portions of the arc specialized for transmission (axons, muscle membrane) the responses are all or none action potentials.

stretch reflex. The stimulus that initiates the reflex is stretch of the muscle, and the response is contraction of the muscle being stretched. The sense organ is the muscle spindle. The impulses originating in the spindle are conducted to the CNS by fast sensory fibers which pass directly to the motor neurons which supply the same muscle. Stretch reflexes are the only monosynaptic reflexes in the body.

Clinical Examples

Tapping the patellar tendon elicits the **knee jerk,** a stretch reflex of the quadriceps femoris muscle, because the tap on the tendon stretches the muscle. A similar contraction is observed if the quadriceps is stretched manually. Stretch reflexes can also be elicited from most of the large muscles of the body. Tapping on the tendon of the triceps brachii, for example, causes an extensor response at the elbow due to reflex contraction of the triceps; tapping on the Achilles tendon causes an ankle jerk due to reflex contraction of the gastrocnemius; and tapping on the side of the face causes a stretch reflex in the masseter. Other examples of stretch reflexes are listed in neurology textbooks.

Structure of Muscle Spindles

Each muscle spindle consists of 2–10 muscle fibers enclosed in a connective tissue capsule. These fibers are more embryonal in character and have less distinct striations than the rest of the fibers in the muscle. They are called **intrafusal fibers** to distinguish them from the **extrafusal fibers,** the regular contractile units of the muscle. The intrafusal fibers are in parallel with the rest of the muscle fibers because the ends of the capsule of the spindle are attached to the tendons at either end of the muscle or to the sides of the extrafusal fibers.

There are 2 types of intrafusal fibers in mammalian muscle spindles. The first type contains many nuclei in a dilated central area and is therefore called a **nuclear bag fiber** (Fig 6–2). The second type, the **nu-**

clear chain fiber, is thinner and shorter and lacks a definite bag. The ends of the nuclear chain fibers connect to the sides of the nuclear bag fibers. The ends of the intrafusal fibers are contractile, whereas the central portions probably are not.

There are 2 kinds of sensory endings in each spindle. The **primary** or **annulospiral endings** are the terminations of rapidly conducting group Ia afferent fibers that wrap around the center of the nuclear bag and nuclear chain fibers. The **secondary** or **flower-spray endings** are terminations of group II sensory fibers and are located nearer the ends of the intrafusal fibers, probably only on nuclear chain fibers.

The spindles have a motor nerve supply of their own. These nerves are 3–6 μm in diameter, constitute about 30% of the fibers in the ventral roots, and belong in Erlanger and Gasser's A γ group. Because of their characteristic size, they are called the **gamma efferents of Leksell,** or the **small motor nerve system.** There also appears to be a sparse innervation of spindles by motor fibers of intermediate size. The function of this **beta innervation** is unknown.

The endings of the gamma efferent fibers are of 2 histologic types. There are motor end plates (**plate endings**) on the nuclear bag fibers, and there are endings that form extensive networks (**trail endings**) primarily on the nuclear chain fibers. It is known that the spindles receive 2 functional types of innervation—dynamic gamma efferents and static gamma efferents (see below)—and it is reasonable to hypothesize that the dynamic gamma efferents terminate at the plate endings while the static gamma efferents terminate at the trail endings.

Central Connections of Afferent Fibers

It can be proved experimentally that the fibers from the primary endings end directly on motor neurons supplying the extrafusal fibers of the same muscle. The time between the application of the stimulus and the response in a reflex is the **reaction time.** In humans, the reaction time for a stretch reflex such as the

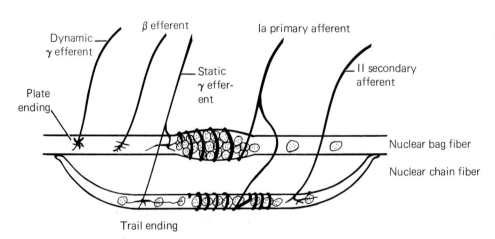

Figure 6–2. Diagram of muscle spindle. (Modified and reproduced, with permission, from Stein RB: Peripheral control of movement. Physiol Rev 54:215, 1974.)

knee jerk is 19—24 msec. Weak stimulation of the sensory nerve from the muscle, known to stimulate only Ia fibers, causes a contractile response with a similar latency. Since the conduction velocity of the afferent and efferent fiber types are known and the distance from the muscle to the spinal cord can be measured, it is possible to calculate how much of the reaction time was taken up by conduction to and from the spinal

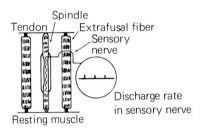

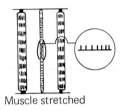

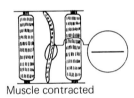

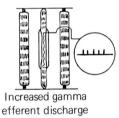

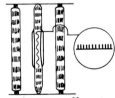

Figure 6—3. Effect of various conditions on muscle spindle discharge. (Drawn in part from Patton, in: *Physiology and Biophysics,* 19th ed. Ruch TC, Patton HD [editors]. Saunders, 1965.)

cord. When this value is subtracted from the reaction time, the remainder, called the **central delay**, is the time taken for the reflex activity to traverse the spinal cord. In humans, the central delay for the knee jerk is 0.6—0.9 msec, and figures of similar magnitude have been found in experimental animals. Since the minimal synaptic delay is 0.5 msec (see Chapter 4), only one synapse could have been traversed. It has been demonstrated that muscle spindles also make connections which cause muscle contraction via polysynaptic pathways.

The afferents from the secondary endings probably make connections that excite extensor muscles.

Function of Muscle Spindles

When the muscle spindle is stretched, the primary endings are distorted and receptor potentials are generated. These in turn set up action potentials in the sensory fibers at a frequency which is proportionate to the degree of stretching. The spindle is in parallel with the extrafusal fibers, and when the muscle is passively stretched the spindles are also stretched. This initiates reflex contraction of the extrafusal fibers in the muscle. On the other hand, the spindle afferents characteristically stop firing when the muscle is made to contract by electrical stimulation of the nerve fibers to the extrafusal fibers because the muscle shortens while the spindle does not (Fig 6—3).

Thus, the spindle and its reflex connections constitute a feedback device which operates to maintain muscle length; if the muscle is stretched, spindle discharge increases and reflex shortening is produced, whereas, if the muscle is shortened without a change in gamma efferent discharge, spindle discharge decreases and the muscle relaxes.

Both primary and secondary endings are stimulated when the spindle is stretched, but the pattern of response differs. The nerve from a primary ending discharges most rapidly while the muscle is being stretched and less rapidly during sustained stretch (Fig 6—4). The nerve from a secondary ending discharges at an increased rate throughout the period when a muscle

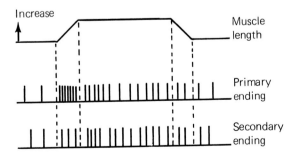

Figure 6—4. Response of spindle afferents to muscle stretch. The bottom 2 lines represent the number of discharges in afferent nerves from the primary and secondary endings as the muscle is stretched and then permitted to return to its original length.

is stretched. Thus, the primary ending responds both to changes in length and changes in the rate of stretching, while the secondary ending responds primarily to length alone. In other words, the primary measures length plus velocity of stretch, and the secondary measures mainly length. The response of the primary ending to the phasic as well as the tonic events in the muscle is important because the prompt, marked phasic response helps to dampen oscillation due to conduction delays in the feedback loop regulating muscle length. There is normally a small oscillation in this feedback loop: this is the physiologic tremor, which has a frequency of approximately 10 Hz. However, the tremor would be worse if it were not for the sensitivity of the spindle to velocity of stretch.

Effects of Gamma Efferent Discharge

Stimulation of the gamma efferent system produces a very different picture from that produced by stimulation of the extrafusal fibers. Such stimulation does not lead directly to detectable contraction of the muscles because the intrafusal fibers are not strong enough or plentiful enough to cause shortening. However, stimulation does cause the contractile ends of the intrafusal fibers to shorten and therefore stretches the nuclear bag portion of the spindles, deforming the annulospiral endings and initiating impulses in the Ia fibers. This in turn can lead to reflex contraction of the muscle. Thus, muscle can be made to contract via stimulation of the α motor neurons that innervate the extrafusal fibers, or the γ efferent neurons which initiate contraction indirectly via the stretch reflex. There is debate at present about how skilled and voluntary movements are brought about, and both α and γ mechanisms may be involved.

When the rate of gamma efferent discharge is increased, the intrafusal fibers are shorter than the extrafusal ones. If the whole muscle is stretched during stimulation of the gamma efferents, additional action potentials are generated owing to the additional stretch of the nuclear bag region, and the rate of discharge in the Ia fibers is further increased (Fig 6–3). Increased gamma efferent discharge thus increases spindle sensitivity, and the sensitivity of the spindles to stretch varies with the rate of gamma efferent discharge.

There is considerable evidence that there is increased gamma efferent discharge along with the increased discharge of the α motor neurons that initiates movements. Because of this "alpha-gamma linkage," the spindle shortens with the muscle, and spindle discharge may continue throughout the contraction. In this way, the spindle remains capable of responding to stretch and reflexly adjusting motor neuron discharge throughout the contraction.

The existence of dynamic and static gamma efferents is mentioned above. Stimulation of the former, which may end via plate endings on nuclear bag fibers, increases spindle sensitivity to rate of change of stretch. Stimulation of the latter, possibly via trail endings on nuclear chain fibers, increases spindle sensitivity to steady, maintained stretch. It is thus possible to adjust separately the spindle responses to phasic and tonic events.

Control of Gamma Efferent Discharge

The motor neurons of the gamma efferent system are regulated to a large degree by descending tracts from a number of areas in the brain. Via these pathways, the sensitivity of the muscle spindles and hence the threshold of the stretch reflexes in various parts of the body can be adjusted and shifted to meet the needs of postural control (see Chapter 12).

Other factors also influence gamma efferent discharge. Anxiety causes an increased discharge, a fact which probably explains the hyperactive tendon reflexes sometimes seen in anxious patients. Stimulation of the skin, especially by noxious agents, increases gamma efferent discharge to ipsilateral flexor muscle spindles while decreasing that to extensors and produces the opposite pattern in the opposite limb. It is well known that having a subject try to pull his hands apart when his flexed fingers are hooked together facilitates his knee jerk reflex (Jendrassik's maneuver), and this may also be due to increased gamma efferent discharge initiated by afferent impulses from the hands.

Reciprocal Innervation

When a stretch reflex occurs, the muscles that antagonize the action of the muscle involved (antagonists) relax. This phenomenon is said to be due to **reciprocal innervation**. Impulses in the Ia fibers from the muscle spindles of the protagonist muscle cause postsynaptic inhibition of the motor neurons to the antagonists. Although there is still some argument on the point, it appears that the pathway mediating this effect is a simple bisynaptic one. A collateral from each Ia fiber passes in the spinal cord to an inhibitory interneuron (Golgi bottle neuron) which synapses directly on one of the motor neurons supplying the antagonist muscles. This example of postsynaptic inhibition is discussed in Chapter 4, and the pathway is illustrated in Fig 4–8.

Inverse Stretch Reflex

Up to a point, the harder a muscle is stretched, the stronger is the reflex contraction. However, when the tension becomes great enough, contraction suddenly ceases and the muscle relaxes. This relaxation in response to strong stretch is called the **inverse stretch reflex**, or **autogenic inhibition**.

The receptor for the inverse stretch reflex is in the **Golgi tendon organ** (Fig 6–5). This organ consists of a net-like collection of knobby nerve endings among the fascicles of a tendon. There are 3–25 muscle fibers per tendon organ. The fibers from the Golgi tendon organs make up the Ib group of myelinated, rapidly conducting sensory nerve fibers. Stimulation of these Ib fibers leads to the production of IPSPs on the motor neurons that supply the muscle from which the fibers arise. The Ib fibers apparently end in the spinal cord on inhibitory interneurons which, in turn, terminate directly on the motor neurons (Fig 6–6). They also

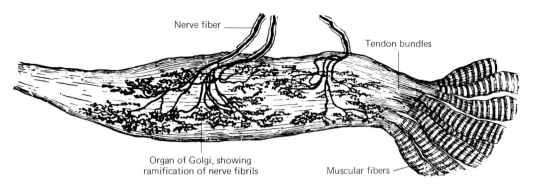

Nerve fiber

Tendon bundles

Organ of Golgi, showing
ramification of nerve fibrils

Muscular fibers

Figure 6–5. Golgi tendon organ. (After Ciaccio. Reproduced, with permission, from: *Gray's Anatomy of the Human Body,* 29th ed. Goss CM [editor]. Lea & Febiger, 1973.)

make excitatory connections with motor neurons supplying antagonists to the muscle.

Since the Golgi tendon organs, unlike the spindles, are in series with the muscle fibers, they are stimulated by both passive stretch and active contraction of the muscle. The threshold of the Golgi tendon organs is low. The degree of stimulation by passive stretch is not great because the more elastic muscle fibers take up much of the stretch, and this is why it takes a strong stretch to produce relaxation. However, discharge is regularly produced by contraction of the

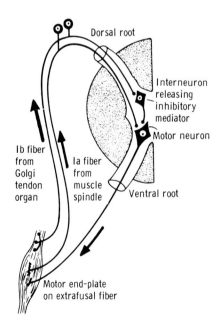

Dorsal root

Interneuron
releasing
inhibitory
mediator

Motor neuron

Ib fiber
from
Golgi
tendon
organ

Ia fiber
from
muscle
spindle

Ventral root

Motor end-plate
on extrafusal fiber

Figure 6–6. Diagram illustrating the pathways responsible for the stretch reflex and the inverse stretch reflex. Stretch stimulates the spindle, and impulses pass up the Ia fiber to excite the motor neuron. It also stimulates the Golgi tendon organ, and impulses passing up the Ib fiber activate the interneuron to release inhibitory mediator. With strong stretch, the resulting hyperpolarization of the motor neuron is so great that it stops discharging.

muscle, and the Golgi tendon organ thus functions as a transducer in a feedback circuit which regulates muscle tension in a fashion analogous to the spindle feedback circuit which regulates muscle length.

The importance of the primary endings in the spindles, the secondary endings in the spindles, and the Golgi tendon organs in regulating the velocity of the muscle contraction, muscle length, and muscle tension, respectively, is illustrated by the fact that section of the afferent nerves to a limb causes the limb to hang loosely at the side in a semiparalyzed state. The organization of the system is shown in Fig 6–7, and the interaction of spindle discharge, tendon organ discharge, and reciprocal innervation in determining the rate of discharge of a motor neuron is shown in Fig 6–8.

Muscle Tone

The resistance of a muscle to stretch is often referred to as its **tone** or **tonus**. If the motor nerve to a muscle is cut, the muscle offers very little resistance and is said to be **flaccid**. A **hypertonic** or **spastic** muscle is one in which the resistance to stretch is high. Somewhere between the states of flaccidity and spasticity is the ill-defined area of normal tone. The muscles are generally **hypotonic** when the rate of gamma efferent discharge is low and hypertonic when it is high.

Lengthening Reaction

When the muscles are hypertonic the sequence of moderate stretch → muscle contraction, strong stretch → muscle relaxation is clearly seen. Passive flexion of the elbow, for example, meets immediate resistance due to the stretch reflex in the triceps muscle. Further stretch activates the inverse stretch reflex. The resistance to flexion suddenly collapses, and the arm flexes. Continued passive flexion stretches the muscle again, and the sequence may be repeated. This sequence of resistance followed by give when a limb is moved passively is known clinically as the **clasp-knife effect** because of its resemblance to the closing of a pocket knife. The physiologic name for it is the **lengthening reaction** because it is the response of a spastic muscle (in the example cited, the triceps) to lengthening.

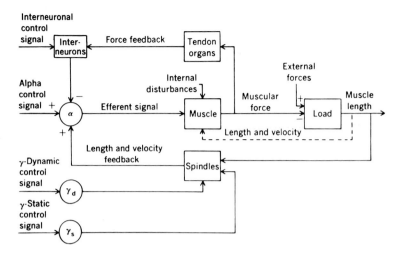

Figure 6–7. Block diagram of peripheral motor control system. The dashed line indicates the nonneural feedback from muscle that limits length and velocity via the inherent mechanical properties of muscle. γd, dynamic gamma motor neurons; γs, static gamma motor neurons. (Reproduced, with permission, from Houk, in: *Medical Physiology,* 13th ed. Mountcastle VB [editor]. Mosby, 1974.)

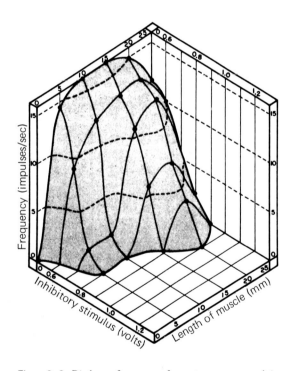

Figure 6–8. Discharge frequency of a motor neuron supplying a leg muscle in a cat. Discharge frequency is plotted against muscle length at various magnitudes of stimulation of the nerve from the antagonist to the muscle. (Reproduced, with permission, from Henneman & others: Excitability and inhibitability of motor neurons of different sizes. J Neurophysiol 28:599, 1965.)

Clonus

Another finding characteristic of states in which increased gamma efferent discharge is present is **clonus**. This neurologic sign is the occurrence of regular, rhythmic contractions of a muscle subjected to sudden, maintained stretch. Ankle clonus is a typical example. This is initiated by brisk, maintained dorsiflexion of the foot, and the response is rhythmic plantar flexion at the ankle. The stretch reflex-inverse stretch reflex sequence described above may contribute to this response. However, it can occur on the basis of synchronized motor neuron discharge without Golgi tendon organ discharge. The spindles of the tested muscle are hyperactive, and the burst of impulses from them discharges all the motor neurons supplying the muscle at once. The consequent muscle contraction stops spindle discharge. However, the stretch has been maintained, and as soon as the muscle relaxes it is again stretched and the spindles stimulated.

POLYSYNAPTIC REFLEXES: THE WITHDRAWAL REFLEX

Polysynaptic reflex paths branch in a complex fashion (Fig 6–9). The number of synapses in each of their branches is variable. Because of the synaptic delay incurred at each synapse, activity in the branches with fewer synapses reaches the motor neurons first, followed by activity in the longer pathways. This causes prolonged bombardment of the motor neurons from a single stimulus and consequently prolonged responses. Furthermore, as shown in Fig 6–9, at least some of the branch pathways turn back on themselves, permitting activity to reverberate until it becomes unable to cause a propagated transsynaptic response

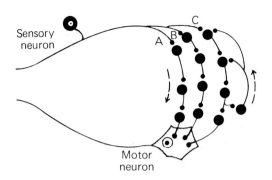

Sensory neuron

Motor neuron

Figure 6–9. Diagram of polysynaptic connections between afferent and efferent neurons in the spinal cord. The dorsal root fiber activates pathway A with 3 interneurons, pathway B with 4 interneurons, and pathway C with 4 interneurons. Note that one of the interneurons in pathway C connects to a neuron which doubles back to other interneurons, forming reverberating circuits.

and dies out. Such **reverberating circuits** are common in the brain and spinal cord.

Withdrawal Reflex

The withdrawal reflex is a typical polysynaptic reflex which occurs in response to a noxious and usually painful stimulation of the skin or subcutaneous tissues and muscle. The response is flexor muscle contraction and inhibition of extensor muscles, so that the part stimulated is flexed and withdrawn from the stimulus. When a strong stimulus is applied to a limb, the response includes not only flexion and withdrawal of that limb but also extension of the opposite limb. This **crossed extensor response** is properly part of the withdrawal reflex. It can also be shown in experimental animals that strong stimuli generate activity in the interneuron pool which spreads to all 4 extremities. This is difficult to demonstrate in normal animals, but is easily demonstrated in an animal in which the modulating effects of impulses from the brain have been abolished by prior section of the spinal cord (**spinal animal**). For example, when the hind limb of a spinal cat is pinched, the stimulated limb is withdrawn, the opposite hind limb extended, the ipsilateral forelimb extended, and the contralateral forelimb flexed. This spread of excitatory impulses up and down the spinal cord to more and more motor neurons is called **irradiation of the stimulus**, and the increase in the number of active motor units is called **recruitment of motor units**.

Importance of the Withdrawal Reflex

Flexor responses can be produced by innocuous stimulation of the skin or by stretch of the muscle, but strong flexor responses with withdrawal are initiated only by stimuli that are noxious or at least potentially harmful to the animal. These stimuli are therefore called **nociceptive stimuli**. Sherrington pointed out the survival value of the withdrawal response. Flexion of

the stimulated limb gets it away from the source of irritation, and extension of the other limb supports the body. The pattern assumed by all 4 extremities puts the animal in position to run away from the offending stimulus. Withdrawal reflexes are **prepotent**, ie, they preempt the spinal pathways from any other reflex activity taking place at the moment.

Many of the characteristics of polysynaptic reflexes can be demonstrated by studying the withdrawal reflex in the laboratory. A weak noxious stimulus to one foot evokes a minimal flexion response; stronger stimuli produce greater and greater flexion as the stimulus irradiates to more and more of the motor neuron pool supplying the muscles of the limb. Stronger stimuli also cause a more prolonged response. A weak stimulus causes one quick flexion movement; a strong stimulus causes prolonged flexion and sometimes a series of flexion movements. This prolonged response is due to prolonged, repeated firing of the motor neurons. The repeated firing is called **after-discharge**, and is due to continued bombardment of motor neurons by impulses arriving by complicated and circuitous polysynaptic paths.

As the strength of a noxious stimulus is increased, the reaction time is shortened. Spatial and temporal facilitation occur at the various synapses in the polysynaptic pathway. Stronger stimuli produce more action potentials per second in the active branches and cause more branches to become active; summation of the EPSPs to the firing level therefore occurs more rapidly.

Local Sign

The exact flexor pattern of the withdrawal reflex

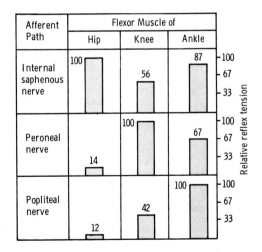

Afferent Path	Flexor Muscle of		
	Hip	Knee	Ankle
Internal saphenous nerve	100	56	87
Peroneal nerve	14	100	67
Popliteal nerve	12	42	100

Relative reflex tension

Figure 6–10. The importance of local sign in determining the character of the withdrawal response in a leg. When afferent fibers in each of the 3 nerves on the left were stimulated, hip, knee, and ankle flexors contracted but the relative tension developed in each case (shaded bars) varied. (Data from Creed & Sherrington: Observations on concurrent contraction of flexor muscles in the flexion reflex. Proc R Soc Lond [Biol] 100:258, 1926.)

in a limb varies with the part of the limb which is stimulated. If the medial surface of the limb is stimulated, for example, the response will include some abduction, whereas stimulation of the lateral surface will produce some adduction with flexion. The reflex response in each case generally serves to effectively remove the limb from the irritating stimulus. This dependence of the exact response on the location of the stimulus is called **local sign.** The degree to which local sign determines the particular response pattern is illustrated in Fig 6–10.

Fractionation & Occlusion

Another characteristic of the withdrawal response is the fact that supramaximal stimulation of any of the sensory nerves from a limb never produces as strong a contraction of the flexor muscles as that elicited by direct electrical stimulation of the muscles themselves. This indicates that the afferent inputs **fractionate** the motor neuron pool, ie, each input goes to only part of the motor neuron pool for the flexors of that particular extremity. On the other hand, if all the sensory inputs are dissected out and stimulated one after the other, the sum of the tension developed by stimulation of each is greater than that produced by direct electrical stimulation of the muscle or stimulation of all inputs at once. This fact indicates that the various afferent inputs share some of the motor neurons, and that occlusion (see Chapter 4) occurs when all inputs are stimulated at once.

Other Polysynaptic Reflexes

There are many polysynaptic reflexes in addition to the withdrawal reflex, all with similar properties. Such reflexes as the abdominal and cremasteric reflexes are forms of the withdrawal reflex. Others include visceral components. Numerous polysynaptic reflexes that relate to specific regulatory functions are described in other sections of this book, and comprehensive lists can be found in neurology textbooks.

GENERAL PROPERTIES OF REFLEXES

It is apparent from the preceding description of the properties of monosynaptic and polysynaptic reflexes that reflex activity is stereotyped and specific in terms of both the stimulus and the response; a particular stimulus elicits a particular response.

Adequate Stimulus

The stimulus that triggers a reflex is generally very precise. This stimulus is called the **adequate stimulus** for the particular reflex. A dramatic example is the scratch reflex in the dog. This spinal reflex is adequately stimulated by multiple linear touch stimuli such as those produced by an insect crawling across the skin. The response is vigorous scratching of the area stimulated. (Incidentally, the precision with which the scratching foot goes to the site of the irritant is a good

example of local sign.) If the multiple touch stimuli are widely separated or are not in a line, the adequate stimulus is not produced and no scratching occurs. Fleas crawl, but they also jump from place to place. This jumping separates the touch stimuli so that an adequate stimulus for the scratch reflex is not produced. It is doubtful if the flea population would long survive without the ability to jump.

Final Common Path

The motor neurons that supply the extrafusal fibers in skeletal muscles are the efferent side of the reflex arc. All neural influences affecting muscular contraction ultimately funnel through them to the muscles, and they are therefore called the **final common paths.** Numerous inputs converge on them. Indeed, it has been reported that the surface of the average motor neuron accommodates 5500 synaptic knobs. There are at least 5 inputs from the same spinal segment to a typical spinal motor neuron. In addition to these, there are excitatory and inhibitory inputs, generally relayed via interneurons, from other levels of the spinal cord and multiple long descending tracts from the brain. All of these pathways converge on and determine the activity in the final common paths.

Central Excitatory & Inhibitory States

The spread up and down the spinal cord of subliminal fringe effects from excitatory stimulation has already been mentioned. Direct and presynaptic inhibitory effects can also be widespread. These effects are generally transient. However, the spinal cord also shows prolonged changes in excitability, possibly because of activity in reverberating circuits or prolonged effects of synaptic mediators. The terms **central excitatory state** and **central inhibitory state** have been used to describe prolonged states in which excitatory influences overbalance inhibitory influences and vice versa. When the central excitatory state is marked, excitatory impulses irradiate not only to many somatic areas of the spinal cord but also to autonomic areas and vice versa. In chronically paraplegic humans, for example, a mild noxious stimulus may cause, in addition to prolonged withdrawal-extension patterns in all 4 limbs, urination, defecation, sweating, and blood pressure fluctuations (**mass reflex**).

In view of the multiple, shifting, and often antagonistic influences which constantly bombard the final common paths, it is surprising that chaos does not result. Yet, as Mountcastle has expressed it, "Order reigns. The end result of reflex action is always one of some functional meaning to the organism, and reflex actions occurring one after the other in time are coordinated in sequences of some purposeful character. Such coordination of neural activity into spatial and sequential patterns which serve a useful end is the essence of the integrative activity of the nervous system."*

*In Bard P (editor): *Medical Physiology,* 11th ed, p 1104. Mosby, 1961.

7...
Cutaneous, Deep, & Visceral Sensation

PATHWAYS

The sense organs for mechanical stimulation (touch and pressure), warmth, cold, and pain have been discussed in Chapter 5, and the types of fibers which carry impulses generated in them to the CNS are listed in Chapter 2. These afferent fibers end on interneurons which make polysynaptic reflex connections to motor neurons at many levels in the spinal cord as well as on the neurons of ascending pathways which relay impulses to the cerebral cortex.

The principal direct pathways to the cerebral cortex for these senses are shown in Fig 7–1. Upon entering the spinal cord, the dorsal root fibers become segregated according to function. Fibers mediating fine touch, pressure, and proprioception ascend in the dorsal columns to the medulla, where they synapse in the gracile and cuneate nuclei. The second order neurons from the gracile and cuneate nuclei cross the midline and ascend in the medial lemniscus to end in the specific sensory relay nuclei of the thalamus. This ascending system is frequently called the **dorsal column** or **lemniscal system**.

Other touch fibers, along with those mediating temperature and pain, synapse on neurons in the dorsal horn. The axons from these neurons cross the midline and ascend in the anterolateral quadrant of the spinal cord, where they form the **anterolateral system** of ascending fibers. In general, touch is associated with the ventral spinothalamic tract whereas pain and temperature are associated with the lateral spinothalamic tract, but there is no rigid localization of function. Some of the fibers of the anterolateral system end in the specific relay nuclei of the thalamus; others project to the midline and intraluminal nonspecific projection nuclei. There is a major input from the anterolateral systems into the mesencephalic reticular formation. Thus, sensory input activates the reticular activating system, which in turn maintains the cortex in the alert state (see Chapter 11).

Collaterals from the fibers that enter the dorsal columns pass to the **substantia gelatinosa**, a lightly staining area that caps each dorsal gray column. Evidence is accumulating that these collaterals can modify the input into other cutaneous sensory systems, including the pain system. The dorsal horn represents a

"gate" in which impulses in the sensory nerve fibers are translated into impulses in ascending tracts, and it now appears that passage through this gate is dependent on the nature and pattern of impulses reaching the substantia gelatinosa. This gate is also affected by impulses in descending tracts from the brain.

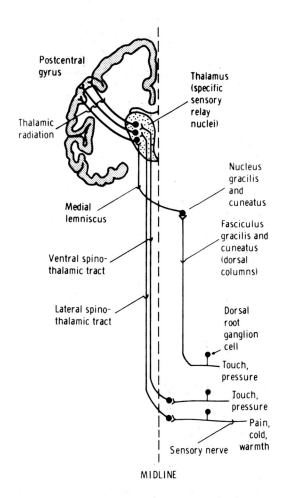

Figure 7–1. Touch, pressure, pain, and temperature pathways. The anterolateral system (ventral and lateral spinothalamic tracts) also projects to the mesencephalic reticular formation and the nonspecific thalamic nuclei. Pathways from the head are not shown.

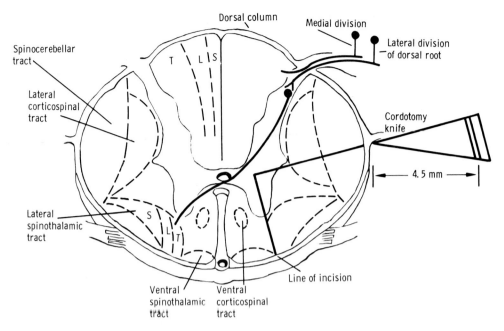

Figure 7–2. Major spinal pathways. The solid line on the right represents the line of incision in performing an anterolateral cordotomy. Note the lamination of the tracts. S, sacral; L, lumbar; T, thoracic.

Axons of the spinothalamic tracts from sacral and lumbar segments of the body are pushed laterally by axons crossing the midline at successively higher levels. On the other hand, sacral and lumbar dorsal column fibers are pushed medially by fibers from higher segments (Fig 7–2). Consequently, both of these ascending systems are laminated, with cervical to sacral segments represented from medial to lateral in the anterolateral pathways and sacral to cervical segments from medial to lateral in the dorsal columns. Because of this lamination, tumors arising outside the spinal cord first compress the spinothalamic fibers from sacral and lumbar areas, causing the early symptom of loss of pain and temperature sensation in the sacral region. Intraspinal tumors cause anesthesia first in higher segments.

The fibers within the lemniscal and anterolateral systems are joined in the brain stem by fibers mediating sensation from the head. Pain and temperature impulses are relayed via the spinal nucleus of the trigeminal nerve, and touch, pressure, and proprioception mostly via the main sensory and mesencephalic nuclei of this nerve.

Cortical Representation

From the specific sensory nuclei of the thalamus, neurons project in a highly specific way to the 2 somatic sensory areas of the cortex: somatic sensory area I (SI) in the postcentral gyrus and somatic sensory area II (SII) in the wall of the sylvian fissure (lateral cerebral sulcus).

The arrangement of the thalamic fibers to SI is such that the parts of the body are represented in order along the postcentral gyrus, with the legs on top

and the head at the foot of the gyrus (Fig 7–3). Not only is there detailed localization of the fibers from the various parts of the body in the postcentral gyrus, but the size of the cortical receiving area for impulses from a particular part of the body is proportionate to the number of receptors in the part. The relative sizes of the cortical receiving areas are shown dramatically in Fig 7–4, in which the proportions of the homunculus have been distorted to correspond to the size of the cortical receiving areas for each. Note that the cortical areas for sensation from the trunk and back are small, whereas very large areas are concerned with impulses from the hand and the parts of the mouth concerned with speech.

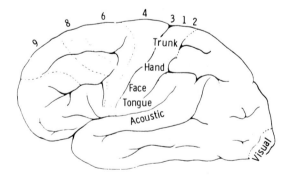

Figure 7–3. Some of the cortical receiving areas for various sensory modalities in the human brain. The numbers are those of Brodmann's cortical areas. The auditory (acoustic) area is actually located in the fissure on the top of the superior temporal gyrus, and is not normally visible. (Reproduced, with permission, from Brazier: *The Electrical Activity of the Nervous System,* 3rd ed. Pitman, 1968.)

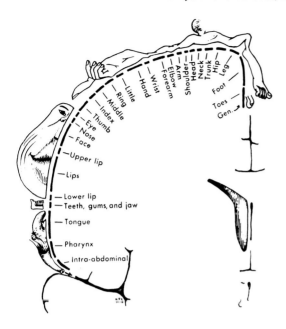

Figure 7–4. Sensory homunculus, drawn overlying a coronal section through the postcentral gyrus. Gen., genitalia. (Reproduced, with permission, from Penfield & Rasmussen: *The Cerebral Cortex of Man.* Macmillan, 1950.)

Studies of the sensory receiving area emphasize the very discrete nature of the point-for-point localization of peripheral areas in the cortex and provide further evidence for the validity of the doctrine of specific nerve energies (see Chapter 5). Stimulation of the various parts of the postcentral gyrus gives rise to sensations projected to appropriate parts of the body. The sensations produced are usually those of numbness, tingling, or a sense of movement, but with fine enough electrodes it has been possible to produce relatively pure sensations of touch, warmth, cold, and pain. The cells in the postcentral gyrus appear to be organized in vertical columns, like cells in the visual cortex (see Chapter 8). The cells in a given column are all activated by afferents from a given part of the body, and all respond to the same sensory modality.

Somatic sensory area II is located in the superior wall of the sylvian fissure. The head is represented at the inferior end of the postcentral gyrus, and the feet at the bottom of the sylvian fissure. The representation of the body parts is not as complete or detailed as it is in the postcentral gyrus. The function of SII is not known, although it may play a role in the perception of pain. Its ablation in animals does not cause any detectable deficit in other sensory modalities.

Effects of Cortical Lesions

In experimental animals and humans, lesions of the postcentral gyrus decrease but do not entirely abolish sensation. Proprioception and fine touch are most affected by cortical lesions. Temperature sensibility is less affected, and pain sensibility is only slightly af-

fected. This suggests that a certain degree of perception is possible in the absence of the cortex. Upon recovery, pain sensibility returns first, followed by temperature sense and, finally, proprioception and fine touch.

Principles of Sensory Physiology

The important general principles that relate to the physiology of sensory systems have been discussed in detail in Chapter 5. Each sense organ is specialized to convert one particular form of energy into action potentials in the sensory nerves. Each modality has a discrete pathway to the brain, and the sensation perceived as well as the part of the body to which it is localized is determined by the particular part of the brain activated. Differences in intensity of a given sensation are signaled in 2 ways: by changes in the frequency of action potentials in the sensory nerves, and by changes in the number of receptors activated. An increase in the intensity of stimulation of a sense organ has very little (if any) effect on the quality of the sensation produced.

Another principle that applies to cutaneous sensation is that of punctate representation. If the skin is carefully mapped, millimeter by millimeter, with a fine hair, a sensation of touch is evoked from spots overlying touch receptors. None is evoked from the intervening areas. Similarly, pain and temperature sensations are produced by stimulation of the skin only over the spots where the sense organs for these modalities are located.

TOUCH

Touch receptor organs adapt rapidly. They are most numerous in the fingers and lips and relatively scarce on the trunk. There are many receptors around hair follicles in addition to those in the subcutaneous tissues of hairless areas. When a hair is moved, it acts as a lever with its fulcrum at the edge of the follicle so that slight movements of the hairs are magnified into relatively potent stimuli to the nerve endings around the follicles. The stiff vibrissae on the snouts of some animals are highly developed examples of hairs that act as levers to magnify tactile stimuli. The pacinian corpuscles, which are also touch receptors, are found in the subcutaneous tissues, muscles, and joints. They also abound in the mesentery, where their function is not known.

The group II sensory fibers that transmit impulses from touch receptors to the CNS are 5–12 μm in diameter and have conduction velocities of 30–70 meters/sec. Some touch impulses are also conducted via C fibers.

Touch information is transmitted in both the lemniscal and anterolateral pathways, so that only very extensive lesions completely interrupt touch sensation. However, there are differences in the type of touch information transmitted in the 2 systems. When the dorsal columns are destroyed, vibratory sensation and proprioception are lost, the touch threshold is elevated, and the number of touch-sensitive areas in the skin is decreased. In addition, localization of touch sensation is impaired. An increase in touch threshold and a decrease in the number of touch spots in the skin are also observed after interrupting the spinothalamic tracts, but the touch deficit is slight and touch localization remains normal. The information carried in the lemniscal system is concerned with the detailed localization, spatial form, and temporal pattern of tactile stimuli. The information carried in the spinothalamic tracts, on the other hand, is concerned with poorly localized, gross tactile sensations.

While lesions limited to the postcentral gyrus produce loss of fine touch discrimination on the opposite side of the body, lesions of the parietal lobe in the representational hemisphere produce contralateral disorders of spatial orientation, and lesions of the parietal lobe in the categorical hemisphere produce agnosias. These abnormalities are discussed in Chapter 16.

PROPRIOCEPTION

Proprioceptive information is transmitted up the spinal cord in the dorsal columns. A good deal of the proprioceptive input goes to the cerebellum, but some passes via the medial lemnisci and thalamic radiations to the cortex. Diseases of the dorsal columns produce ataxia because of the interruption of proprioceptive input to the cerebellum.

There is some evidence that proprioceptive information passes to consciousness in the anterolateral columns of the spinal cord. Since stimulation of group I fibers produces no electrical response in the cerebral cortex, impulses initiated in the muscle spindles and Golgi tendon organs apparently do not reach consciousness. Conscious awareness of the position of the various parts of the body in space depends instead upon impulses from sense organs in and around the joints. The organs involved are slowly adapting "spray" endings, structures that resemble Golgi tendon organs, and probably pacinian corpuscles in the synovia and ligaments. Impulses from these organs and those from touch receptors in other tissue are synthesized in the cortex into a conscious picture of the position of the body in space. Microelectrode studies indicate that many of the neurons in the sensory cortex respond to particular movements, not just to touch or static position. In this regard, the sensory cortex is organized like the visual cortex (see Chapter 8).

TEMPERATURE

There are 2 types of temperature sense organs: those responding maximally to temperatures slightly above body temperature, and those responding maximally to temperatures slightly below body temperature. The former are the sense organs for what we call warmth, and the latter for what we call cold. However, the adequate stimuli are actually 2 different degrees of warmth, since cold is not a form of energy.

Mapping experiments show that there are discrete cold-sensitive and warmth-sensitive spots in the skin. There are 4–10 times as many cold spots as warm. The temperature sense organs are naked nerve endings that respond to absolute temperature, not the temperature gradient across the skin. The afferents are small myelinated fibers 2–5 μm in diameter in Erlanger and Gasser's A δ group (group III fibers; see Chapter 2). Impulses in them pass to the postcentral gyrus via the lateral spinothalamic tract and the thalamic radiation.

Because the sense organs are located subepithelially, it is the temperature of the subcutaneous tissues that determines the responses. Cool metal objects feel colder than wooden objects of the same temperature because the metal conducts heat away from the skin more rapidly, cooling the subcutaneous tissues to a greater degree. Below a skin temperature of 20° and above 40° C, there is no adaptation, but between 20° and 40° C there is adaptation, so that the sensation produced by a temperature change gradually fades to one at thermal neutrality. In humans, the intensities of warm or cold sensations are related by a power function to the temperature of the stimulus (see Chapter 5). Above 45° C, tissue damage begins to occur and the sensation becomes one of pain.

PAIN

The sense organs for pain are the naked nerve endings found in almost every tissue of the body. Pain impulses are transmitted to the CNS by 2 fiber systems. One system is made up of small myelinated A δ fibers, 2–5 μm in diameter, which conduct at rates of 12–30 meters/sec. The other consists of unmyelinated C fibers, 0.4–1.2 μm in diameter. These latter fibers are found in the lateral division of the dorsal roots, and are often called dorsal root C fibers. They conduct at the slow rate of 0.5–2 meters/sec. Both fiber groups end on the lateral spinothalamic tract neurons, and pain impulses ascend via this tract to the ventral posteromedial and posterolateral nuclei of the thalamus. From there, they relay to the postcentral gyri of the cerebral cortex.

Although there are no pain fibers in the dorsal columns, section of the dorsal column fibers may make painful stimuli more severe and unpleasant (see below).

Fast & Slow Pain

The presence of 2 pain pathways, one slow and one fast, explains the physiologic observation that there are 2 kinds of pain. A painful stimulus causes a "bright," sharp, localized sensation followed by a dull, aching, diffuse, and unpleasant feeling. These 2 sensations are variously called fast and slow pain or first and second pain. The farther from the brain the stimulus is applied, the greater the temporal separation of the 2 components. This and other evidence make it clear that fast pain is due to activity in the A δ pain fibers, while slow pain is due to activity in the C pain fibers.

Subcortical Perception & Affect

There is considerable evidence that sensory stimuli are perceived in the absence of the cerebral cortex, and this is especially true of pain. The cortical receiving areas are apparently concerned with the discriminative, exact, and meaningful interpretation of pain, but perception alone does not require the cortex.

Pain was called by Sherrington the "psychical adjunct of an imperative protective reflex." Stimuli which are painful generally initiate potent withdrawal and avoidance responses. Furthermore, pain is peculiar among the senses in that it is associated with a strong emotional component. Information transmitted via the special senses may secondarily evoke pleasant or unpleasant emotions, depending largely upon past experience, but pain alone has a "built-in" unpleasant affect. Present evidence indicates that this affective response depends upon connections of the pain pathways in the thalamus. Damage to the thalamus may be associated with a peculiar over-reaction to painful stimuli known as the **thalamic syndrome**. In this condition, usually due to blockage of the thalamogeniculate branch of the posterior cerebral artery with consequent damage to the posterior thalamic nuclei, minor stimuli lead to prolonged, severe, and very unpleasant pain. Such bouts of pain may occur spontaneously, or at least without evident external stimuli. Another interesting fact is that at least in some cases pain can be dissociated from its unpleasant subjective affect by cutting the deep connections between the frontal lobes and the rest of the brain (**prefrontal lobotomy**). After this operation patients report that they feel pain but that it "doesn't bother" them. The operation is sometimes useful in the treatment of intractable pain caused by terminal cancer.

Lobotomy is, of course, only one of the many neurosurgical procedures employed to relieve intractable pain in terminal cancer patients, and it produces extensive personality changes (see Chapter 16). Other operations are summarized in Fig 7–5. One of the most extensively used is **anterolateral cordotomy**. In this procedure, a knife is inserted into the lateral aspect of the spinal cord and swept anteriorly and laterally as shown in Fig 7–2. When properly performed, this procedure cuts the lateral spinothalamic pain fibers while leaving some of the ventral spinothalamic touch fibers intact. Even if there is extensive damage to the touch fibers in the anterolateral quad-

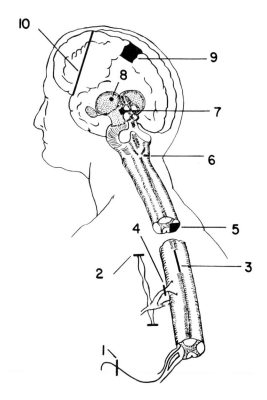

Figure 7–5. Diagram of various surgical procedures designed to alleviate pain. 1, nerve section; 2, sympathectomy (for visceral pain); 3, myelotomy to section spinothalamic fibers in anterior white commissure; 4, posterior rhizotomy; 5, anterolateral cordotomy; 6, medullary tractotomy; 7, mesencephalic tractotomy; 8, thalamotomy; 9, gyrectomy; 10, prefrontal lobotomy. (Modified from MacCarty & Drake: Neurosurgical procedures for the control of pain. Proc Staff Meet Mayo Clin 31:208, 1956.)

rants, touch is very little impaired because the dorsal column touch system is intact.

Deep Pain

The main difference between superficial and deep sensibility is the different nature of the pain evoked by noxious stimuli. Unlike superficial pain, deep pain is poorly localized, nauseating, and frequently associated with sweating and changes in blood pressure. Pain can be elicited experimentally from the periosteum and ligaments by injecting hypertonic saline into them. The pain produced in this fashion initiates reflex contraction of nearby skeletal muscles. This reflex contraction is similar to the muscle spasm associated with injuries to bones, tendons, and joints. The steadily contracting muscles become ischemic, and ischemia stimulates the pain receptors in the muscles (see below). The pain in turn initiates more spasm, and a vicious cycle is set up.

Adequate Stimulus

Pain receptors are specific, and pain is not produced by overstimulation of other receptors. On the other hand, the adequate stimulus for pain receptors is not as specific as that for others because they can be stimulated by a variety of strong stimuli. For example, pain receptors respond to warmth, but it has been calculated that their threshold for thermal energy is over 100 times that of the warmth receptors. Pain receptors also respond to electrical, mechanical, and, especially, chemical energy.

It has been suggested that pain is chemically mediated, and that stimuli which provoke it have in common the ability to liberate a chemical agent which stimulates the nerve endings. The chemical agent might be a kinin. The kinins are polypeptides that are liberated from proteins by proteolytic enzymes. They are known to be liberated in tissues by noxious stimuli, and they are capable of producing severe pain. However, the pain produced by injected kinins is usually transient. Histamine has also been suspected of being a chemical mediator of pain, but there is some evidence that it causes local liberation of kinins when it is injected into the tissues.

Muscle Pain

If a muscle contracts rhythmically in the presence of an adequate blood supply, pain does not usually result. However, if the blood supply to a muscle is occluded, contraction soon causes pain. The pain persists after the contraction until blood flow is reestablished. If a muscle with a normal blood supply is made to contract continuously without periods of relaxation, it also begins to ache because the maintained contraction compresses the blood vessels supplying the muscle.

These observations are difficult to interpret except in terms of the release during contraction of a chemical agent (Lewis' "P factor") that causes pain when its local concentration is high enough. When the blood supply is restored, the material is washed out or metabolized. The identity of the P factor is not settled, but it could be K^+ or possibly a kinin.

Clinically, the substernal pain that develops when the myocardium becomes ischemic during exertion (angina pectoris) is a classic example of the accumulation of P factor in a muscle. Angina is relieved by rest because this decreases the myocardial O_2 requirement and permits the blood supply to remove the factor. Intermittent claudication, the pain produced in the leg muscles of persons afflicted with occlusive vascular disease, is another example. It characteristically comes on while the patient is walking and disappears when he rests.

Hyperalgesia

In pathologic conditions the sensitivity of the pain receptors is altered. There are 2 important types of alteration, primary and secondary hyperalgesia. In the area surrounding an inflamed or injured area, the threshold for pain is lowered so that trivial stimuli cause pain. This phenomenon, **primary hyperalgesia**, is seen in the area of the **flare**, the region of vasodilatation around the injury. In the area of actual tissue damage, the vasodilation and, presumably, the pain are due to substances liberated from injured cells, but the flare in surrounding undamaged tissue is due to a chemical agent liberated by antidromic impulses in sensory nerve fibers. This agent is postulated to be a proteolytic enzyme which causes the liberation of vasodilator kinins in the tissues. The kinins also lower the threshold of the pain fibers in the area and may themselves produce pain. Evidence for this hypothesis is the observation that stimulation of the peripheral end of a cut dorsal root produces vasodilatation in the area served by the root, and if the subcutaneous tissues are perfused during such stimulation, the perfusate contains a peptide that causes pain upon injection into innervated skin.

Another aberration of sensation following injury is **secondary hyperalgesia**. In the area affected, the threshold for pain is actually elevated but the pain produced is unpleasant, prolonged, and severe. The area from which this response is obtained extends well beyond the site of injury, and the condition does not last as long as primary hyperalgesia. It is probably due to some sort of central facilitation by impulses from the injured area of the pathways responsible for the unpleasant affect component of pain. Such facilitation or alteration of pathways may be a spinal subliminal fringe effect, or it may occur at the thalamic or even the cortical level.

DIFFERENCES BETWEEN SOMATIC & VISCERAL SENSORY MECHANISMS

The autonomic nervous system, like the somatic, has afferent components, central integrating stations, and effector pathways. The visceral afferent mechanisms play a major role in homeostatic adjustments. In the viscera there are a number of special receptors— osmoreceptors, baroreceptors, chemoreceptors, etc— which respond to changes in the internal environment. The afferent nerves from these receptors make reflex connections that are intimately concerned with regulating the function of the various systems with which they are associated, and their physiology is discussed in the chapters on these systems.

The receptors for pain and the other sensory modalities present in the viscera are similar to those in skin, but there are marked differences in their distribution. There are no proprioceptors in the viscera, and few temperature and touch sense organs. If the abdominal wall is infiltrated with a local anesthetic, the abdomen can be opened and the intestines can be handled, cut, and even burned without eliciting any discomfort. Pain receptors are present in the viscera, however, and although they are more sparsely distributed than in somatic structures, certain types of stimuli cause severe pain. There are many pacinian corpuscles in the mesentery, but their function in this location is not known.

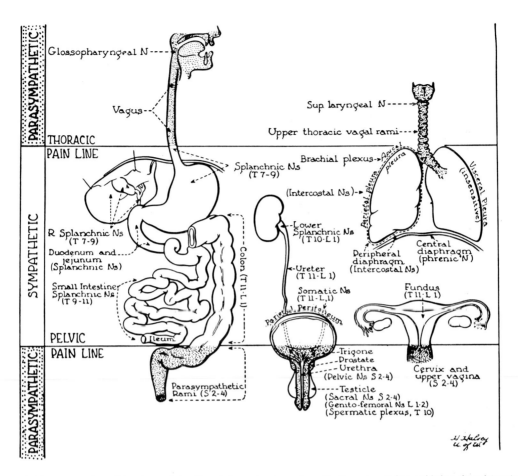

Figure 7—6. Pain innervation of the viscera. Pain afferents from structures above the thoracic pain line and below the pelvic pain line traverse parasympathetic pathways. (After White. Reproduced, with permission, from Ruch, in: *Physiology and Biophysics*, 19th ed. Ruch TC, Patton HD [editors]. Saunders, 1965.)

Afferent fibers from visceral structures reach the CNS via sympathetic and parasympathetic pathways. Their cell bodies are located in the dorsal roots and the homologous cranial nerve ganglia. Specifically, there are visceral afferents in the facial, glossopharyngeal, and vagus nerves, in the thoracic and upper lumbar dorsal roots, and in the sacral roots (Fig 7—6). There may also be visceral afferent fibers from the eye in the trigeminal nerve. There are A β and A δ afferent fibers in the splanchnic nerves, but only A δ fibers in the pelvic and vagus nerves. Visceral sensation travels along the same pathways as somatic sensation in the spinothalamic tracts and thalamic radiations, and the cortical receiving areas for visceral sensation are intermixed with the somatic receiving areas in the postcentral gyri.

VISCERAL PAIN

Pain from visceral structures is poorly localized, unpleasant, associated with nausea and autonomic symptoms, and often radiates or is referred to other areas.

Stimulation of Pain Fibers

Because there are relatively few pain receptors in the viscera, visceral pain is poorly localized. However, as almost everyone knows from personal experience, visceral pain can be very severe. The receptors in the walls of the hollow viscera are especially sensitive to distention of these organs. Such distention can be produced experimentally in the gastrointestinal tract by inflation of a swallowed balloon attached to a tube. This produces pain which waxes and wanes (intestinal colic) as the intestine contracts and relaxes on the balloon. Similar colic is produced in intestinal obstruction by the contractions of the dilated intestine above the obstruction. When a viscus is inflamed or hyperemic, relatively minor stimuli cause severe pain. This is probably a form of primary hyperalgesia similar to that which occurs in somatic structures. Traction on the mesentery is also claimed to be painful, but the significance of this observation in the production of visceral pain is not clear. Visceral pain is particularly unpleasant not only because of the affective component it has in common with all pain but also because so many visceral afferents excited by the same process that causes the pain have reflex connections that initiate nausea, vomiting, and other autonomic effects.

Pathways

Pain impulses from the thoracic and abdominal viscera are almost exclusively conducted through the sympathetic nervous system and the dorsal roots of the first thoracic to the second lumbar spinal nerves. This is why sympathectomy effectively abolishes pain from the heart, stomach, and intestines. However, pain impulses from the esophagus, trachea, and pharynx are mediated via vagal afferents, and pain from the structures deep in the pelvis is transmitted in the sacral parasympathetic nerves (Fig 7–6).

Muscle Spasm & Rigidity

Visceral pain, like deep somatic pain, initiates reflex contraction of nearby skeletal muscle. This reflex spasm is usually in the abdominal wall, and makes the abdominal wall rigid. It is most marked when visceral inflammatory processes involve the peritoneum. However, it can occur without such involvement. The anatomic details of the reflex pathways by which impulses from diseased viscera initiate skeletal muscle spasm are still obscure. The spasm protects the underlying inflamed structures from inadvertent trauma. Indeed, this reflex spasm is sometimes called "guarding."

The classical signs of inflammation in an abdominal viscus are pain, tenderness, autonomic changes such as hypotension and sweating, and spasm of the abdominal wall. From the preceding discussion, the genesis of each of these signs is apparent. The tenderness is due to the heightened sensitivity of the pain receptors in the viscus, the autonomic changes due to activation of visceral reflexes, and the spasm due to reflex contraction of skeletal muscle in the abdominal wall.

REFERRAL & INHIBITION OF PAIN

Referred Pain

Irritation of a viscus frequently produces pain which is felt not in the viscus but in some somatic structure that may be a considerable distance away. Such pain is said to be **referred** to the somatic structure. Deep somatic pain may also be referred, but superficial pain is not. When visceral pain is both local and referred, it sometimes seems to spread or **radiate** from the local to the distant site.

Obviously, a knowledge of referred pain and the common sites of pain referral from each of the viscera is of great importance to the physician. Perhaps the best-known example is referral of cardiac pain to the inner aspect of the left arm. Other dramatic examples

include pain in the tip of the shoulder due to irritation of the central portion of the diaphragm and pain in the testicle due to distention of the ureter. Additional instances abound in the practice of medicine, surgery, and dentistry. However, sites of reference are not stereotyped, and unusual reference sites occur with considerable frequency. Heart pain, for instance, may be purely abdominal, may be referred to the right arm, and may even be referred to the neck. Referred pain can be produced experimentally by stimulation of the cut end of a splanchnic nerve.

Dermatomal Rule

When pain is referred it is usually to a structure that developed from the same embryonic segment or dermatome as the structure in which the pain originates. This principle is called the **dermatomal rule**. For example, the diaphragm migrates from the neck region during embryonic development to its adult location in the abdomen and takes its nerve supply, the phrenic nerve, with it. One-third of the fibers in the phrenic nerve are afferent, and they enter the spinal cord at the level of the second to fourth cervical segments, the same location at which afferents from the tip of the shoulder enter. Similarly, the heart and the arm have the same segmental origin, and the testicle has migrated with its nerve supply from the primitive urogenital ridge from which the kidney and ureter also developed.

Role of Convergence in Referred Pain

Not only do the nerves from the visceral structures and the somatic structures to which pain is referred enter the nervous system at the same level, but

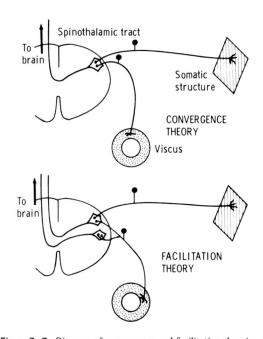

Figure 7–7. Diagram of convergence and facilitation theories of referred pain.

there are many more sensory fibers in the peripheral nerves than there are axons in the lateral spinothalamic tracts. Therefore, a considerable degree of convergence of peripheral sensory fibers on the spinothalamic neurons must occur. One theory of the mechanism underlying referred pain is based on this fact. It holds that somatic and visceral afferents converge on the same spinothalamic neurons (Fig 7–7). Since somatic pain is much more common than visceral pain, the brain has "learned" that activity arriving in a given pathway is due to a pain stimulus in a particular somatic area. When the same pathway is stimulated by activity in visceral afferents, the signal reaching the brain is no different and the pain is projected to the somatic area.

Past experience does play an important role in referred pain. Although pain originating in an inflamed abdominal viscus is usually referred to the midline, in patients who have had previous abdominal surgery the pain of abdominal disease is frequently referred to their surgical scars. Pain originating in the maxillary sinus is usually referred to nearby teeth, but in patients with a history of traumatic dental work such pain is regularly referred to the previously traumatized teeth. This is true even when the teeth are a considerable distance away from the sinus.

Facilitation Effects

Another theory of the origin of referred pain holds that, owing to subliminal fringe effects, incoming impulses from visceral structures lower the threshold of spinothalamic neurons receiving afferents from somatic areas, so that minor activity in the pain pathways from the somatic areas—activity which would normally die out in the spinal cord—passes on to the brain.

If convergence alone were the explanation for referred pain, anesthetizing the somatic area of reference with procaine should have no effect on the pain, whereas if subliminal fringe effects were responsible the pain should disappear. The effects of local anesthesia in the area of reference vary. When the pain is severe, it is usually unaffected, but when the pain is mild it may be completely abolished. Therefore, it appears that both convergence and facilitation play a role in the pathogenesis of referred pain.

Central Inhibition & Counterirritants

It is of course well known that soldiers wounded in the heat of battle may feel no pain until the battle is over. Many people have learned from practical experience that touching or shaking an injured area decreases the pain of the injury. Acupuncture has been used for 4000 years to prevent or relieve pain, and, using this technic, it is possible in some instances to perform major surgery without any other type of anesthesia. These and other observations make it clear that pain transmission and perception are subject to inhibition or modification.

Experimental evidence for the modifiability of pain transmission is provided by the observation that the potentials evoked in the cerebral cortex by stimulation of the splanchnic nerves disappear if the stimulation is preceded or accompanied by stimulation of somatic afferents. Another fact that suggests that central inhibition occurs in afferent systems is the experimental observation that if an area of secondary hyperalgesia is repeatedly stimulated it shrinks in size.

One site of inhibition of pain transmission is probably the substantia gelatinosa, the "gate" through which pain impulses reach the lateral spinothalamic system. Stimulation of large fiber afferents from an area from which pain is being initiated reduces the pain. Collateral fibers from the dorsal column touch fibers enter the substantia gelatinosa, and it has been postulated that impulses in these collaterals or interneurons on which they end inhibit transmission from the dorsal root pain fibers to the spinothalamic neurons. The mechanism involved appears to be presynaptic inhibition (see Chapter 4) of the endings of the primary afferents that transmit pain impulses.

It is well known that morphine relieves pain and produces euphoria. There are receptors for morphine in the brain, spinal cord, and gastrointestinal tract, and it has now been demonstrated that a variety of naturally occurring peptides bind to these receptors. The larger peptides are called endorphins; the smaller ones are called enkephalins (see Chapter 15). There is some evidence that acupuncture causes release of these peptides, possibly in the substantia gelatinosa. However, their exact function in sensory physiology is as yet unknown.

It has been claimed that transmission in the substantia gelatinosa can be inhibited by impulses in the pathways descending from the brain. Chronic stimulation of the dorsal columns with an implanted stimulator has been used clinically as a method of relieving intractable pain. The pain relief could be due to antidromic conduction to the "gate" in the substantia gelatinosa or to orthodromic conduction to a similar gate somewhere in the brain stem. However, an action at the dorsal horn level seems likely since section of the dorsal columns may cause enhancement of the response to noxious stimuli.

Inhibition in central sensory pathways may explain the efficacy of counterirritants. Stimulation of the skin over an area of visceral inflammation produces some relief of the pain due to the visceral disease. The old-fashioned mustard plaster works on this principle. Some similar mechanism may explain the "anesthesia" produced in dental patients by loud sound, although much of this effect is admittedly due to suggestion.

Itch & Tickle

Itching is probably produced by repetitive low-frequency stimulation of C fibers. Very mild stimulation of this system, especially if produced by something that moves across the skin, produces tickle. Itch spots can be identified on the skin by careful mapping; like the pain spots, they are in regions in which there are many naked endings of unmyelinated fibers. Itch persists along with burning pain in nerve block experiments when only C fibers are conducting, and itch, like pain, is abolished by section of the spinothalamic tracts. However, the distribution of itch and pain are different; itching occurs only in the skin, the eyes, and certain mucous membranes, and not in the deep tissues or viscera. Furthermore, low-frequency stimulation of pain fibers generally produces pain, not itch, and high-frequency stimulation of itch spots on the skin may merely increase the intensity of the itching without producing pain. These observations suggest that the C fiber system responsible for itching is not the same as that responsible for pain. It is interesting that a tickling sensation is usually regarded as pleasurable, whereas itching is at least annoying, and pain is unpleasant.

Itching can be produced not only by repeated local mechanical stimulation of the skin but by a variety of chemical agents. Histamine produces intense itching, and various injuries cause its liberation in the skin. However, in most instances of itching, histamine does not appear to be the responsible agent; doses of histamine that are too small to produce itching still produce redness and swelling on injection into the skin, and severe itching frequently occurs without any visible change in the skin. The kinins cause severe itching, and it may be that they are the chemical mediators responsible for the sensation. It is interesting in this regard that itch powder, which is made up of the spicules from the pods of the tropical plant cowhage, contains a proteolytic enzyme, and the powder presumably acts by liberating itch-producing peptides.

OTHER SENSATIONS

"Synthetic Senses"

The cutaneous senses for which separate receptors exist are touch, warmth, cold, pain, and possibly itching. Combinations of these sensations plus, in some cases, cortical components are synthesized into the sensations of vibratory sensation, 2-point discrimination, and stereognosis.

Vibratory Sensibility

When a vibrating tuning fork is applied to the skin, a buzzing or thrill is felt. The sensation is most marked over bones, but it can be felt when the tuning fork is placed in other locations. The receptors involved are the pressure receptors, but a time factor is also necessary. A pattern of rhythmic pressure stimuli is interpreted as vibration. The impulses responsible for the vibrating sensation are carried in the dorsal columns. Degeneration of this part of the spinal cord occurs in poorly controlled diabetes, pernicious anemia, some vitamin deficiencies, and occasionally in other conditions, and depression of the threshold for vibratory stimuli is an early symptom of this degeneration. Vibratory sensation and proprioception are closely related; when one is depressed, so is the other.

Two-Point Discrimination

The minimal distance by which 2 touch stimuli must be separated to be perceived as separate is called the **2-point threshold**. It depends upon touch plus the cortical component of identifying 1 rather than 2 stimuli. Its magnitude varies from place to place on the body, and is smallest where the touch receptors are most abundant. Points on the back, for instance, must be separated by 65 mm or more before they can be distinguished as separate points, whereas on the fingers 2 stimuli can be resolved if they are separated by as little as 3 mm. On the hands, the magnitude of the 2-point threshold is approximately the diameter of the area of skin supplied by a single sensory unit. However, the peripheral neural basis of discriminating 2 points is not completely understood, and in view of the extensive interdigitation and overlapping of the sensory units, it is probably complex.

Stereognosis

The ability to identify objects by handling them without looking at them is called **stereognosis**. Normal persons can readily identify objects such as keys and coins of various denominations. This ability obviously depends upon relatively intact touch and pressure sensation, but it also has a large cortical component. Impaired stereognosis is an early sign of damage to the cerebral cortex, and sometimes occurs in the absence of any defect in touch and pressure sensation when there is a lesion in the parietal lobe posterior to the postcentral gyrus.

8 ...
Vision

ANATOMIC CONSIDERATIONS

The eyes are complex sense organs that have evolved from primitive light-sensitive spots on the surface of invertebrates. Within its protective casing, each eye has a layer of receptors, a lens system for focusing light on these receptors, and a system of nerves for conducting impulses from the receptors to the brain. The principal structures are shown in Fig 8–1. The outer protective layer of the eyeball, the **sclera**, is modified anteriorly to form the transparent **cornea**, through which light rays enter the eye. Inside the sclera is the **choroid**, a pigmented layer that contains many of the blood vessels which nourish the structures in the eyeball. Lining the posterior two-thirds of the choroid is the **retina**, the neural tissue containing the receptor cells.

The **crystalline lens** is a transparent structure held in place by a circular **lens ligament**, or **zonule**. The zonule is attached to the thickened anterior part of the choroid, the **ciliary body**. The ciliary body contains circular muscle fibers and longitudinal fibers which attach near the corneoscleral junction. In front of the

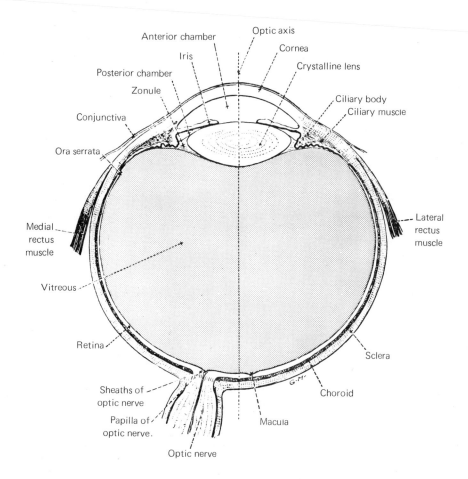

Figure 8–1. Section through right eye in horizontal plane magnified about 4 times. (After Eycleshymer & Jones. Reproduced, with permission, from Jones & Shepard: *A Manual of Surgical Anatomy*. Saunders, 1945.)

lens is the pigmented and opaque **iris**, the colored portion of the eye. The iris contains circular muscle fibers which constrict and radial fibers which dilate the **pupil**. Variations in the diameter of the pupil can produce up to 5-fold changes in the amount of light reaching the retina.

The anterior chamber of the eye between the cornea and the lens is filled with the **aqueous humor**, a fluid with a low protein content which is formed partly by diffusion and partly by active transport of components from the plasma. The space between the lens and the retina is filled with a clear gelatinous material called the **vitreous (vitreous humor)**.

Retina

The retina is a complex 10-layered structure which extends anteriorly almost to the ciliary body. It contains the visual receptors, the **rods and cones**, and 4 types of neurons: **bipolar cells, ganglion cells, horizontal cells,** and **amacrine cells** (Fig 8–2). The rods and cones, which are next to the choroid, synapse with bipolar cells, and the bipolar cells synapse with ganglion cells. The axons of the ganglion cells converge

and leave the eye as the optic nerve. Horizontal cells connect receptor cells to other receptor cells, and amacrine cells connect ganglion cells to one another. There is considerable overall convergence of receptors on bipolar cells and bipolar cells on ganglion cells (see below). Since the receptor layer of the retina is apposed to the choroid, light rays must pass through the ganglion cell and bipolar cell layers to reach the rods and cones. The pigmented layer of choroid next to the retina absorbs light rays, preventing the reflection of rays back through the retina. Such reflection would produce blurring of the visual images.

The cells of the retina are arranged in orderly layers (Fig 8–2). The neural elements are bound together by glial cells called Müller cells. The processes of these cells form an internal limiting membrane on the inner surface of the retina and an external limiting membrane in the receptor layer.

The optic nerve leaves the eye and the retinal blood vessels enter it at a point 3 mm medial to and slightly above the posterior pole of the globe. This region is visible through the ophthalmoscope as the **optic disk** (Fig 8–3). There are no visual receptors

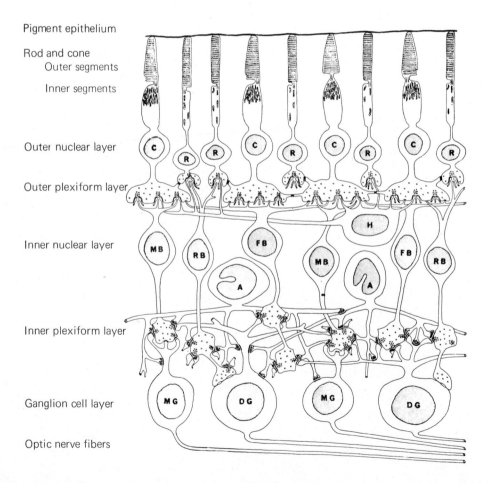

Pigment epithelium

Rod and cone
   Outer segments

   Inner segments

Outer nuclear layer

Outer plexiform layer

Inner nuclear layer

Inner plexiform layer

Ganglion cell layer

Optic nerve fibers

Figure 8–2. Neural components of the retina. C, cone; R, rod; MB, RB, and FB, midget, rod, and flat bipolar cells; DG and MG, diffuse and midget ganglion cells; H, horizontal cells; A, amacrine cells. (Reproduced, with permission, from Dowling & Boycott: Organization of the primate retina: Electron microscopy. Proc R Soc Lond [Biol] 166:80, 1966.)

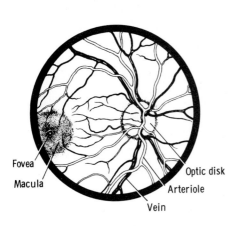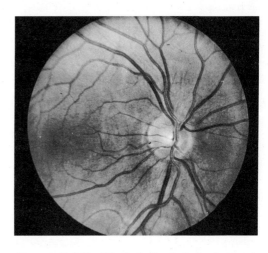

Figure 8–3 Retina seen through the ophthalmoscope in a normal human. Diagram at left identifies the landmarks in the photograph on the right. (Reproduced, with permission, from Vaughan & Asbury: *General Ophthalmology*, 8th ed. Lange, 1977.)

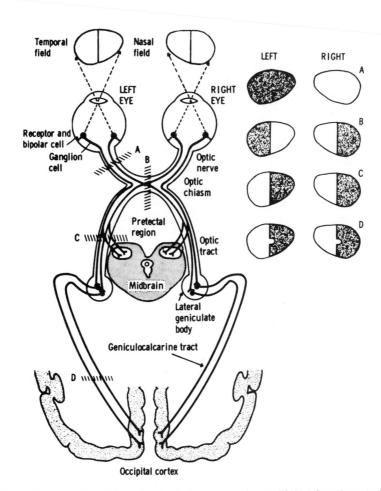

Figure 8–4. Visual pathways. Lesions at the points marked by the letters cause the visual field defects shown in the diagrams on the right (see text). Occipital lesions may spare the fibers from the macula (as in D) because of the separation in the brain of these fibers from the others subserving vision.

overlying the disk, and consequently this spot is blind (the **blind spot**). At the posterior pole of the eye there is a yellowish pigmented spot, the **macula lutea**. This marks the location of the **fovea centralis**, a thinned-out, rod-free portion of the retina where the cones are densely packed and there are very few cells and no blood vessels overlying the receptors. The fovea is highly developed in humans. It is the point where visual acuity is greatest. When attention is attracted to or fixed on an object, the eyes are normally moved so that light rays coming from the object fall on the fovea.

The arteries, arterioles, and veins in the superficial layers of the retina near its vitreous surface can be seen through the ophthalmoscope. Since this is the one place in the body where arterioles are readily visible, ophthalmoscopic examination is of great value in the diagnosis and evaluation of diabetes mellitus, hypertension, and other diseases that affect the blood vessels. The retinal vessels supply the bipolar and ganglion cells, but the receptors are nourished for the most part by the capillary plexus in the choroid. This is why retinal detachment is so damaging to the receptor cells.

Neural Pathways

The axons of the ganglion cells pass caudally in the **optic nerve** and **optic tract** to end in the **lateral geniculate body**, a part of the thalamus. The fibers from each nasal hemiretina decussate in the **optic chiasm**. In the geniculate body, the fibers from the nasal half of one retina and the temporal half of the other synapse in a highly specific fashion on the cells whose axons form the **geniculocalcarine tract**. This tract passes to the occipital lobe of the cerebral cortex. The primary visual receiving area, or **visual cortex** (Brodmann's area 17), is located principally on the sides of the calcarine fissure. Some of the optic nerve fibers, or possibly their collaterals, pass from the optic tract to the pretectal region of the midbrain and the superior colliculus, where they form connections which mediate visual reflexes (Fig 8–4).

Receptors

Each rod and cone is divided into an inner and an outer segment, a nuclear region, and a synaptic zone (Fig 8–5). The outer segments are modified cilia, and are made up of regular stacks of flattened saccules composed of membrane. These saccules contain the photosensitive pigment. The inner segments are rich in mitochondria. The rods are named for the thin, rod-like appearance of their outer segments. Cones generally have thick inner segments and conical outer segments, although their morphology varies from place to place in the retina.

Rod outer segments are being constantly renewed by formation of new saccules at the inner edge of the segment and phagocytosis of old saccules from the outer tip by cells of the pigment epithelium. In the disease retinitis pigmentosa, the phagocytic process is defective and a layer of debris accumulates between the receptors and the pigment epithelium. Cone re-

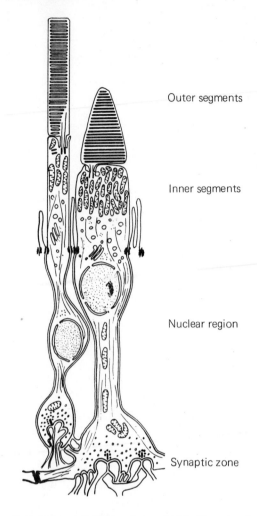

Outer segments

Inner segments

Nuclear region

Synaptic zone

Figure 8–5. Human rod *(left)* and cone *(right)*. (Reproduced, with permission, from Missotten: *The Ultrastructure of the Human Retina.* Editions Arscia, 1965.)

newal is a more diffuse process and appears to occur at multiple sites in the outer segments.

The fovea contains no rods, and each foveal cone has a single bipolar cell connecting it to a single ganglion cell, so that each foveal cone is connected to a single fiber in the optic nerve. In other portions of the retina, rods predominate (Fig 8–6), and there is a good deal of convergence. Since there are approximately 6 million cones and 120 million rods in each human eye, but only 1.2 million nerve fibers in each optic nerve, the overall convergence of receptors through bipolar cells on ganglion cells is about 105:1. In the peripheral portions of the retina, rods and cones often converge on the same ganglion cell.

The rods are extremely sensitive to light and are the receptors for night vision (**scotopic vision**). The scotopic visual apparatus is not capable of resolving the details and boundaries of objects or determining their color. The cones have a much higher threshold, but the cone system has a much greater acuity and is the sys-

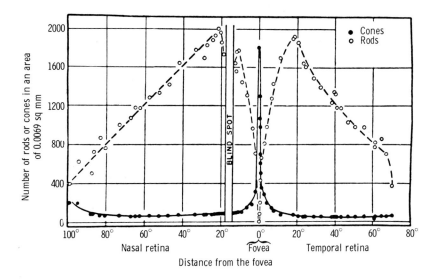

Figure 8—6. Rod and cone density along the horizontal meridian through the human retina. A plot of the relative acuity of vision in the various parts of the light-adapted eye would parallel the cone density curve; a similar plot of relative acuity of the dark-adapted eye would parallel the rod density curve. (Modified and reproduced, with permission, from Osterberg: Topography of the rods and cones in the human retina. Acta Ophthalmol [Suppl] [Kbh] 16, 1935.)

tem responsible for vision in bright light (**photopic vision**) and for color vision. There are thus 2 kinds of inputs to the CNS from the eye: input from the rods and input from the cones. The existence of these 2 kinds of inputs, each working maximally under different conditions of illumination, is called the **duplicity theory**.

Eye Muscles

The eye is moved within the orbit by 6 ocular muscles (Fig 8—7). These are innervated by the oculomotor, trochlear, and abducens nerves. The muscles and the directions in which they move the eyeball are discussed at the end of this chapter.

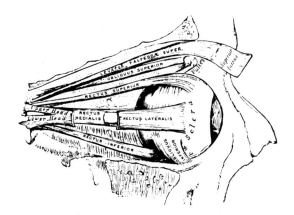

Figure 8—7. Muscles of the right orbit. The 6 muscles that move the eyeball and the levator palpebrae superioris, which raises the upper lid, are shown. (Reproduced, with permission, from: *Gray's Anatomy of the Human Body,* 29th ed. Goss CM [editor] . Lea & Febiger, 1973.)

Protection

The eye is well protected from injury by the bony walls of the orbit. The cornea is moistened and kept clear by tears which course from the **lacrimal gland** in the upper portion of each orbit across the surface of the eye to empty via the **lacrimal duct** into the nose. Blinking helps keep the cornea moist.

THE IMAGE-FORMING MECHANISM

The eyes convert energy in the visible spectrum into action potentials in the optic nerve. The wavelengths of visible light are approximately 397—723 nm. The images of objects in the environment are focused on the retina. The light rays striking the retina generate potentials in the rods and cones. Impulses initiated in the retina are conducted to the cerebral cortex, where they produce the sensation of vision.

Principles of Optics

Light rays are bent, or refracted, when they pass from one medium into a medium of a different density, except when they strike perpendicular to the interface. Parallel light rays striking a biconvex lens (Fig 8—8) are refracted to a point, or **principal focus,** behind the lens. The principal focus is on a line passing through the centers of curvature of the lens, the **principal axis**. The distance between the lens and the principal focus is the **principal focal distance**. For practical purposes, light rays from an object that strike a lens more than 20 ft away are considered to be parallel. The rays from an object closer than 20 ft are diverging, and are therefore brought to a focus farther back on

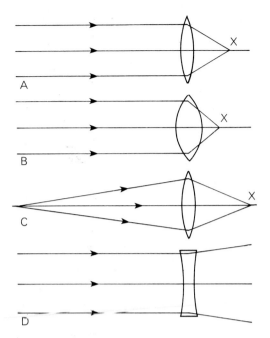

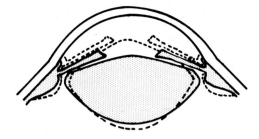

Figure 8–9. Accommodation. The solid lines represent the shape of the lens. iris, and ciliary body at rest and the dotted lines represent the shape during accommodation.

Figure 8–8. Refraction of light rays by lenses. *A:* Biconvex lens. *B:* Biconvex lens of greater strength than *A. C:* Same lens as *A,* showing effect on light rays from a near point. *D:* Biconcave lens. The center line in each case is the principal axis. X is the principal focus.

the principal axis than the principal focus (Fig 8–8). Biconcave lenses cause light rays to diverge.

The greater the curvature of a lens, the greater its refractive power. The refractive power of a lens is conveniently measured in **diopters,** the number of diopters being the reciprocal of the principal focal distance in meters. For example, a lens with a principal focal distance of 0.25 meter has a refractive power of 1/0.25, or 4 diopters. The human eye has a refractive power of approximately 66.7 diopters at rest.

Accommodation

When the ciliary muscle is relaxed, parallel light rays striking the optically normal (**emmetropic**) eye are brought to a focus on the retina. As long as this relaxation is maintained, rays from objects closer to the observer are brought to a focus behind the retina, and consequently the objects appear blurred. The problem of bringing diverging rays from objects closer than 6 meters (20 ft) to a focus on the retina can be solved by increasing the distance between the lens and the retina or by increasing the curvature or refractive power of the lens. In bony fish, the problem is solved by increasing the length of the eyeball, a solution analogous to the manner in which the images of objects closer than 6 meters are focused on the film of a camera by moving the lens away from the film. In mammals, the problem is solved by increasing the curvature of the lens.

The process by which the curvature of the lens is increased is called **accommodation**. At rest, the lens is

held under tension by the lens ligaments. Because the lens substance is malleable and the lens capsule has considerable elasticity, the lens is pulled into a flattened shape. When the gaze is directed at a near object, the ciliary muscle contracts. This decreases the distance between the edges of the ciliary body and relaxes the lens ligaments, so that the lens springs into a more convex shape. This change in shape may add as many as 12 diopters to the refractive power of the eye. The relaxation of the lens ligaments produced by contraction of the ciliary muscle is due partly to the sphincter-like action of the circular muscle fibers in the ciliary body and partly to the contraction of longitudinal muscle fibers that attach anteriorly, near the corneoscleral junction. When these fibers contract, they pull the whole ciliary body forward and inward. This motion brings the edges of the ciliary body closer together.

The change in lens curvature during accommodation affects principally the anterior surface of the lens (Fig 8–9). This can be demonstrated by a simple experiment first described many years ago. If an observer holds an object in front of the eyes of an individual who is looking into the distance, 3 reflections of the object are visible in the subject's eye. A clear, small upright image is reflected from the cornea; a larger, fainter upright image is reflected from the anterior surface of the lens; and a small inverted image is reflected from the posterior surface of the lens. If the subject then focuses his vision on something nearby, the large, faint upright image becomes smaller and moves toward the other upright image whereas the other 2 images change very little. The change in size of the image is due to the increase in curvature of the reflecting surface, the anterior surface of the lens (Fig 8–9). The fact that the small upright image does not change and the inverted image changes very little shows that the corneal curvature is unchanged and that the curvature of the posterior lens surface is changed very little by accommodation.

Near Point

Accommodation is an active process, requiring muscular effort, and can therefore be tiring. Indeed, the ciliary muscle is one of the most used muscles in the body. The degree to which the lens curvature can be increased is, of course, limited, and light rays from an object very near the individual cannot be brought to a focus on the retina even with the greatest effort. The nearest point to the eye at which an object can be brought into clear focus by accommodation is called the **near point of vision**. The near point recedes throughout life, slowly at first and then rapidly with advancing age. For example, at age 8 the average normal near point is 8.6 cm from the eye and at age 20 it is 10.4 cm from the eye; but at age 60 it is 83.3 cm from the eye. This recession of the near point is due principally to increasing hardness of the lens substance, with a resulting steady decrease in the degree to which the curvature of the lens can be increased. By the time the normal individual reaches the age of 40–45, the near point often recedes far enough so that reading and close work become difficult. This condition, which is known as **presbyopia**, can be corrected by wearing glasses with convex lenses (see below).

The Near Response

In addition to accommodation, the visual axes converge and the pupil constricts when an individual looks at a near object. This 3-part response—accommodation, convergence, and pupillary constriction—is called the **near response**.

Other Pupillary Reflexes

When light is directed into one eye, the pupil constricts (**pupillary light reflex**). The pupil of the other eye also constricts (**consensual light reflex**). The optic nerve fibers that carry the impulses initiating pupillary responses end in the pretectal region and the superior colliculi. The pathway for the light reflex, which presumably passes from the pretectal region to the oculomotor nuclei (Edinger-Westphal nuclei) bilaterally, is different from that for accommodation. In some pathologic conditions, notably neurosyphilis, the pupillary response to light may be absent while the response to accommodation remains intact. This phenomenon, the so-called **Argyll Robertson pupil**, is said to be due to a destructive lesion in the tectal region.

Retinal Image

In the eye, light is actually refracted at the anterior surface of the cornea and at the anterior and posterior surfaces of the lens. The process of refraction can be represented diagrammatically, however, without introducing any appreciable error, by drawing the rays of light as if all refraction occurs at the anterior surface of the cornea. Fig 8–10 is a diagram of such a "reduced" or "schematic" eye. In this diagram, the **nodal point** or optical center of the eye coincides with the junction of the middle and posterior third of the lens, 15 mm from the retina. This is the point through which the light rays from an object pass without refraction. All other rays entering the pupil from each point on the object are refracted and brought to a focus on the retina. If the height of the object (**AB**), and its distance from the observer (**Bn**) are known, the size of its retinal image can be calculated because **AnB**

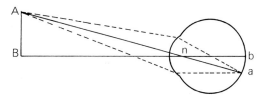

Figure 8–10. Reduced eye. n, nodal point. AnB and anb are similar triangles. In this reduced eye, the nodal point is 15 mm from the retina. All refraction is assumed to take place at the surface of the cornea, 5 mm from the nodal point, between a medium of density 1.000 (air) and a medium of density 1.333 (water). The dotted lines represent rays of light diverging from A and refracted at the cornea so that they are focused on the retina at a.

and **anb** in Fig 8–10 are similar triangles. The angle AnB is the **visual angle** subtended by object AB. It should be noted that the retinal image is inverted. The connections of the retinal receptors are such that from birth any inverted image on the retina is viewed right side up and projected to the visual field on the side opposite to the retinal area stimulated. This perception is innate. It is present in infants and when vision is restored in previously blind individuals who have had congenital cataracts removed surgically. If retinal images are turned right side up by means of special lenses, the objects viewed look as if they were upside down.

Common Defects of the Image-Forming Mechanism

In some individuals, the eyeball is shorter than normal and parallel rays of light are brought to a focus behind the retina. This abnormality is called **hyperopia**, or farsightedness (Fig 8–11). Sustained accommodation, even when viewing distant objects, can partially compensate for the defect, but the prolonged muscular effort is tiring and may cause headaches and blurring of vision. The prolonged convergence of the visual axes associated with the accommodation may lead eventually to squint, or **strabismus** (see below). The use of glasses with convex lenses to aid the refractive power of the eye in shortening the focal distance corrects the defect.

In **myopia**, or nearsightedness, the anteroposterior diameter of the eyeball is too long. This defect can be corrected by the use of glasses with biconcave lenses so that parallel light rays are made to diverge slightly before they strike the eye.

Astigmatism is a common condition in which the curvature of the cornea is not uniform. When the curvature in one meridian is different from that in others, light rays in that meridian are refracted to a different focus so that part of the retinal image is blurred. A similar defect may be produced if the lens is pushed out of alignment or the curvature of the lens is not uniform, but these conditions are rare. Astigmatism can usually be corrected with cylindric lenses placed in such a way that they equalize the refraction in all meridians. **Presbyopia** has been mentioned above.

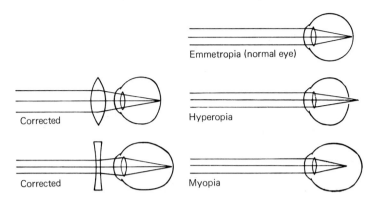

Figure 8–11. Common defects of the optical system of the eye. In hyperopia the eyeball is too short, and light rays come to a focus behind the retina. A biconvex lens corrects this by adding to the refractive power of the lens of the eye. In myopia the eyeball is too long, and light rays focus in front of the retina. Placing a biconcave lens in front of the eye causes the light rays to diverge slightly before striking the eye, so that they are brought to a focus on the retina.

THE PHOTORECEPTOR MECHANISM: GENESIS OF NEURAL ACTIVITY

The potential changes that initiate action potentials in the retina are generated by the action of light on photosensitive compounds in the rods and cones. When light is absorbed by these substances, their structure changes, and this change is responsible for initiating neural activity.

The photosensitive compounds in the eyes of humans and most other mammals are made up of a protein, called an **opsin**, and **retinene$_1$**, the aldehyde of vitamin A_1. The term retinene$_1$ is used to distinguish this compound from retinene$_2$, which is found in the eyes of some animal species. Since the retinenes are aldehydes, they are also called **retinals**. The A vitamins themselves are alcohols and are therefore called **retinols**.

Rhodopsin

The photosensitive pigment in the rods is called **rhodopsin, or visual purple.** Its opsin is called **scotopsin.** Light bleaches rhodopsin by breaking the retinene-scotopsin bond, the reaction proceeding through a series of short-lived intermediates to retinene and scotopsin.

The mechanism of action of light on rhodopsin is shown diagrammatically in Fig 8–12. The retinene in rhodopsin is in the form of the 11-cis isomer. The only action of light is conversion of the retinene to the all-trans isomer, forming **prelumirhodopsin.** This

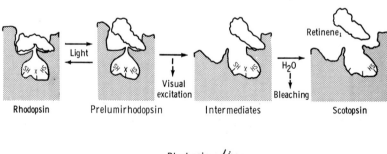

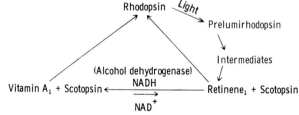

Figure 8–12. *Top:* Diagrammatic representation of events believed to occur in rods. Light converts retinene from the cis to the trans isomer, straightening out the molecule and permitting the opsin to open up. SH, HS, and X represent hypothetical active groups in the opsin that are exposed by the straightening of the retinene molecule. *Bottom:* Rhodopsin cycle in humans. The iodopsin cycle is presumably similar. (Modified from Brown in: *Medical Physiology,* 13th ed. Mountcastle VB [editor]. Mosby, 1974.)

straightens out the retinene and permits the spontaneous occurrence of the next step, a change in the shape of the opsin. The opening up of the opsin may expose reactive groups which catalyze the reactions producing electrical activity. The last step in the sequence of reactions is the bleaching proper, the separation of the retinene from the opsin by hydrolysis. Some of the rhodopsin is regenerated directly, while some of the retinene$_1$ is reduced by the enzyme alcohol dehydrogenase in the presence of NADH to vitamin A$_1$, and this in turn reacts with scotopsin to form rhodopsin.

All of these reactions except the formation of prelumirhodopsin are independent of light, proceeding equally well in light or darkness. The amount of rhodopsin in the receptors therefore varies inversely with the incident light.

In vitro, solutions of rhodopsin absorb light maximally at a wavelength of 505 nm (Fig 8–13). The curve relating the sensitivity in dim light of the intact eye to light of different wavelengths also reaches a maximum at 505 nm. The fact that this **scotopic visibility curve** and the absorption curve of rhodopsin in vitro coincide is strong evidence that the rod pigment responsible for dim light vision is indeed rhodopsin.

Cone Pigments

There are 3 different types of cones in primates (see below), and there are 3 different cone pigments. One cone pigment, **iodopsin**, has been isolated from chicken retinas. It is also found in human cones, and appears to be the pigment most sensitive to red light. It is made up of retinene$_1$ and **photopsin**, a protein which is different from scotopsin. The other cone pigments also contain retinene$_1$ and the differences between them are due to differences in the structures of the opsins. The **photopic visibility curve** (Fig 8–13) is the composite curve of the 3 cone systems.

Receptor Potentials

The rods and cones do not generate action potentials, and they are unique among the sensory receptors that have been studied in that their response to their adequate stimulus, light, is a hyperpolarization rather than a depolarization. The cone receptor potential has a sharp onset and a sharp offset (Fig 8–14), whereas the rod receptor potential has a sharp onset and a slow offset. In the dark, there is a steady current flow from the inner to the outer segments of the rods and presumably of the cones, and light decreases this current flow. The resulting hyperpolarization generates graded responses in the bipolar cells (see below).

The details of the mechanism by which the straightening of retinene by light leads to hyperpolarization is still a subject of debate, but current evidence indicates that this event triggers a decrease in the Na$^+$ conductance in the outer segments. This conductance change could be due to release of a substance that blocks the Na$^+$ channels in the membranes of the sacs. The neural events from the receptor potentials to the brain are described below.

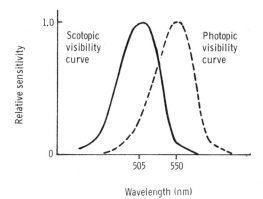

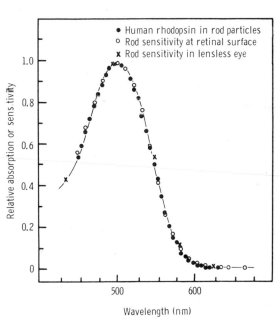

Figure 8–13. *Top:* Scotopic and photopic visibility curves. Both curves are adjusted so that at peak sensitivity they have a relative sensitivity value of 1.0. In terms of absolute values, rod (scotopic) sensitivity is, of course, much greater than cone (photopic) sensitivity. *Bottom:* Correspondence between absorption of human rhodopsin and rod sensitivity. The rod sensitivity curves have been plotted with and without the lens. (Reproduced, with permission, from Wald & Brown: Human rhodopsin. Science 127:222, 1958.)

The receptor potentials of both rods and cones have been shown to be preceded by an earlier biphasic electrical response. This response has no latency detectable by presently available methods and has been named the **early receptor potential.** It is closely associated with rapid molecular events that follow the absorption of light by the photopigment. It provides a convenient method for recording these rapid events, and its amplitude indicates accurately the concentration of photopigment. However, it is not part of the direct sequence of excitatory events in retinal photoreceptors.

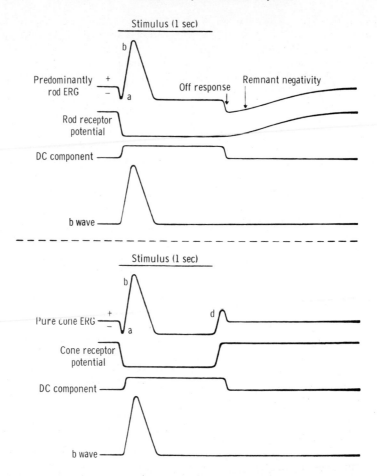

Figure 8—14. Receptor potentials and other components in relation to the electroretinogram (ERG). The c wave is omitted. The ERG and the components are all plotted on the same time scale. The plus and minus signs indicate that positive deflections are plotted upward and negative deflections downward. (Reproduced, with permission, from Brown: The electroretinogram: Its components and their origins. Vision Res 8:633, 1968.)

Dark Adaptation

If an individual who has spent considerable time in a brightly lighted environment is placed in dim light, his retina slowly becomes more sensitive to light as, to use the layman's term, he "becomes accustomed to the dark." This decline in visual threshold is known as **dark adaptation**. It is nearly maximal in about 20 minutes, although there is some further decline over longer periods. On the other hand, when one passes suddenly from a dim to a brightly lighted environment, the light seems intensely and even uncomfortably bright until the eyes adapt to the increased illumination and the visual threshold rises. This adaptation occurs over a period of about 5 minutes, and is called **light adaptation** although, strictly speaking, it is merely the disappearance of dark adaptation.

There are actually 2 components to the dark adaptation response (Fig 8—15). The first drop in visual threshold, rapid but small in magnitude, is known to be due to dark adaptation of the cones because when only the foveal, rod-free portion of the retina is tested the decline proceeds no further. In the

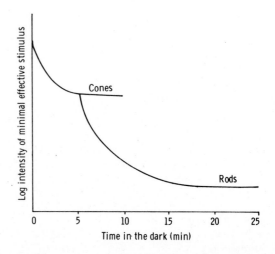

Figure 8—15. Dark adaptation. The curve shows the change in the intensity of a stimulus necessary to just excite the retina in dim light as a function of the time the observer has been in the dark.

peripheral portions of the retina, a further drop occurs due to adaptation of the rods. The total change in threshold between the light-adapted and the fully dark-adapted eye is very great.

Radiologists, aircraft pilots, and others who need maximal visual sensitivity in dim light can avoid having to wait 20 minutes in the dark to become dark-adapted if they wear red goggles when in bright light. Light wavelengths in the red end of the spectrum stimulate the rods to only a slight degree while permitting the cones to function reasonably well (Fig 8–13). Therefore, a person wearing red glasses can see in bright light while his rods are becoming dark-adapted.

The time required for dark adaptation is determined in part by the time required to build up the rhodopsin stores. In bright light, much of the pigment is continuously being broken down, and some time is required in dim light for accumulation of the amounts necessary for optimal rod function. However, dark adaptation also occurs in the cones, and additional factors are undoubtedly involved.

Effect of Vitamin Deficiencies on the Eye

In view of the importance of vitamin A in the synthesis of rhodopsin and iodopsin, it is not surprising that avitaminosis A produces visual abnormalities. Among these, one of the earliest is night blindness, or **nyctalopia**. This fact first called attention to the role of vitamin A in rod function, but it is now clear that concomitant cone degeneration occurs as vitamin A deficiency develops when dietary intake of this fat-soluble vitamin is reduced or its intestinal absorption is depressed. Prolonged deficiency is associated with anatomic changes in the rods and cones followed by degeneration of the neural layers of the retina. Treatment with vitamin A can restore retinal function if given before the receptors are destroyed.

Other vitamins, especially those of the B complex, are necessary for the normal functioning of the retina and other neural tissues. Nicotinamide is part of the nicotinamide adenine dinucleotide (NAD^+) molecule, and this coenzyme plays a role in the interconversion of retinene and vitamin A in the rhodopsin cycle.

NEURAL RESPONSES

Responses of Bipolar, Amacrine, & Horizontal Cells

Intracellular recording from bipolar cells has been accomplished, and it has been found that the bipolar cells, like the photoreceptors, do not generate action potentials. Instead, they generate relatively steady hyperpolarizing potentials or depolarizing potentials of up to 10 mV. In some cells, hyperpolarizing potentials are produced by a spot of light, whereas depolarizing potentials are produced by an annulus. Cells with opposite patterns are also observed, ie, depolarization in response to a spot and hyperpolarization in response to an annulus. Thus, the receptive fields of the bipolar

cells appear to be organized into central and peripheral portions which elicit opposing reactions. The **receptive field** of a particular cell is the area from which a stimulus produces a response in that cell. If the periphery and the center are stimulated at the same time, the activities tend to cancel out.

The horizontal cells produce only graded hyperpolarizing and depolarizing responses. These cells integrate rod and cone responses and, among other things, appear to play a role in color coding (see below). They also increase retinal sensitivity by improving contrast.

The amacrine cells, on the other hand, produce transient depolarizing responses at the onset and offset of a visual stimulus. They are the first cells in the visual pathway capable of generating impulses, and these impulses are initiated during the depolarizations. Thus, the amacrine cells appear to be concerned with registering changes in illumination rather than steady levels of illumination.

Response Patterns of Ganglion Cells

Ganglion cells generate action potentials which are transmitted along their axons to the lateral geniculate body. The extensive convergence and divergence of neural pathways in the retina have been described above. This permits considerable organization and structuring of visual information before it leaves the retina. The characteristic patterns of ganglion cell responses are shown in Fig 8–16. Ganglion cells generally discharge at a slow rate in the absence of stimulation. Some cells respond with increased discharge when a small, more or less circular beam of light is shined on their receptive fields ("on" center cells), and some cells respond with inhibition of discharge ("off" center

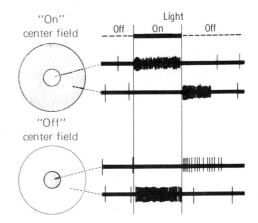

Figure 8–16. Organization of "on" center and "off" center receptive fields of ganglion cells. In the former case, stimulation of the center increases the number of action potentials generated (upper oscilloscope trace), while stimulation of the surrounding zone inhibits discharge but is followed by an "off" burst (lower oscilloscope trace). In the case of the "off" center field, the response patterns are reversed. (Reproduced, with permission, from Hubel: The visual cortex of the brain. Scientific American 209:54, Nov 1963. Copyright © 1963 by Scientific American, Inc. All rights reserved.)

cells). This inhibition is followed by a burst of impulses when the stimulus is turned off.

If the light is shined on the area surrounding the retinal spot where stimulation produced an "on" response, the ganglion cell discharge is inhibited; conversely, if a light is shined on the area surrounding the retinal spot where stimulation produced an "off" response, the ganglion cell discharge rate is increased. Thus, the responses of the ganglion cells are reminiscent of the responses of the bipolar cells. The inhibitory interaction is an example of **lateral** or **afferent inhibition**—that form of inhibition in which activation of a particular neural unit is associated with inhibition of the activity of surrounding units. It is a general phenomenon in mammalian sensory systems and helps to sharpen the edges of a stimulus and improve discrimination.

Some ganglion cells respond to steady illumination; others respond only to changes in illumination. These latter cells are affected most by the amacrine cells. Some ganglion cells respond most markedly to stimulus motion in a particular direction.

Electroretinogram

The electrical activity of the eye has been studied by recording fluctuations in the potential difference between an electrode in the eye and another on the back of the eye. At rest there is a 6 mV potential difference between the front and the back of the eye, with the front positive. When light strikes the eye, a characteristic sequence of potential changes follows. The record of this sequence is known as the **electroretinogram (ERG)**. Turning on the light stimulus elicits the **a** and **b** waves, as shown in Fig 8–17, and also the **c** wave, which is so slow that with short stimuli its peak occurs after the stimulus. When the stimulus is turned off, a negative off-deflection occurs.

Through careful analysis of the effects of drugs and records obtained with microelectrodes inserted to varying depths in the retina, the ERG has been resolved into its components. The **c** wave is generated in

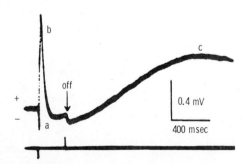

Figure 8–17. Electroretinogram recorded with an electrode in the vitreous humor of a cat. Note that, by convention in electroretinography, positive deflections are upward. The onset and termination of the stimulus are indicated by the vertical lines in the lower record. (Reproduced, with permission, from Brown: The electroretinogram: Its components and their origins. Vision Res 8:633, 1968.)

the pigment epithelium. The neural components which summate to give the other deflections of the ERG are summarized in Fig 8–14. The negative **rod receptor potential** has a sudden onset, the leading edge of which is seen as the **a** wave, whereas the slow decay of this receptor potential produces the **remnant negativity** that appears in the ERG of a predominantly rod retina. A component that arises in the inner nuclear layer has been called the DC component because of its resemblance to a direct current pulse, and its decay creates the simple **off response** that is typical of the rod ERG. The **b** wave also comes from the inner nuclear layer. The ERG from retinas containing only cones is similar, except that the **cone receptor potential** has a faster decay. Since this decay precedes that of the oppositely directed DC component, a positive deflection called the **d** wave occurs after the stimulus.

The exact cells that generate the **b** wave and DC component are not known. The **b** wave may result from activity in bipolar cells, and glial cells may also be involved.

Electroretinograms can be recorded in humans with one electrode on the cornea and the other on the skin of the head. Electroretinographic records are helpful in the diagnosis of certain ophthalmologic disorders, but most of these diseases are more readily diagnosed by simpler methods.

Synaptic Mediators in the Retina

There is evidence that acetylcholine is a transmitter at some of the synaptic junctions in the retina. The retina also contains relatively large amounts of dopamine, 5-hydroxytryptamine, gamma-aminobutyric acid (GABA), melatonin, and the polypeptide, substance P. The evidence that most of these substances are synaptic mediators in the brain is discussed in Chapter 15. Evidence that GABA is an important transmitter in the eye includes the observation that injection of the GABA antagonist picrotoxin into the blood supply of the eye abolishes the directional sensitivity of ganglion cells that normally respond to changes in the direction of a stimulus. The presence of dopamine in some of the neurons in the retina has been established by histochemical technics. It has been reported that one of the drugs which inhibits monoamine oxidase impairs red-green color discrimination. Monoamine oxidase is the enzyme that catalyzes the oxidation of 5-hydroxytryptamine and dopamine (see Chapter 15).

Activity of Neurons in the Brain

The ganglion cell axons project an accurate spatial representation of the retina on the lateral geniculate body, and the body projects a similar point for point representation on the visual cortex. There appear to be about twice as many fibers projecting from the lateral geniculate body to the visual cortex as there are reaching the body. In the visual cortex, there are many nerve cells associated with each fiber.

The receptive fields of the neurons in the lateral geniculate body are similar to those of the ganglion cells except that they respond more to the peripheral portions of their fields. In the visual cortex, however, single cells respond to lines and edges in their receptive fields rather than to circular spots. On the basis of the characteristics of their responses, the cells have been classified as simple, complex, or hypercomplex.

The **simple cells** respond maximally to slits of light, dark lines, or edges, but a particular cell responds only when the stimulus has a particular orientation. The farther the stimulating line is turned from the optimal orientation, the less the discharge it creates (Fig 8–18), and discharge is minimal when it is perpendicular to the optimal orientation. Like the ganglion cells, the simple cells show patterns of on-off interaction in their receptive fields. Typically, a long narrow "on" area is sandwiched between 2 "off" areas. Other patterns are also found, but the organization is always linear. Simple cells respond to movement of the stimulus, but with only a transient burst of activity.

The **complex cells** also respond to edges and lines in a particular orientation, but they discharge in a sustained fashion when the stimulus is moved. An appreciable number of the neurons in the visual cortex are directionally sensitive in this fashion. **Hypercomplex cells** resemble complex cells, but their response is dependent on the length of the edge or line. Simple cells are stellate neurons, whereas complex and hypercomplex cells are larger pyramidal neurons. Since these various types of cells in the visual cortex respond to one or another of the features of the stimulus, they have been called **feature detectors**. Feature detectors are also found in the cortical areas for other sensory modalities.

The visual cortex, like the other primary sensory areas in the cortex, is organized in vertically oriented columns of cells. Many simple cells project onto each complex cell. Presumably, among the many millions of neurons in the visual cortex there are simple cells with maximum rates of discharge for all the possible orientations in all the portions of the visual field. The complex cells integrate the discharges of the simple cells and the output of the complex cells is in turn elaborated by as yet unknown mechanisms into the sensation of vision.

Physiologic Nystagmus

Even when a subject stares fixedly at a stationary object, the eyeballs are not still; there are continuous jerky motions and other movements. This **physiologic nystagmus** appears to have an important function. Although individual visual receptors do not adapt rapidly to constant illumination, their neural connections do. Indeed, it has been shown that if, by means of an optical lever system, the image of an object is fixed so that it falls steadily on the same spot in the retina, the object disappears from view. Continuous visualization of objects apparently requires that the retinal images be continuously and rapidly shifted from one receptor to another.

Visual Acuity

Physiologic nystagmus is one of the many factors that determine **visual acuity**. This parameter of vision should not be confused with **visual threshold**. Visual threshold is the minimal amount of light that elicits a sensation of light; visual acuity is the degree to which the details and contours of objects are perceived. Although there is evidence that other measures are more accurate, visual acuity is usually defined in terms of the **minimum separable**—ie, the shortest distance by which 2 lines can be separated and still be perceived as 2 lines. Clinically, visual acuity is often determined by use of the familiar Snellen letter charts viewed at a distance of 20 ft (6 meters). The individual being tested reads aloud the smallest line he can distinguish. The results are expressed as a fraction. The numerator of the fraction is 20, the distance at which the subject reads the chart. The denominator is the greatest distance from the chart at which a normal individual can read the smallest line the subject can read. Normal visual acuity is 20/20; a subject with 20/15 visual acuity has better than normal vision (not farsightedness); and one with 20/100 visual acuity has subnormal vision. The Snellen charts are designed so that the height of the letters in the smallest line a normal individual can read at 20 ft subtends a visual angle of 5 min. Each line in the letters subtends 1 min of arc, and the lines in the letters are separated by 1 min of arc. Thus the minimum separable in a normal individual corresponds to a visual angle of about 1 min.

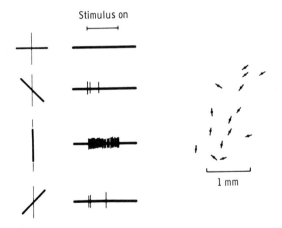

Stimulus on

1 mm

Figure 8–18. *Left:* Diagrammatic representation of the response of a single neuron in the occipital cortex to a linear visual stimulus with various orientations. The records show the number of action potentials generated when the eye was stimulated. Discharge was maximal when the orientation of the stimulus was vertical, as indicated on the left, and nil when it was horizontal. (Data from Hubel & Wiesel: Receptive fields of single neurons in the cat's striate cortex. J Physiol [Lond] 148:574, 1959.) *Right:* Receptive field orientation of superficial neurons in a small portion of the occipital cortex. The locations of the neurons are indicated by the dots on this map of the cortical surface, and the orientation of the stimulus to which each neuron responded maximally is indicated by the line through the dot. (Data from Hubel & Wiesel: Shape and arrangement of columns in cat's striate cortex. J Physiol [Lond] 165:559, 1963.)

Visual acuity is a complex phenomenon, and is influenced by a large variety of factors. These include optical factors such as the state of the image-forming mechanisms of the eye, retinal factors such as the state of the cones, and stimulus factors including the illumination, brightness of the stimulus, contrast between the stimulus and background, and the length of time the subject is exposed to the stimulus.

Critical Fusion Frequency

The time-resolving ability of the eye is determined by measuring the **critical fusion frequency (CFF)**, the rate at which stimuli can be presented and still be perceived as separate stimuli. Stimuli presented at a more rapid rate than the CFF are perceived as a continuous stimulus. Motion pictures move because the frames are presented at a rate above the CFF. Consequently, movies begin to flicker when the projector slows down.

Visual Fields & Binocular Vision

The visual field of each eye is the portion of the external world visible out of that eye. Theoretically it should be circular, but actually it is cut off medially by the nose and superiorly by the roof of the orbit (Fig 8–19). Mapping the visual fields is important in neurologic diagnosis. The peripheral portions of the visual fields are mapped with an instrument called a **perimeter**, and the process is referred to as **perimetry**. One eye is covered while the other is fixed on a central point. A small target is moved toward this central point along selected meridians, and, along each, the location where it first becomes visible is plotted in degrees of arc away from the central point (Fig 8–19). The central visual fields are mapped with a **tangent screen**, a black felt screen across which a white target is

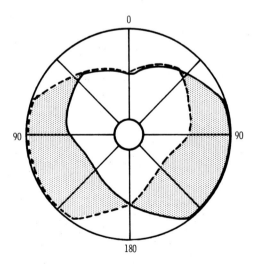

Figure 8–19. Monocular and binocular visual fields. The dotted line encloses the visual field of the left eye; the solid line that of the right eye. The common area (heart-shaped clear zone in the center) is viewed with binocular vision. The shaded areas are viewed with monocular vision.

moved. By noting the locations where the target disappears and reappears, the blind spot and any **scotomas** (blind spots due to disease) can be outlined.

The central parts of the visual fields of the 2 eyes coincide; therefore, anything in this portion of the field is viewed with **binocular vision**. The impulses set up in the 2 retinas by light rays from an object are fused at the cortical level into a single image (**fusion**). The points on the retina on which the image of an object must fall if it is to be seen binocularly as a single object are called **corresponding points**. If one eye is gently pushed out of line while staring fixedly at an object in the center of the visual field, double vision (**diplopia**) results; the image on the retina of the eye that is displaced no longer falls on the corresponding point. When visual images chronically fall on noncorresponding points in the 2 retinas in children under the age of 6, one is eventually suppressed and diplopia disappears. This suppression is a cortical phenomenon, and it usually does not develop in adults.

Binocular vision is often assigned an important role in the perception of depth. Actually, depth perception is to a large degree monocular, depending upon the relative sizes of objects, their shadows, and, in the case of moving objects, their movement relative to one another (movement parallax). However, binocular vision does add some appreciation of depth and proportion.

Effect of Lesions in the Optic Pathways

The anatomy of the pathways from the eyes to the brain is shown in Fig 8–4. Lesions along these pathways can be localized with a high degree of accuracy by the effects they produce in the visual fields.

The fibers from the nasal half of each retina decussate in the optic chiasm, so that the fibers in the optic tracts are those from the temporal half of one retina and the nasal half of the other. In other words, each optic tract subserves half of the field of vision. Therefore, a lesion that interrupts one optic nerve causes blindness in that eye, but a lesion in one optic tract causes blindness in half of the visual field (Fig 8–4). This defect is classified as a **homonymous** (same side of both visual fields) **hemianopsia** (half-blindness). Lesions affecting the optic chiasm, such as pituitary tumors expanding out of the sella turcica, cause destruction of the fibers from both nasal hemiretinas, and produce a **heteronymous** (opposite sides of the visual fields) **hemianopsia**. Since the fibers from the maculas are located posteriorly in the optic chiasm, hemianopsic scotomas develop before there is complete loss of vision in the 2 hemiretinas. Selective visual field defects are further classified as bitemporal, binasal, and right or left.

The optic nerve fibers from the upper retinal quadrants subserving vision in the lower half of the visual field terminate in the medial half of the lateral geniculate body, while the fibers from the lower retinal quadrants terminate in the lateral half. The geniculocalcarine fibers from the medial half of the lateral geniculate terminate on the superior lip of the calca-

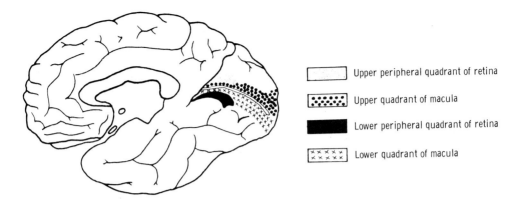

Upper peripheral quadrant of retina

Upper quadrant of macula

Lower peripheral quadrant of retina

Lower quadrant of macula

Figure 8–20. Medial view of human cerebral hemisphere showing projection of the retina on the calcarine fissure. (Redrawn and reproduced, with permission, from Brouwer: Projection of the retina on the cortex in man. Res Publ Assoc Res Nerv Ment Dis 13:529, 1934.)

rine fissure, while those from the lateral half terminate on the inferior lip. Furthermore, the fibers from the lateral geniculate body which subserve macular vision separate from those which subserve peripheral vision and end more posteriorly on the lips of the calcarine fissure (Fig 8–20). Because of this anatomic arrangement, occipital lobe lesions may produce discrete quadrantic visual field defects (upper and lower quadrants of each half visual field). **Macular sparing**, ie, loss of peripheral vision with intact macular vision, is also common with occipital lesions (Fig 8–4) because the macular representation is separate from that of the peripheral fields and very large relative to that of the peripheral fields. Therefore, occipital lesions must extend considerable distances to destroy macular as well as peripheral vision.

Bilateral destruction of the occipital cortex in humans causes essentially complete blindness, although in lower mammals considerable vision (especially rod vision) remains. The primary visual receiving area, Brodmann's area 17, also plays a role in visual discrimination. Areas 18 and 19, the so-called visual association areas, are apparently concerned with visual orientation, depth perception, and the relay of information from the visual cortex to other parts of the brain.

The fibers subserving the reflex pupillary constriction produced by shining a light into the eye leave the optic tracts in front of the geniculate bodies to enter the pretectal region. Therefore, blindness with preservation of the pupillary light reflex is almost invariably due to a lesion behind the optic tracts.

COLOR VISION

Characteristics of Color

Colors have 3 attributes: **hue, intensity,** and **saturation,** or degree of freedom from dilution with white. For any color there is a **complementary color**

which, when properly mixed with it, produces a sensation of white. Black is the sensation produced by the absence of light, but it is probably a positive sensation because the blind eye does not "see black"; it "sees nothing." Such phenomena as successive and simultaneous contrasts, optical tricks which produce a sensation of color in the absence of color, negative and positive after-images, and various psychologic aspects of color vision are also pertinent. Detailed discussion of these phenomena can be found in textbooks of physiologic optics.

Another observation of basic importance is the demonstration that the sensation of any spectral color, white, and even the extraspectral color, purple, can be produced by mixing various proportions of red light (wavelength 723–647 nm), green light (575–492 nm), and blue light (492–450 nm). Red, green, and blue are therefore called the **primary colors.**

Retinal Mechanisms

Before the turn of the century, color vision was believed to be subserved by 3 types of cones, each type containing a different photosensitive substance and being maximally sensitive to one of the 3 primary colors. This view, generally called the **Young-Helmholtz theory,** also held that the sensation of any given color was determined by the relative frequency of the impulses reaching the brain from each of the 3 cone systems.

The existence of 3 types of cones in the eyes of fish, monkeys, and humans has been proved by measuring the absorption spectrums of individual cones (Fig 8–21). One type of human cone absorbs light maximally in the blue-violet portion of the spectrum; the second absorbs maximally in the green portion; and the third absorbs maximally in the yellow portion. Blue, green, and red are the primary colors, but the cones with their maximal sensitivity in the yellow portion of the spectrum are sensitive enough in the red portion to respond to red light at a lower threshold than green. This is all the Young-Helmholtz theory re-

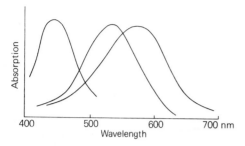

Figure 8—21. Absorption spectrums of the 3 cone pigments in the human retina. The pigment that peaks at 445 nm senses blue and the pigment that peaks at 535 nm senses green. The remaining pigment peaks in the yellow portion of the spectrum, at 570 nm, but its spectrum extends far enough into the long wavelengths to sense red. (Reproduced, with permission, from Michael: Color vision. N Engl J Med 288:729, 1973.)

quires. Thus, the 3-receptor theory of color vision is established.

On the other hand, current evidence does not support the view that there are separate pathways from each of the cone systems to the brain. There is instead a coding process in the retina that converts color information into "on" and "off" responses in individual optic nerve fibers. In fish retinas, certain horizontal cells receive a depolarizing input from red and a hyperpolarizing input from green cells. Thus, the size and polarity of the potential in each of these horizontal cells depends on the degree of simultaneous stimulation of the red and green cones to which it is connected. Other horizontal cells are depolarized by yellow light and hyperpolarized by blue light. They are attached to red and green cones, both of which are stimulated by yellow light, and to blue cones. Their response depends on the relative proportions of yellow and blue light striking the receptor field. Thus, color is coded in terms of the magnitude and polarity of the horizontal cell potentials along a yellow-blue spectrum and red-green spectrum. Responses in the human retina are presumably similar. Such an arrangement would explain the fact that the 4 main subjective hues of the spectrum are yellow, red, green, and blue. It would also explain the fact that red and green are **complementary colors** which, when mixed in appropriate amounts, lead to cancellation of color sensation. Similarly, yellow and blue are complementary colors. The way these graded horizontal cell potentials are coded in ganglion cell action potentials is not settled, but the effect appears to be an on-off code; certain ganglion cells appear to be red-on, green-off cells; others are green-on, red-off cells; etc.

Color Blindness

There are numerous tests for detecting color blindness. The most commonly used routine tests are the yarn matching test and the Ishihara charts. In the former test the subject is presented with a skein of yarn and asked to pick out the ones which match it from a pile of variously colored skeins. The Ishihara

charts and similar polychromatic plates are plates on which are printed figures made up of colored spots on a background of similarly shaped colored spots. The figures are intentionally made up of colors that are liable to look the same as the background to an individual who is color blind.

The most common classification of the types of color blindness is based on the 3-receptor theory. Some individuals are unable to distinguish certain colors, whereas others have only a color weakness. The suffix -anomaly denotes color weakness and the suffix -anopia color blindness. The prefixes prot-, deuter-, and trit- refer to defects of the red, green, and blue cone systems, respectively. Individuals with normal color vision and those with protanomaly, deuteranomaly, and tritanomaly are called **trichromats**; they have all 3 cone systems, but one may be weak. **Dichromats** are individuals with only 2 cone systems; they may have protanopia, deuteranopia, or tritanopia. **Monochromats** have only one cone system. Dichromats can match their color spectrum by mixing only 2 primary colors, and monochromats match theirs by varying the intensity of only one. Apparently monochromats see only black and white and shades of gray.

Inheritance of Color Blindness

Abnormal color vision is present in the human population in about 8% of males and 0.4% of females. Some cases arise as a complication of various eye diseases, but most are inherited. Deuteranomaly is the most common form, followed by deuteranopia, protanopia, and protanomaly. These abnormalities are inherited as recessive and X-linked characteristics, ie, they are due to a mutant gene on the X chromosome. Since all of the male's cells except germ cells contain one X and one Y chromosome in addition to the 44 somatic chromosomes (see Chapter 23), color blindness is present in males if the X chromosome has the abnormal gene. On the other hand, the normal female's cells have 2 X chromosomes, one from each parent, and since color blindness is recessive, females show the defect only when both X chromosomes contain the abnormal gene. However, female children of a color blind male are carriers of color blindness, and pass the defect on to half of their sons. Therefore, color blindness skips generations and appears in males of every second generation. Hemophilia, Duchenne muscular dystrophy, and a variety of other inherited disorders are caused by mutant genes on the X chromosome.

EYE MOVEMENTS

The direction in which each of the eye muscles moves the eye and the definitions of the terms used in describing eye movements are summarized in Table 8–1. Since the oblique muscles pull medially (Fig 8–7), their actions vary with the position of the eye. When the eye is turned nasally, the obliques elevate

Table 8—1. Actions of the external ocular muscles.*

Muscle	Primary Action	Secondary Action
Lateral rectus	Abduction	None
Medial rectus	Adduction	None
Superior rectus	Elevation	Adduction, intorsion
Inferior rectus	Depression	Adduction, extorsion
Superior oblique	Depression	Intorsion, abduction
Inferior oblique	Elevation	Extorsion, abduction

*Abduction and adduction refer to rotation of the eyeball around the vertical axis with the pupil moving away from or toward the midline, respectively; elevation and depression refer to rotation around the transverse horizontal axis, with the pupil moving up or down; and torsion refers to rotation around the anteroposterior horizontal axis with the top of the pupil moving toward the nose (intorsion) or away from the nose (extorsion). (Reproduced, with permission, from Vaughan & Asbury: *General Ophthalmology,* 8th ed. Lange, 1977.)

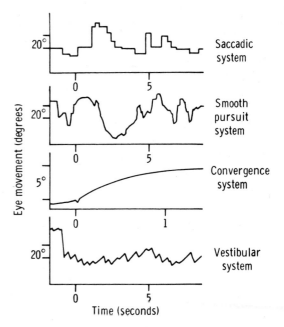

Figure 8—22. Types of eye movements. (Modified and reproduced, with permission, from Robinson: Eye movement control in primates. Science 161 [No. 3847]:1219—1224, 1968. Copyright 1968 by the American Association for the Advancement of Science.)

and depress it, whereas the superior and inferior recti rotate it; when the eye is turned temporally, the superior and inferior recti elevate and depress it and the obliques rotate it.

Since much of the visual field is binocular, it is clear that a very high order of coordination of the movements of the 2 eyes is necessary if visual images are to fall at all times on corresponding points in the 2 retinas and diplopia is to be avoided.

There are 4 types of eye movements, each controlled by a different neural system but sharing the same final common path, the motor neurons that supply the external ocular muscles (Fig 8—22). **Saccades,** sudden jerky movements, occur as the gaze shifts from one object to another. **Smooth pursuit movements** are tracking movements of the eyes as they follow moving objects. **Vestibular movements,** adjustments which occur in response to stimuli initiated in the semicircular canals, maintain visual fixation as the head moves. **Convergence movements** bring the visual axes toward each other as attention is focused on objects near the observer. The similarity to a man-made tracking system on an unstable platform such as a ship is apparent; saccadic movements seek out visual targets, pursuit movements follow them as they move about, and ves-

tibular movements stabilize the tracking device as the platform on which the device is mounted (ie, the head) moves about.

Strabismus

Abnormalities of the coordinating mechanisms can be due to a variety of causes. When the visual axes no longer are maintained in a position that keeps the visual images on corresponding retinal points, **strabismus** or squint is said to be present. Successful treatment of some types of strabismus is possible by careful surgical shortening of some of the eye muscles, by eye muscle training exercises, and by the use of glasses with prisms which bend the light rays sufficiently to compensate for the abnormal position of the eyeball.

9...
Functions of the Ear

ANATOMIC CONSIDERATIONS

Receptors for 2 sensory modalities, hearing and equilibrium, are housed in the ear. The external ear, the middle ear, and the cochlea of the inner ear are concerned with hearing. The semicircular canals, the utricle, and probably the saccule of the inner ear are concerned with equilibrium.

EXTERNAL & MIDDLE EAR

The external ear funnels sound waves into the **external auditory meatus.** In some animals the ears can be moved like radar antennas to seek out sound. From the meatus, the **external auditory canal** passes inward to the **tympanic membrane,** or ear drum (Fig 9–1).

The middle ear is an air-filled cavity in the temporal bone that opens via the eustachian tube into the nasopharynx and through the nasopharynx to the exterior. The tube is usually closed, but during swallowing, chewing, and yawning it opens, keeping the air pressure on the 2 sides of the ear drum equalized. The 3 **auditory ossicles,** the **malleus, incus,** and **stapes,** are located in the middle ear. The **manubrium,** or handle of the malleus, is attached to the back of the tympanic membrane. Its head is attached to the wall of the middle ear and its short process is attached to the incus, which in turn articulates with the head of the stapes. The stapes is named for its resemblance to a stirrup. Its **foot plate** is attached by an annular ligament to the walls of the **oval window** (Fig 9–2). Two small skeletal muscles, the **tensor tympani** and the **stapedius,** are also located in the middle ear. Contraction of the former pulls the manubrium of the malleus medially and decreases the vibrations of the tympanic membrane; contraction of the latter pulls the foot plate of the stapes out of the oval window.

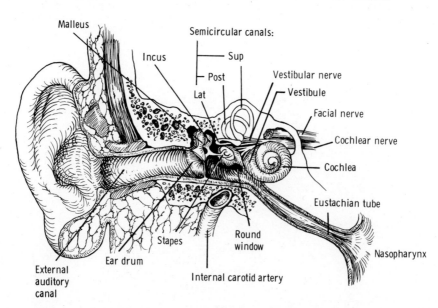

Figure 9–1. The human ear. To make the relationships clear, the cochlea has been turned slightly and the middle ear muscles have been omitted. Sup, superior; Post, posterior; Lat, lateral. (Modified and redrawn from Brödel: *Three Unpublished Drawings of The Anatomy of The Human Ear.* Saunders, 1946.)

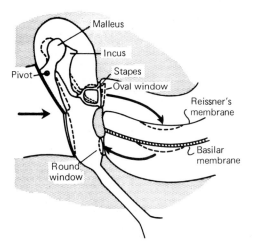

Figure 9–2. Schematic representation of the auditory ossicles and the way their movement translates movements of the tympanic membrane into a wave in the fluid of the inner ear. The wave is dissipated at the round window. The movements of the ossicles, the membranous labyrinth, and the round window are indicated by dashed lines. (Redrawn from an original by Netter in Ciba Clinical Symposia, copyright © 1962, Ciba Pharmaceutical Co. Reproduced with permission.)

INNER EAR

The inner ear, or **labyrinth**, is made up of 2 parts, one within the other. The **bony labyrinth** is a series of channels in the petrous portion of the temporal bone. Inside these channels, surrounded by a fluid called **perilymph**, is the **membranous labyrinth**. The mem-

branous labyrinth more or less duplicates the shape of the bony channels (Fig 9–3). It is filled with a fluid called **endolymph**, and there is no communication between the spaces filled with endolymph and those filled with perilymph.

Cochlea

The cochlear portion of the labyrinth is a coiled tube, 35 mm long, which in humans makes 2¾ turns. Throughout its length the basilar membrane and Reissner's membrane divide it into 3 chambers, or **scalae** (Fig 9–4). The upper **scala vestibuli** and the lower **scala tympani** contain perilymph and communicate with each other at the apex of the cochlea through a small opening called the **helicotrema**. At the base of the cochlea, the scala vestibuli ends at the oval window, which is closed by the foot plate of the stapes. The scala tympani ends at the **round window**, a foramen on the medial wall of the middle ear which is closed by the flexible **secondary tympanic membrane**. The **scala media**, the middle cochlear chamber, is continuous with the membranous labyrinth and does not communicate with the other 2 scalae. It contains endolymph (Figs 9–3 and 9–4).

Organ of Corti

Located on the basilar membrane is the organ of Corti, the structure that contains the auditory receptor cells. This organ extends from the apex to the base of the cochlea, and consequently has a spiral shape. The auditory receptors are hair cells arranged in 2 rows (Fig 9–4), with their processes piercing the tough, membrane-like **reticular lamina**. There are 3500 inner and 20,000 outer hair cells in each human cochlea. The reticular lamina is supported by the **rods of Corti**. Covering the rows of hair cells is a thin,

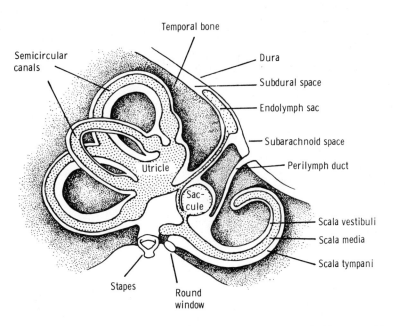

Figure 9–3. Relationship between the membranous and osseous labyrinths (diagrammatic).

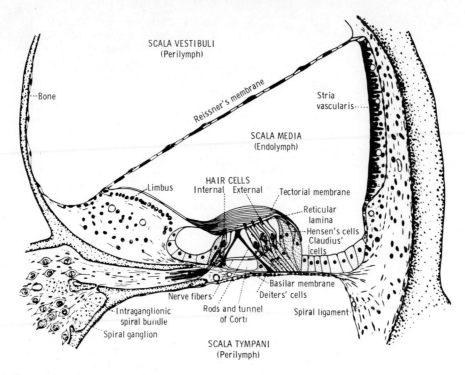

Figure 9—4. Cross-section of one turn of the cochlea of a guinea pig. (Reproduced, with permission, from Davis & others: Acoustic trauma in the guinea pig. J Acoust Soc Am 25:1180, 1953.)

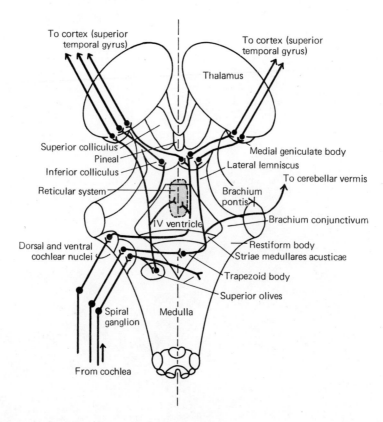

Figure 9—5. Simplified diagram of main auditory pathways superimposed on a dorsal view of the brain stem. Cerebellum and cerebral cortex removed.

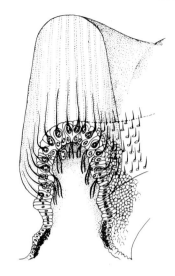

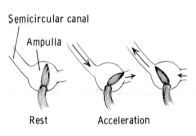

Semicircular canal

Ampulla

Rest   Acceleration

Figure 9–6. Ampullar crista. *Above:* Schematic 3-dimensional drawing of a cross-section of an ampullar crista. *Below:* Movements of cupula in ampullary crista during rotational acceleration. Arrows indicate direction of fluid movement. (Redrawn and reproduced, with permission, from Wersäll: Studies on the structure and innervation of the sensory epithelium of the cristae ampullares in the guinea pig. Acta Otolaryngol [Suppl] [Stockh] 126:1, 1956.)

viscous but elastic **tectorial membrane** in which the tips of the hair cell processes are embedded. The cell bodies of the afferent neurons that arborize extensively around the hair cells are located in the **spiral ganglion** within the **modiolus,** the bony core around which the cochlea is wound. Their axons form the auditory division of the acoustic nerve and terminate in the **dorsal** and **ventral cochlear nuclei** of the medulla oblongata. There are approximately 28,000 fibers in each auditory nerve, and so there is no net convergence of receptors on first order neurons; most of the fibers, however, supply more than one cell and, conversely, most cells are supplied by more than one fiber.

Central Auditory Pathways

From the cochlear nuclei, axons carrying auditory impulses pass via a variety of pathways to the **inferior colliculi,** the centers for auditory reflexes; and via the **medial geniculate body** in the thalamus to the **auditory cortex.** Others enter the reticular formation (Fig 9–5). Information from both ears converges on each superior olive, and at all higher levels most of the neurons re-

spond to inputs from both sides. In humans, the primary auditory cortex, Brodmann's area 41, is located in the superior portion of the temporal lobe, buried in the floor of the lateral cerebral fissure (Fig 7–3). There is reason to believe that there are several additional auditory receiving areas, just as there is a secondary receiving area for cutaneous sensation (see Chapter 7). The auditory association areas adjacent to the primary auditory receiving area are widespread, extending onto the insula. The **olivocochlear bundle** is a prominent bundle of efferent fibers in each auditory nerve which arises in the olivary nucleus of the opposite side and ends around the bases of the hair cells of the organ of Corti.

Semicircular Canals

On each side of the head, the semicircular canals are perpendicular to each other so that they are oriented in the 3 planes of space. Inside the bony canals, the membranous canals are suspended in perilymph. A receptor structure, the **crista ampullaris,** is located in the expanded end or **ampulla** of each of the membranous canals. Each crista consists of hair cells and sustentacular cells surmounted by a gelatinous partition, or **cupula,** that closes off the ampulla like a swinging door (Fig 9–6). Endings of the afferent fibers of the vestibular division of the acoustic nerve are in close contact with the hair cells.

Utricle & Saccule

Within each membranous labyrinth, on the floor of the utricle, there is an **otolithic organ** or **macula.** Another macula is located on the wall of the saccule, tilted 30° from the vertical plane. The maculas contain sustentacular cells and hair cells, surmounted by a membrane in which are embedded crystals of calcium carbonate, the **otoliths** (Fig 9–7). In the maculas and cristae, there are hair cells surrounded by nerve fibers (type I) and hair cells with nerve fibers only at the base (type II). However, the functional difference between

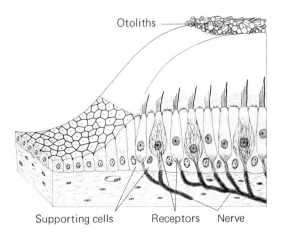

Otoliths

Supporting cells   Receptors   Nerve

Figure 9–7. Otolithic organ. (Reproduced, with permission, from Junqueira, Carneiro, & Contopoulos: *Basic Histology,* 2nd ed. Lange, 1977.)

the 2 types is uncertain. The nerve fibers from the hair cells join those from the cristae.

Neural Pathways

The cell bodies of the 19,000 neurons supplying the cristae and maculas on each side are located in the vestibular ganglion. Each vestibular nerve terminates in the ipsilateral 4-part vestibular nucleus and in the flocculonodular lobe of the cerebellum. Second order neurons pass down the spinal cord from the vestibular nuclei in the vestibulospinal tracts and ascend through the **medial longitudinal fasciculi** to the motor nuclei of the cranial nerves concerned with the control of eye movement. There are also anatomically poorly defined pathways by which impulses from the vestibular receptors are relayed via the thalamus to the cerebral cortex (Fig 9–8).

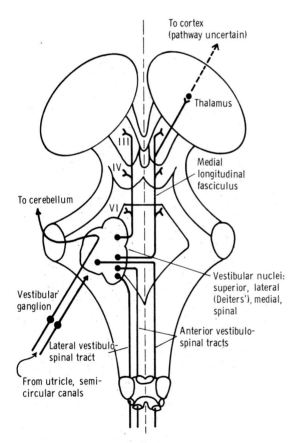

Figure 9–8. Principal vestibular pathways superimposed on a dorsal view of the brain stem. Cerebellum and cerebral cortex removed.

HEARING

AUDITORY RESPONSES

Sound Waves

Sound is the sensation produced when longitudinal vibrations of the molecules in the external environment, ie, alternate phases of condensation and rarefaction of the molecules, strike the tympanic membrane. A plot of these movements as changes in pressure on the tympanic membrane per unit of time is a series of waves (Fig 9–9), and such movements in the environment are generally called sound waves. The waves travel through air at a speed of approximately 344 meters/sec (770 miles/hour) at 20° C at sea level. The speed of sound increases with temperature and with altitude. Other media in which humans occasionally find themselves also conduct sound waves, but at different speeds. For example, the speed of sound in water is 1428 meters/sec (3194 miles/hour).

Generally speaking, the **loudness** of a sound is correlated with the **amplitude** of a sound wave and its **pitch** with the **frequency**, or number of waves per unit of time. The greater the amplitude, the louder the sound; and the greater the frequency, the higher the pitch. However, pitch is determined by other poorly understood factors in addition to frequency, and frequency affects loudness since the auditory threshold is lower at some frequencies than others (see below).

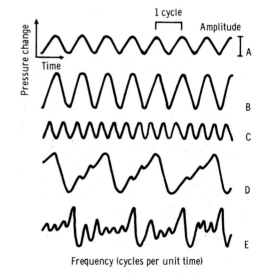

Figure 9–9. Characteristics of sound waves. *A* is the record of a pure tone. *B* has a greater amplitude and is louder than A. *C* has the same amplitude as A but a greater frequency, and its pitch is higher. *D* is a complex wave form which is regularly repeated. Such patterns are perceived as musical sounds, whereas waves like that shown in *E,* which have no regular pattern, are perceived as noise.

Sound waves that have repeating patterns, even though the individual waves are complex, are perceived as musical sounds; aperiodic nonrepeating vibrations cause a sensation of noise. Most musical sounds are made up of a wave with a primary frequency which determines its pitch plus a number of harmonic vibrations, or **overtones,** which give the sound its characteristic **timbre** or quality. Variations in timbre permit us to identify the sounds of the various musical instruments even though they are playing notes of the same pitch.

The amplitude of a sound wave can be expressed in terms of the maximum pressure change or the root mean square pressure at the ear drum, but a relative scale is more convenient. The **decibel scale** is such a scale. The intensity of a sound in **bels** is the logarithm of the ratio of the intensities of that sound and a standard sound:

$$\text{bel} = \log \frac{\text{intensity of sound}}{\text{intensity of standard sound}}$$

The intensity is proportionate to the square of the sound pressure. Therefore,

$$\text{bel} = 2 \log \frac{\text{pressure of sound}}{\text{pressure of standard sound}}$$

A decibel is 0.1 bel. The standard sound reference level adopted by the Acoustical Society of America corresponds to 0 decibels at a pressure level of 0.000204 dyne/sq cm, a value that is just at the auditory threshold for the average human. In Fig 9–10, the decibel levels of various common sounds are compared. It is important to remember that the decibel scale is a log scale. Therefore, a value of 0 decibels does not mean

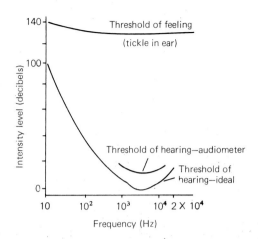

Figure 9–11. Human audibility curve. The middle curve is that obtained by audiometry under the usual conditions. The lower curve is that obtained under ideal conditions. At about 140 decibels (top curve), sounds are felt as well as heard. (Redrawn and reproduced, with permission, from Licklider, in *Handbook of Experimental Psychology.* Stevens SS [editor] . Wiley, 1951.)

the absence of sound but a sound level of an intensity equal to that of the standard. Furthermore, the 0–140 decibel range from threshold intensity to an intensity that is potentially damaging to the organ of Corti actually represents a 10^{14} (100 trillion)-fold variation in sound intensity.

The sound frequencies audible to the human range from about 20 to a maximum of 20,000 cycles per second (cps or Hz). In other animals, notably bats and dogs, much higher frequencies are audible. The threshold of the human ear varies with the pitch of the sound (Fig 9–11), the greatest sensitivity being in the 1000–4000 Hz range. The pitch of the average male voice in conversation is about 120 Hz and that of the average female voice about 250 Hz. The number of pitches that can be distinguished by an average individual is about 2000, but trained musicians can improve on this figure considerably. Pitch discrimination is best in the 1000–3000 Hz range and is poor at high and low pitches.

Masking

It is common knowledge that the presence of one sound decreases an individual's ability to hear other sounds. This phenomenon is known as **masking.** It is believed to be due to the relative or absolute refractoriness of previously stimulated auditory receptors and nerve fibers to other stimuli. The degree to which a given tone masks other tones is related to its pitch. The masking effect of the background noise in all but the most carefully soundproofed environments raises the auditory threshold a definite and measurable amount.

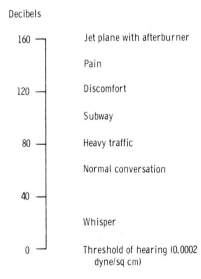

Figure 9–10. Decibel scale for common sounds. The reference standard is that adopted by the Acoustical Society of America, 10^{-16} watt/sq cm. (Modified from Stevens: Some similarities between hearing and seeing. Laryngoscope 68:512, 1958.)

SOUND TRANSMISSION

The ear converts sound waves in the external environment into action potentials in the auditory nerves. The waves are transformed by the ear drum and auditory ossicles into movements of the foot plate of the stapes. These movements set up waves in the fluid of the inner ear. The action of the waves on the organ of Corti generates action potentials in the nerve fibers.

Functions of the Tympanic Membrane & Ossicles

In response to the pressure changes produced by sound waves on its external surface, the tympanic membrane moves in and out. The membrane therefore functions as a **resonator** which reproduces the vibrations of the sound source. It stops vibrating almost immediately when the sound wave stops, ie, it is very nearly **critically damped**. The motions of the tympanic membrane are imparted to the manubrium of the malleus. The malleus rocks on an axis through the junction of its long and short processes, so that the short process transmits the vibrations of the manubrium to the incus. The incus moves in such a way that the vibrations are transmitted to the head of the stapes. Movements of the head of the stapes swing its foot plate to and fro like a door hinged at the posterior edge of the oval window. The auditory ossicles thus function as a lever system which converts the resonant vibrations of the tympanic membrane into movements of the stapes against the perilymph-filled scala vestibuli of the cochlea (Figs 9–2 and 9–12). This system increases the sound pressure which arrives at the oval window because the lever action of the malleus and incus multiplies the force 1.3 times and the area of the tympanic membrane is much greater than the area of the foot plate of the stapes. There are losses of sound energy due to resistance, but it has been calculated that, at frequencies below 3000 Hz, 60% of the sound

energy incident on the tympanic membrane is transmitted to the fluid in the cochlea.

Tympanic Reflex

When the middle ear muscles—the tensor tympani and the stapedius—contract, they pull the manubrium of the malleus inward and the foot plate of the stapes outward. This decreases sound transmission. Loud sounds initiate a reflex contraction of these muscles generally called the **tympanic reflex**. Its function is protective, preventing strong sound waves from causing excessive stimulation of the auditory receptors. However, the reaction time for the reflex is 40–160 msec, so it does not protect against brief intense stimulation such as that produced by gunshots.

Bone & Air Conduction

Conduction of sound waves to the fluid of the inner ear via the tympanic membrane and the auditory ossicles is called **ossicular conduction**. Sound waves also initiate vibrations of the secondary tympanic membrane that closes the round window. This process, unimportant in normal hearing, is called **air conduction**. A third type of conduction, **bone conduction**, is the transmission of vibrations of the bones of the skull to the fluid of the inner ear. When tuning forks or other vibrating bodies are applied directly to the skull, considerable conduction occurs in this fashion, and this route also plays some role in the transmission of extremely loud sounds.

Traveling Waves

The movements of the foot plate of the stapes set up a series of traveling waves in the perilymph of the scala vestibuli. A diagram of such a wave is shown in

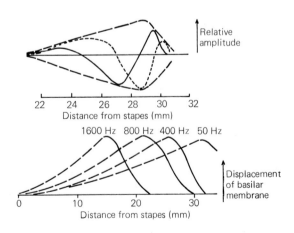

Figure 9–13. Traveling waves. *Above:* The solid and the short-dashed lines represent the wave at 2 instants of time. The long-dashed line shows the "envelope" of the wave formed by connecting the wave peaks at successive instants. *Below:* Displacement of the basilar membrane by the waves generated by stapes vibration of the frequencies shown at the top of each curve. (Data from Bekesy & Rosenblith, in: *Handbook of Experimental Psychology.* Stevens SS [editor]. Wiley, 1951.)

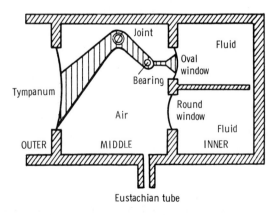

Figure 9–12. Diagrammatic representation of the transmission of vibrations from the outer to the inner ear. (Reproduced, with permission, from Lippold & Winton: *Human Physiology,* 6th ed. Churchill, 1972.)

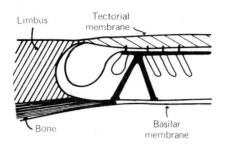
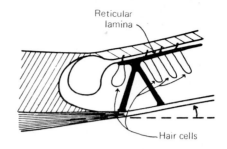

Figure 9–14. Effect of movement on the organ of Corti. The shearing action between 2 stiff structures, the tectorial membrane and the reticular lamina, bends the processes of the hair cells. (Reproduced, with permission, from Davis, in: *Physiological Triggers and Discontinuous Rate Processes.* Bullock TH [editor]. American Physiological Society, 1957.)

Fig 9–13. As the wave moves up the cochlea, its height increases to a maximum and then drops off rapidly. The distance from the stapes to this point of maximum height varies with the frequency of the vibrations initiating the wave. High-pitched sounds generate waves that reach maximum height near the base of the cochlea; low-pitched sounds generate waves that peak near the apex. The bony walls of the scala vestibuli are rigid, but Reissner's membrane is flexible. The basilar membrane is not under tension, and it also is readily depressed into the scala tympani by the peaks of waves in the scala vestibuli. Displacements of the fluid in the scala tympani are dissipated into air at the round window. Therefore, sound produces distortion of the basilar membrane, and the site at which this distortion is maximal is determined by the frequency of the sound wave. The tops of the hair cells in the organ of Corti are held rigid by the reticular lamina, and their hairs are embedded in the tectorial membrane (Figs 9–4 and 9–14). When the basilar membrane is depressed, the motion of the tectorial membrane relative to the reticular lamina bends the hairs. This bending in some way generates action potentials in the auditory nerves.

ELECTRICAL PHENOMENA

Endocochlear Potential

At rest, there is a steady 80 mV potential difference, the **endocochlear potential**, between the endolymph of the scala media and the perilymph. The endolymph is positive to the perilymph, whereas the interiors of the large cells of the organ of Corti, including the hair cells, are 65–75 mV negative to the perilymph. The total potential difference between the cells and the endolymph is therefore 150 mV. The boundaries of the space from which the endocochlear potential can be recorded are shown in Fig 9–15. The tunnel of Corti and the bases of the hair cells, which are bathed in perilymph, are outside this space. The ionic compositions of endolymph and perilymph are very different, endolymph being the only ECF in the body

Table 9–1. Composition of endolymph, perilymph, and spinal fluid.*

	Endolymph	Perilymph	Spinal Fluid
K^+	144.8	4.8	4.2
Na^+	15.8	150.3	150.0
Cl^-	107.1	121.5	122.4
Protein	15.0	50.0	21.0

*Data from Smith & others: Laryngoscope 64:141, 1954. K^+, Na^+, Cl^-, mEq/liter; protein, mg/dl.

with a high K^+ content (Table 9–1). The significance of this fact in terms of potential differences is unsettled; the difference in ionic composition exists not only in the cochlea, where the potential difference between endolymph and perilymph is 80 mV, but in the utricle, where the potential difference between the 2 is only 5 mV. However, it seems clear that the endo-

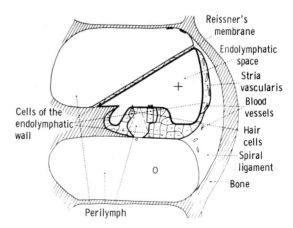

Figure 9–15. Distribution of the positive endocochlear potential (the area within the heavy black line). This potential is positive (+) relative to the perilymph (0). The minus signs inside the cells indicate that they are negative relative to the perilymph. (Reproduced, with permission, from Tasaki & others: Exploration of cochlear potentials in guinea pig with a microelectrode. J Acoust Soc Am 26:765, 1954.)

cochlear potential is generated by and depends upon an ion pump in the stria vascularis. A sodium-potassium activated adenosine triphosphatase system (see Chapter 1) has been demonstrated in this structure.

Cochlear Microphonic & Summating Potentials

One of the electrical responses of the cochlea to sound is the **cochlear microphonic**, a potential fluctuation that can be recorded between an electrode on or near the cochlea and an indifferent electrode. It is generated by deformation of the processes of the hair cells, and is linearly proportionate to the magnitude of the basement membrane displacement. Consequently, it reproduces the wave form of the sound stimulus. Indeed, the reproduction of the frequency and amplitude of the sound is so faithful that if music is played into an experimental animal's ear a faithful rendition of the song can be produced by simply feeding the cochlear microphonic into an audio amplifier. The microphonic can be recorded from the auditory nerve close to the cochlea, and it is probably produced by mechanical distortion (**piezoelectric effect**) affecting the hair cells or some other structure in the cochlea. Two additional potentials, the **negative** and **positive summating potentials**, are generated when sound strikes the ear. They are principally direct current baseline shifts on which the cochlear microphonic is superimposed.

Action Potentials in Auditory Nerve Fibers

The frequency of the action potentials in single auditory nerve fibers is proportionate to the loudness of the sound stimuli. At low sound intensities, each axon discharges to sounds of only one frequency, and this frequency varies from axon to axon depending upon the part of the cochlea from which the fiber

comes. At higher sound intensities, the individual axons discharge to a wider spectrum of sound frequencies (Fig 9–16)—particularly to frequencies lower than that at which threshold stimulation occurs. The "response area" of each unit, the area above the line that defines its threshold at various frequencies, resembles the shape of the traveling wave in the cochlea.

Genesis of Action Potentials

The way the various cochlear potentials are interrelated in the genesis of action potentials in the afferent nerves is still unsettled. Apparently the cochlear microphonic, possibly in association with the negative summating potential, serves as the generator potential. The endocochlear potential probably keeps the receptors in a ready state by maintaining the potential difference between the hair cells and their processes.

The major determinant of the pitch perceived when a sound wave strikes the ear is the place in the organ of Corti that is maximally stimulated. The traveling wave set up by a tone produces peak depression of the basilar membrane, and consequently maximal receptor stimulation, at one point. The distance between this point and the stapes is inversely related to the pitch of the sound, low tones producing maximal stimulation at the apex of the cochlea and high tones producing maximal stimulation at the base. The pathways from the various parts of the cochlea to the brain are distinct. An additional factor involved in pitch perception at sound frequencies of less than 2000 Hz may be the pattern of the action potentials in the auditory nerve. When the frequency is low enough, the nerve fibers begin to respond with an impulse to each cycle of a sound wave. The importance of this **volley effect**, however, is limited; and the frequency of the action potentials in a given auditory nerve fiber determines principally the loudness, rather than the pitch, of a sound.

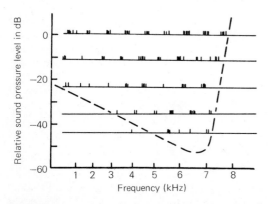

Figure 9–16. Responses (vertical lines) of a guinea pig single auditory nerve fiber to tones of different frequencies and intensities. The sound intensity is expressed in decibels below an arbitrary standard. The dotted line encloses the "response area" of this fiber. Note the sharp cut-off at higher frequencies and the relatively greater response spectrum at higher sound intensities on the low-frequency side. (Reproduced, with permission, from Tasaki: Nerve impulses in individual auditory nerve fibers of guinea pig. J Neurophysiol 17:97, 1954.)

BRAIN MECHANISMS

Auditory Responses of Neurons in the Medulla Oblongata

The responses of individual second order neurons in the cochlear nuclei to sound stimuli are like those of the individual auditory nerve fibers. The frequency at which sounds of lowest intensity evoke a response varies from unit to unit; with increased sound intensities, the band of frequencies to which a response occurs becomes wider. The major difference between the responses of the first and second order neurons is the presence of a sharper "cut-off" on the low-frequency side in the medullary neurons (Fig 9–17). This greater specificity of the second order neurons is probably due to some sort of inhibitory process in the brain stem, but how it is achieved is not known.

Although the pitch of a sound depends primarily

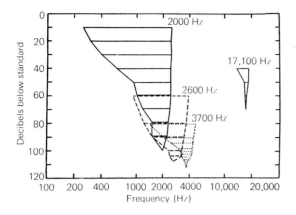

Figure 9–17. "Response areas" of 4 second order auditory neurons in the cochlear nuclei of the cat. The sound intensity is expressed in decibels below an arbitrary standard. Compare with Fig 9–16. (Reproduced, with permission, from Galambos & Davis: The response of single auditory nerve fibers to acoustic stimulation. J Neurophysiol 6.39, 1943.)

on the frequency of the sound wave, loudness also plays a part; low tones (below 500 Hz) seem lower, and high tones (above 4000 Hz) seem higher as their loudness increases. Duration also affects pitch to a minor degree. The pitch of a tone cannot be perceived unless it lasts for more than 0.01 sec, and with durations between 0.01 and 0.1 sec pitch rises as duration increases.

Auditory Cortex

The pathways from the cochlea to the auditory cortex are described in the first section of this chapter. Impulses ascend from the dorsal and ventral cochlear nuclei through complex paths that are both crossed and uncrossed. In animals, there is an organized pattern of tonal localization in the primary auditory cortex, as if the cochlea had been unrolled upon it. In humans, low tones are represented anterolaterally and high tones posteromedially in the auditory cortex. However, individual neurons in the auditory cortex respond to such parameters as the onset, duration, and repetition rate of an auditory stimulus and particularly to the direction from which it came. In this way, they are analogous to some of the neurons in the visual cortex (see Chapter 8). Many animal species have better hearing than humans in the absence of any auditory cortex. In the common laboratory mammals, destruction of the auditory cortex not only fails to cause deafness but also fails to obliterate established conditioned responses to sound of a given frequency. On the other hand, responses to a given sequence of 3 or more tones are absent. All of this suggests that the auditory cortex is concerned with recognition of tonal patterns, with analysis of properties of sounds, and with sound localization.

Sound Localization

Determination of the direction from which a

sound emanates depends upon detecting the difference in time between the arrival of the stimulus in the 2 ears and the consequent difference in phase of the sound waves on the 2 sides, as well as upon the fact that the sound is louder on the side closest to the source. The time difference is said to be the most important factor at frequencies below 3000 Hz, and the loudness difference the most important at frequencies above 3000 Hz. Many neurons in the auditory cortex receive input from both ears, and they respond maximally or minimally when the time of arrival of a stimulus at one ear is delayed by a fixed time period relative to the time of arrival at the other ear. This fixed time period varies from neuron to neuron. Sounds coming from directly in front of the individual presumably differ in quality from those coming from behind, because the external ears are turned slightly forward. Sound localization is markedly disrupted by lesions of the auditory cortex in many experimental animals and in man.

Inhibitory Mechanisms

Stimulation of the efferent olivocochlear bundle in the auditory nerve decreases the neural response to auditory stimuli, by liberating a hyperpolarizing mediator, possibly acetylcholine, from the endings of the olivocochlear fibers. Other mechanisms inhibit transmission at the synaptic relays in the brain stem. These and similar mechanisms which operate as "volume controls" in all the specific sensory systems are discussed in detail in Chapter 11.

DEAFNESS

Clinical deafness may be due to impaired sound transmission in the external or middle ear (**conduction deafness**) or to damage to the neural pathways (**nerve deafness**). Among the causes of conduction deafness are plugging of the external auditory canals with wax or foreign bodies, destruction of the auditory ossicles, thickening of the ear drum following repeated middle ear infections, and abnormal rigidity of the attachments of the stapes to the oval window. Causes of nerve deafness include toxic degeneration of the acoustic nerve produced by streptomycin, tumors of the acoustic nerve and cerebellopontine angle, and vascular damage in the medulla.

Conduction and nerve deafness can be distinguished by a number of simple tests with a tuning fork. Three of these tests, named for the men who developed them, are outlined in Table 9–2. The Weber and Schwabach tests demonstrate the important masking effect of environmental noise on the auditory threshold.

Audiometry

Auditory acuity is commonly measured with an audiometer. This device presents the subject with pure tones of various frequencies through earphones. At

Table 9–2. Common tests with a tuning fork to distinguish between
nerve and conduction deafness.

	Weber	Rinne	Schwabach
Method	Base of vibrating tuning fork placed on vertex of skull.	Base of vibrating tuning fork placed on mastoid process until subject no longer hears it, then held in air next to ear.	Bone conduction of patient compared to that of normal subject.
Normal	Hears equally on both sides.	Hears vibration in air after bone conduction is over.	
Conduction deafness (one ear)	Sound louder in diseased ear because masking effect of environmental noise is absent on diseased side.	Does not hear vibrations in air after bone conduction is over.	Bone conduction better than normal (conduction defect excludes masking noise).
Nerve deafness (one ear)	Sound louder in normal ear.	Hears vibration in air after bone conduction is over.	Bone conduction less than normal.

each frequency, the threshold intensity is determined and plotted on a graph as a percentage of normal hearing. This provides an objective measurement of the degree of deafness and a picture of the tonal range most affected.

Fenestration Procedures

A common form of conduction deafness is that due to **otosclerosis,** a disease in which the attachments of the foot plate of the stapes to the oval window become abnormally rigid. In patients with this disease, air conduction (see above) can be utilized to bring about some restoration of hearing. A membrane-covered outlet from the bony labyrinth is created so that waves set up by vibrations of the secondary tympanic membrane can be dissipated. In the "fenestration operation," an outlet is created by drilling a hole in the horizontal semicircular canal and covering it with skin.

produces displacement of the endolymph in the direction of the rotation, and the cupula swings in a direction opposite to that during acceleration. It returns to midposition in 25–30 sec. Movement of the cupula in one direction commonly causes increased impulse traffic in single nerve fibers from its crista, whereas movement in the opposite direction commonly inhibits neural activity (Fig 9–18).

Rotation causes maximal stimulation of the semicircular canals most nearly in the plane of rotation. Since the canals on one side of the head are a mirror image of those on the other side, the endolymph is displaced toward the ampulla on one side and away from it on the other. The pattern of stimulation reaching the brain therefore varies with the direction as well as the plane of rotation. Linear acceleration probably fails to displace the cupula and therefore does not stimulate the cristae. However, there is considerable evidence that when one part of the labyrinth is destroyed other parts take over its functions. Experi-

VESTIBULAR FUNCTION

RESPONSES TO ROTATIONAL & LINEAR ACCELERATION

Semicircular Canals

Rotational acceleration in the plane of a given semicircular canal stimulates its crista. The endolymph, because of its inertia, is displaced in a direction opposite to the direction of rotation. The fluid pushes on the cupula and swings it like a door (Fig 9–6), bending the processes of the hair cells. When a constant speed of rotation is reached, the fluid spins at the same rate as the body and the cupula swings back into the upright position. When rotation is stopped, deceleration

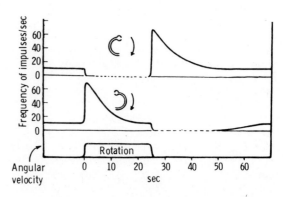

Figure 9–18. Ampullary responses to rotation. Average time course of impulse discharge from ampulla of 2 semicircular canals during rotational acceleration, steady rotation, and deceleration. (Reproduced, with permission, from Adrian: Discharges from vestibular receptors in the cat. J Physiol [Lond] 101:389, 1943.)

mental localization of labyrinthine functions is therefore difficult.

The tracts that descend from the vestibular nuclei into the spinal cord are concerned primarily with postural adjustments (see Chapter 12); the ascending connections to cranial nerve nuclei are largely concerned with eye movements.

Nystagmus

The characteristic jerky movement of the eye observed at the start and end of a period of rotation is called **nystagmus**. It is actually a reflex which maintains visual fixation on stationary points while the body rotates, although it is not initiated by visual impulses and is present in blind individuals. When rotation starts, the eyes move slowly in a direction opposite to the direction of rotation. When the limit of this movement is reached, the eyes quickly snap back to a new fixation point and then again move slowly in the other direction. The slow component is initiated by impulses from the labyrinths; the quick component is triggered by a center in the brain stem. Nystagmus is frequently horizontal, ie, the eyes move in the horizontal plane; but it can also be vertical, when the head is tipped sidewise during rotation, or rotatory, when the head is tipped forward. By convention, the direction of eye movement in nystagmus is identified by the direction of the quick component. The direction of the quick component during rotation is the same as that of the rotation, but the **postrotatory nystagmus** that occurs due to displacement of the cupula when rotation is stopped is in the opposite direction.

Macular Responses

In mammals, the utricular and saccular maculas respond to linear acceleration. The otoliths are more dense than the endolymph, and acceleration in any direction causes them to be displaced in the opposite direction, distorting the hair cells and generating activity in the nerve fibers. The maculas also discharge tonically in the absence of head movement, because of the pull of gravity on the otoliths. The impulses generated from these receptors are partly responsible for reflex righting of the head and other important postural adjustments discussed in Chapter 12.

Although most of the responses to stimulation of the maculas are reflex in nature, vestibular impulses also reach the cerebral cortex. These impulses are presumably responsible for conscious perception of motion and supply part of the information necessary for orientation in space. The nausea, blood pressure changes, sweating, pallor, and vomiting that are the well-known accompaniments of excessive vestibular stimulation are probably due to reflexes mediated via vestibular connections in the brain stem. **Vertigo** is the sensation of rotation in the absence of actual rotation.

Caloric Stimulation

The semicircular canals can be stimulated by instilling water that is hotter or colder than body temperature into the external auditory meatus. The temperature difference sets up convection currents in the endolymph, with consequent motion of the cupula. This technic of **caloric stimulation**, which is sometimes used diagnostically, causes some nystagmus, vertigo, and nausea. To avoid these symptoms, it is important when irrigating the ear canals in the treatment of ear infections to be sure that the fluid used is at body temperature.

ORIENTATION IN SPACE

Orientation in space depends in large part upon input from the vestibular receptors, but visual cues are also important. When the horizon is manipulated so that the vestibular and visual cues are conflicting, women are said to place more reliance on their visual sensations and men on their vestibular. Pertinent information is also supplied by impulses from proprioceptors in joint capsules, which supply data about the relative position of the various parts of the body, and impulses from cutaneous exteroceptors, especially touch and pressure receptors. These 4 inputs are synthesized at a cortical level into a continuous picture of the individual's orientation in space.

EFFECTS OF LABYRINTHECTOMY

The effects of unilateral labyrinthectomy are presumably due to unbalanced discharge from the remaining normal side. They vary from species to species and with the speed at which the labyrinth is destroyed. Rats develop abnormal body postures and roll over and over as they continuously attempt to right themselves. Postural changes are less marked in humans, but the symptoms are distressing. Motion aggravates the symptoms, but efforts to minimize stimulation by lying absolutely still are constantly thwarted by waves of nausea, vomiting, and even diarrhea. Fortunately, compensation for the loss occurs, and after 1–2 months the symptoms disappear completely.

Symptoms of this type are absent after bilateral destruction of the labyrinths, but defects in orientation are present. For this reason, diving is hazardous for persons who lack vestibular function. The only means these individuals have of finding the surface is vision, because in the water the pressure sensed by the cutaneous exteroceptors is equal all over the body. If for any reason vision is obscured, a person whose vestibular apparatus is impaired has no mechanism for orienting himself. Therefore, he may swim away from rather than toward the surface and, consequently, he may drown.

10 . . .
Smell & Taste

Smell and taste are generally classified as visceral senses because of their close association with gastrointestinal function. Physiologically, they are related to each other. The flavors of various foods are in large part a combination of their taste and smell. Consequently, foods may taste "different" if one has a cold which depresses his sense of smell. Both taste and smell receptors are chemoreceptors which are stimulated by molecules in solution in the fluids of the nose and mouth. However, these 2 senses are anatomically quite different. The smell receptors are distance receptors (teleceptors); the smell pathways have no relay in the thalamus; and there is no neocortical projection area for olfaction. The taste pathways pass up the brain stem to the thalamus and project to the postcentral gyrus along with those for touch and pressure sensibility from the mouth.

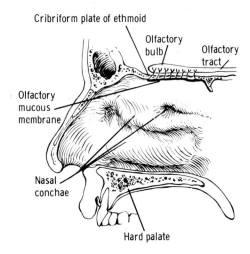

Figure 10—1. Olfactory mucous membrane. (Reproduced, with permission, from Chusid: *Correlative Neuroanatomy & Functional Neurology,* 16th ed. Lange, 1976.)

SMELL

RECEPTORS & PATHWAYS

Olfactory Mucous Membrane

The olfactory receptors are located in a specialized portion of the nasal mucosa, the yellowish-pigmented **olfactory mucous membrane**. In dogs and other animals in which the sense of smell is highly developed (macrosmatic animals), the area covered by this membrane is large; in microsmatic animals such as humans, it is small, covering an area of 5 sq cm in the roof of the nasal cavity near the septum (Fig 10—1). The supporting cells secrete the layer of mucus which constantly overlies the epithelium and send many microvilli into this mucus. Interspersed among the supporting cells of this mucous membrane are 10—20 million receptor cells. Each olfactory receptor is a neuron, and the olfactory mucous membrane is said to be the place in the body where the nervous system is closest to the external world. The neurons have short, thick dendrites with expanded ends called olfactory rods (Fig 10—2). From these rods cilia project to the

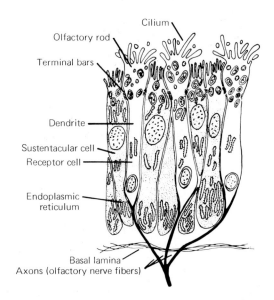

Figure 10—2. Structure of the olfactory mucous membrane. (Reproduced, with permission, from de Lorenzo, in: *Olfaction and Taste.* Zotterman Y [editor]. Macmillan, 1963.)

surface of the mucus. The cilia are unmyelinated processes, about 2 μm long and 0.1 μm in diameter. There are 10–20 cilia per receptor neuron. The axons of the olfactory receptor neurons pierce the cribriform plate of the ethmoid bone and enter the olfactory bulbs.

Olfactory Bulbs

In the olfactory bulbs the axons of the receptors terminate among the dendrites of the **mitral** and **tufted cells** (Fig 10–3) to form the complex globular synapses called **olfactory glomeruli**. An average of 26,000 receptor cell axons converge on each glomerulus. The axons of the tufted cells pass posteriorly through the **medial olfactory stria**, cross the midline in the **anterior commissure**, and enter the opposite olfactory bulb. The functional significance of this peculiar fiber arrangement is not known. In experimental animals, section of the anterior commissure apparently produces considerable olfactory deficit, but destruction of one olfactory bulb produces only unilateral loss of olfaction (**anosmia**).

Another group of fibers passes through the **intermediate olfactory stria** to end in the **anterior perforated substance** and the **area of the diagonal band**. Impulses concerned with olfactory reflexes pass from this region to the rest of the limbic system and hypothalamus. A third band of fibers, mostly axons of mitral cells, passes from the glomeruli through the **lateral olfactory stria** to the cortical and medial portions of the ipsilateral **amygdaloid nucleus** and to the prepiriform and periamygdaloid cortex. There are no

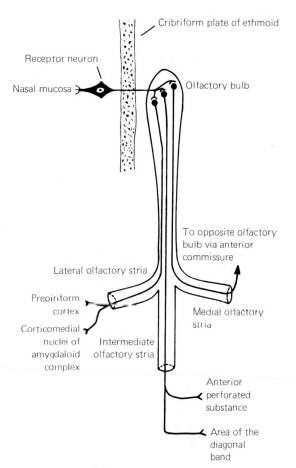

Figure 10–4. Diagram of olfactory pathways.

direct connections to the hippocampal formation or the hippocampal gyrus, and the **cortical olfactory area** is in the prepiriform and periamygdaloid cortex (Fig 10–4). Evoked potentials have been recorded in the amygdaloid nuclei in response to olfactory stimuli in humans.

Limbic System

The inferior frontal and perihilar portions of the cerebral cortex and the associated deep nuclei in these regions have been called the **rhinencephalon** because this part of the brain was presumed to subserve only olfactory functions. In mammals and man, only a small part of the rhinencephalon is directly concerned with olfaction. The rest of the rhinencephalon is concerned with the emotional responses, instincts, and complex neuroendocrine regulatory functions discussed in Chapter 15. For this reason, the term rhinencephalon has generally been dropped and this part of the brain is now called the **limbic system** or **limbic lobe** (Fig 15–1).

Inhibitory Pathways

There are efferent fibers in the olfactory striae, and stimulation of these fibers decreases the electrical

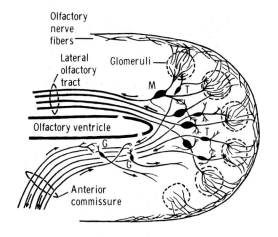

Figure 10–3. Neural pathways in the olfactory bulb. Olfactory nerve fibers enter the glomeruli from the surface. They synapse there with the dendrites of mitral cells (M) and tufted cells (T). The axons of the mitral cells form the lateral olfactory tract, while those of the tufted cells form primarily the medial olfactory tract to the opposite bulb via the anterior commissure. Fibers from the opposite olfactory bulb end on granule cells (G). The olfactory ventricle is a projection of the cerebral ventricles present in lower animals but absent in humans. (Reproduced, with permission, from Adey, in: *Handbook of Physiology*. Field J, Magoun HW [editors]. Washington: The American Physiological Society, 1959. Section 1, pp 535–548.)

activity of the olfactory bulbs. Presumably, therefore, inhibitory mechanisms analogous to those in the eye, ear, and other sensory systems exist in the olfactory system.

PHYSIOLOGY OF OLFACTION

Stimulation of Receptors

Olfactory receptors respond only to substances that are in contact with the olfactory epithelium and are dissolved in the thin layer of mucus that covers it. The olfactory thresholds for the representative substances shown in Table 10–1 illustrate the remarkable sensitivity of the olfactory receptors to some substances. For example, methyl mercaptan, the substance that gives garlic its characteristic odor, can be smelled at a concentration of less than one-millionth of a milligram per liter of air. On the other hand, discrimination of differences in the intensity of any given odor is poor. The concentration of an odor-producing substance must be changed by about 30% before a difference can be detected. The comparable visual discrimination threshold is a 1% change in light intensity.

When odoriferous molecules react with a receptor, they generate a receptor potential; but the mechanism by which the molecules generate the potential is not known. Odor-producing molecules are generally those containing from 3–4 up to 18–20 carbon atoms, and molecules with the same number of carbon atoms but different structural configurations have different odors. Relatively high water and lipid solubility are characteristic of substances with strong odors. One theory holds that odoriferous molecules inactivate enzyme systems in the epithelium, altering its chemical reactions. Another theory holds that the molecules alter the surface of the receptor cells, thus changing their electrical state. A third theory holds that the molecules simply alter the Na^+ permeability of the receptor membrane.

Discrimination of Different Odors

Humans can distinguish between 2000 and 4000

different odors. The physiologic basis of this olfactory discrimination is not known. A number of attempts have been made to divide olfactory receptors into different fundamental types, but they have not been very successful. There is some evidence that odor discrimination depends on the spatial pattern of receptors stimulated in the mucous membrane. The direction from which a smell comes appears to be indicated by the slight difference in the time of arrival of odoriferous molecules in the 2 nostrils.

There is a close relationship between smell and sexual function in animals, and the perfume ads are ample evidence that a similar relationship exists in humans. The sense of smell is generally more acute in women than in men, and in women it is most acute at the time of ovulation. Olfaction and taste are both hypersensitive in patients with adrenocortical insufficiency.

Sniffing

The portion of the nasal cavity containing the olfactory receptors is poorly ventilated. Most of the air normally moves quietly through the lower part of the nose with each respiratory cycle, although eddy currents, probably set up by convection as cool air strikes the warm mucosal surfaces, pass some air over the olfactory mucous membrane. The amount of air reaching this region is greatly increased by sniffing, an action which includes contraction of the lower part of the nares on the septum to help deflect the air stream upward. Sniffing is a semireflex response that usually occurs when a new odor attracts attention.

Role of Pain Fibers in the Nose

Naked endings of many trigeminal pain fibers are found in the olfactory mucous membrane. They are stimulated by irritating substances, and an irritative, trigeminally mediated component is part of the characteristic "odor" of such substances as peppermint, menthol, and chlorine. These endings are also responsible for initiating sneezing, lacrimation, respiratory inhibition, and other reflex responses to nasal irritants.

Adaptation

It is common knowledge that when one is continuously exposed to even the most disagreeable odor, perception of the odor decreases and eventually ceases. This sometimes beneficent phenomenon is due to the fairly rapid adaptation which occurs in the olfactory system. It is specific for the particular odor being smelled, and the threshold for other odors is unchanged. Olfactory adaptation is in part a central phenomenon, but it is also due to a change in the receptors.

Table 10–1. Some olfactory thresholds.*

Substance	mg/liter of Air
Ethyl ether	5.83
Chloroform	3.30
Pyridine	0.03
Oil of peppermint	0.02
Iodoform	0.02
Butyric acid	0.009
Propyl mercaptan	0.006
Artificial musk	0.00004
Methyl mercaptan	0.0000004

*Data from Allison & Katz: J Ind Chem 11:336, 1919.

TASTE

RECEPTOR ORGANS & PATHWAYS

Taste Buds

The taste buds, the sense organs for taste, are ovoid bodies measuring 50–70 µm. Each taste bud is made up of supporting cells and 5–18 hair cells, the **gustatory receptors.** The receptor cells each have a number of hairs projecting into the **taste pore,** the opening at the epithelial surface of the taste bud (Fig 10–5). The unmyelinated ends of the sensory nerve fibers are wrapped around the receptor cells in intimate fashion. Each taste bud is innervated by about 50 nerve fibers, and, conversely, each nerve fiber receives input from an average of 5 taste buds. If the sensory nerve is cut, the taste buds it innervates degenerate and eventually disappear. However, if the nerve regenerates, the cells in the neighborhood become organized into new taste buds, presumably as a result of some sort of chemical inductive effect from the regenerating fiber.

The taste buds are located in the mucosa of the epiglottis, palate, and pharynx and in the walls of the **fungiform** and **vallate papillae** of the tongue. The fungiform papillae are rounded structures most numerous near the tip of the tongue; the vallate papillae are prominent structures arranged in a V on the back of the tongue. There are up to 5 taste buds per fungiform papilla, and they are usually located at the top of the papilla. The larger vallate papillae each contain up to 100 taste buds, usually located along the sides of the papillae. The small conical **filiform papillae** which cover the dorsum of the tongue do not usually contain

taste buds. There are a total of about 10,000 taste buds in humans.

Taste Pathways

The sensory nerve fibers from the taste buds on the anterior two-thirds of the tongue travel in the chorda tympani branch of the facial nerve. The fibers from the posterior third of the tongue reach the brain stem via the glossopharyngeal nerve. The fibers from areas other than the tongue reach the brain stem via the vagus nerve. On each side, the myelinated but relatively slow-conducting taste fibers in these 3 nerves unite in the medulla oblongata to form the **tractus solitarius** (Fig 10–6). The second order neurons are located in the nucleus of this tract, and their axons cross the midline and join the medial lemniscus, ending with the fibers for touch, pain, and temperature sensibility in the specific sensory relay nuclei of the thalamus. Impulses are relayed from there to the taste projection area in the cerebral cortex at the foot of the postcentral gyrus. Taste does not have a separate cortical projection area, but is represented in the portion of the postcentral gyrus that subserves cutaneous sensation from the face.

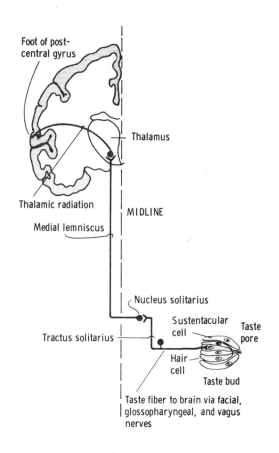

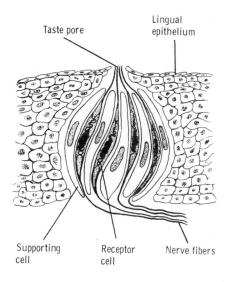

Figure 10–5. Taste bud.

Figure 10–6. Diagram of taste pathways.

PHYSIOLOGY OF TASTE

Receptor Stimulation

Taste receptors are chemoreceptors that respond to substances dissolved in the oral fluids bathing them. These substances appear to evoke generator potentials, but how the molecules in solution interact with the receptor cells to produce these potentials is not known. There is evidence that the taste-producing molecules act on the membranes of the receptor cells or their processes. One theory is based on the hypothesis that the receptor hairs have a polyelectrolyte surface film. According to this theory, binding of ions to this film causes a distortion in the spatial arrangement of the film with a consequent change in the distribution of charge density. There is also evidence that taste-provoking molecules bind to specific proteins in taste buds. The binding of substances to the receptors must be weak because it usually takes relatively little washing with water to abolish a taste.

Basic Taste Modalities

In humans there are 4 basic tastes: sweet, sour, bitter, and salt. Bitter substances are tasted on the back of the tongue, sour along the edges, sweet at the tip, and salt on the dorsum anteriorly (Fig 10–7). Sour and bitter substances are also tasted on the palate along with some sensitivity to sweet and salt. All 4 modalities can be sensed on the pharynx and epiglottis. Anesthetizing the palate increases the threshold for sour and bitter tastes, whereas anesthetizing the tongue elevates the threshold for salt and sweet tastes. The taste buds are not histologically different in the different areas, but the existence of physiologic differences

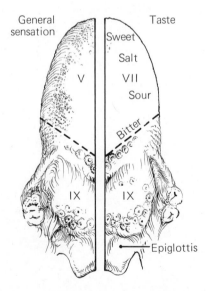

Figure 10–7. Sensory innervation of the tongue. The numbers refer to cranial nerves. (Modified and reproduced, with permission, from Chusid: *Correlative Neuroanatomy & Functional Neurology,* 16th ed. Lange, 1976.)

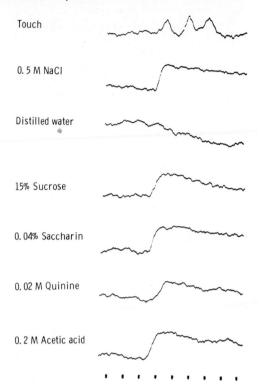

Figure 10–8. Integrated responses of the whole human chorda tympani to various solutions poured over the tongue. The height of each curve is proportionate to the firing rate. The dots at the bottom are at 1-second intervals. (Reproduced, with permission, from Zotterman: The nervous mechanism of taste. Ann NY Acad Sci 81:358, 1959.)

has been demonstrated by recording the electrical activity of nerve fibers from single taste buds in animals. These studies show that some taste buds respond only to bitter stimuli whereas others respond only to salt, sweet, or sour stimuli. Some respond to more than one modality, but none to all four. A curious finding of unknown physiologic significance is the demonstration that in cats, dogs, pigs, and rhesus monkeys there are taste buds that respond to the application of distilled water. Presumably, therefore, these animals can "taste water." Taste buds of this type are absent in rats and humans (Fig 10–8).

Taste Thresholds & Intensity Discriminations

The ability of humans to discriminate differences in the intensity of tastes, like intensity discrimination in olfaction, is relatively crude. A 30% change in the concentration of the substance being tasted is necessary before an intensity difference can be detected. The threshold concentrations of substances to which the taste buds respond vary with the particular substance (Table 10–2). These thresholds are lowered in patients with adrenocortical insufficiency.

Substances Evoking Primary Taste Sensations

Acids taste sour. The H^+, rather than the asso-

Table 10–2. Some taste thresholds.

Substance	Taste	Threshold Concentration (mols/liter)
Hydrochloric acid	Sour	0.0001
Sodium chloride	Salt	0.02
Strychnine hydrochloride	Bitter	0.0000016
Glucose	Sweet	0.08
Sucrose	Sweet	0.01
Saccharin	Sweet	0.000023

ciated anion, stimulates the receptors. For any given acid, sourness is generally proportionate to the H^+ concentration, but organic acids are often more sour for a given H^+ concentration than are mineral acids. This is probably because they penetrate cells more rapidly than the mineral acids.

A **salty** taste is produced by the anion of inorganic salts. The halogens are particularly effective, but some organic compounds also taste salty.

The substance usually used to test the **bitter** taste is quinine sulfate. This compound can be detected in a concentration of 0.000008 mols, although the threshold for strychnine hydrochloride is even lower (Table 10–2). Other organic compounds, especially morphine, nicotine, caffeine, and urea, taste bitter. Inorganic salts of magnesium, ammonium, and calcium also taste bitter. The taste is due to the cation. Thus, there is no readily apparent common feature of the molecular structure of substances that taste bitter.

Most **sweet** substances are organic. Sucrose, maltose, lactose, and glucose are the most familiar examples, but polysaccharides, glycerol, some of the alcohols and ketones, and a number of compounds with no apparent relation to any of these, such as chloroform, beryllium salts, and various amides of aspartic acid also taste sweet. So do some proteins, including 2 that are 100,000 times as sweet as sucrose. Saccharin is in demand as a sweetening agent in reducing diets because it produces satisfactory sweetening in an amount that is a minute fraction of the amount of calorie-rich sucrose required for the same purpose. Lead salts also taste sweet, which is why a cloying sweet taste is common when one is spray painting with lead-containing paints.

Flavor

The almost infinite variety of tastes so dear to the gourmet are mostly synthesized from the 4 basic taste components. In some cases a desirable taste includes an element of pain stimulation (eg, "hot" sauces). In addition, smell plays an important role in the overall sensation produced by food, and the consistency (or texture) and temperature of foods also contribute to their "flavor."

Taste Variation & After-Effects

There is considerable variation in the distribution of the 4 basic taste buds in various species and, within a given species, from individual to individual. In humans, there is an interesting variation in ability to taste **phenylthiocarbamide (PTC).** In dilute solution, PTC tastes sour to about 70% of the Caucasian population but is tasteless to the other 30%. Inability to taste PTC is inherited as an autosomal recessive trait. Testing for this trait is of considerable value in studies of human genetics.

Taste exhibits after-reactions and contrast phenomena that are similar in some ways to visual afterimages and contrasts. Some of these are chemical "tricks," but others may be true central phenomena. A taste modifier protein, **miraculin,** has been discovered in a plant. When applied to the tongue, this protein makes acids taste sweet.

Animals, including humans, form particularly strong aversions to novel foods if eating the food is followed by illness. The survival value of such aversions is apparent in terms of avoiding poisons. The facility with which this type of learning occurs is so great that it has led some investigators to argue that its occurrence is reason to challenge classical learning theory.

11...

The Reticular Activating System, Sleep, & the Electrical Activity of the Brain

THE RETICULAR FORMATION & THE RETICULAR ACTIVATING SYSTEM

The various sensory pathways described in Chapters 7–10 relay impulses from sense organs via 3- and 4-neuron chains to particular loci in the cerebral cortex. The impulses are responsible for perception and localization of individual sensations. Impulses in these systems also relay via collaterals to the **reticular activating system (RAS)** in the brain stem reticular formation. Activity in this system produces the conscious, alert state that makes perception possible.

The **reticular formation**, the phylogenetically old reticular core of the brain, occupies the midventral portion of the medulla and midbrain. It is made up of myriads of small neurons arranged in complex, intertwining nets. Located within it are centers which regulate respiration, blood pressure, heart rate, and other vegetative functions. In addition, it contains ascending and descending components that play important roles in the adjustment of endocrine secretion, the formation of conditioned reflexes, and the regulation of sensory input, learning, and consciousness. The components concerned with consciousness and the modulation of sensory input are discussed in this chapter. The vegetative functions of the reticular core are considered in physiology texts that deal with these systems. The functions related to learning are discussed in Chapter 16, "Higher Functions of the Nervous System."

The reticular activating system is a complex polysynaptic pathway. Collaterals funnel into it not only from the long ascending sensory tracts but also from the trigeminal, auditory, and visual systems and the olfactory system. The complexity of the neuron net and the degree of convergence in it abolish modality specificity, and most reticular neurons are activated with equal facility by different sensory stimuli. The system is therefore **nonspecific**, whereas the classical sensory pathways are **specific** in that the fibers in them are activated only by one type of sensory stimulation. Activity in the RAS percolates upward, and part of it bypasses the thalamus to project diffusely to the cortex. Another part of the RAS ends in the intralaminar and related thalamic nuclei, and from them is projected diffusely and nonspecifically to the whole neocortex (Fig 11–1). The RAS is intimately concerned with the electrical activity of the cortex.

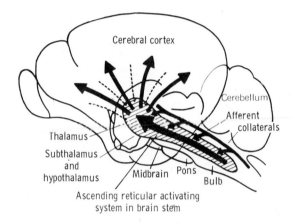

Ascending reticular activating system in brain stem

Figure 11–1. Diagram of ascending reticular system projected on a sagittal section of the cat brain. (Reproduced, with permission, from Starzl & others: Collateral afferent excitation of reticular formation of brain stem. J Neurophysiol 14:479, 1951.)

THE THALAMUS & THE CEREBRAL CORTEX

Thalamic Nuclei

On developmental and topographic grounds, the thalamus can be divided into 3 parts: the epithalamus, the dorsal thalamus, and the ventral thalamus. The **epithalamus** has connections to the olfactory system, and the projections and functions of the **ventral thalamus** are undetermined. The **dorsal thalamus** can be divided into nuclei which project diffusely to the whole neocortex and nuclei which project to specific discrete portions of the neocortex and limbic system. The nuclei which project to all parts of the neocortex are the midline and intralaminar nuclei. They are called collectively the **nonspecific projection nuclei**. They receive input from the reticular activating system. Impulses responsible for the diffuse secondary response and the alerting effect of reticular activation (see below) are relayed through them. The nuclei of the dorsal thalamus that project to specific areas can be divided into 3 groups: the specific sensory relay nuclei, the nuclei concerned with efferent control mechanisms, and the nuclei concerned with complex integrative functions. The **specific sensory relay nuclei** include the medial and lateral geniculate bodies that relay auditory and visual impulses to the auditory and visual cortices and the ventrobasal group of nuclei that relay somatesthetic information to the postcentral gyrus. The **nuclei concerned with efferent control mechanisms** include several nuclei that are concerned with motor function. They receive input from the basal ganglia and the cerebellum and project to the motor cortex. Also included in this group are the anterior nuclei, which receive afferents from the mammillary bodies and project to the limbic cortex as part of the limbic circuit which appears to be concerned with recent memory and emotion (see Chapters 15 and 16). The **nuclei concerned with complex integrative functions** are the dorsolateral nuclei that project to the cortical association areas and are concerned primarily with functions such as language.

Cortical Organization

The neocortex is generally arranged in 6 layers (Fig 11–2). The neurons are mostly pyramidal cells with extensive vertical dendritic trees (Figs 11–2, 11–3) that may reach to the cortical surface. The axons of these cells usually give off recurrent collaterals which turn back and synapse on the superficial portions of the dendritic trees. Afferents from the specific nuclei of the thalamus terminate primarily in cortical layer IV, whereas the nonspecific afferents are distributed to all cortical layers.

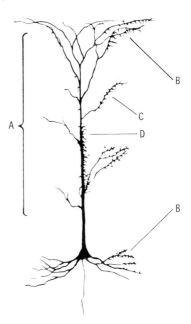

Figure 11–3. Cortical pyramidal cell, showing the distribution of presynaptic terminals. *A*, nonspecific afferents from the reticular formation and the thalamus; *B*, recurrent collaterals of pyramidal cell axons; *C*, commissural fibers from mirror image sites in contralateral hemisphere; *D*, specific afferents from thalamic sensory relay nuclei. (Reproduced, with permission, from Chew & Leiman: The structural and functional organization of the neocortex. Neurosci Res Program Bull 8:157, 1970.)

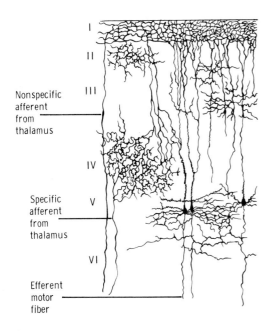

Figure 11–2. Neuronal connections in the neocortex. On the left are afferent fibers from the thalamus. The numbers identify the cortical layers. Note the extensive dendritic processes of the cells, especially those in the deep layers. (Based on drawing of Lorente de No, in Fulton: *Physiology of the Nervous System.* Oxford Univ Press, 1943.)

EVOKED CORTICAL POTENTIALS

The electrical events that occur in the cortex after stimulation of a sense organ can be monitored with an exploring electrode connected to another electrode at an indifferent point some distance away. A characteristic response is seen in animals under barbiturate anesthesia. If the exploring electrode is over the primary receiving area for the particular sense, a surface-positive wave appears with a latency of 5–12 msec. This is followed by a small negative wave and then by a larger, more prolonged positive deflection with a latency of 20–80 msec. This sequence of potential changes is illustrated in Fig 11–4. The first positive-negative wave sequence is the **primary evoked potential**; the second is the **diffuse secondary response.**

Primary Evoked Potential

The primary evoked potential is highly specific in its location and can be observed only where the pathways from a particular sense organ end. Indeed, it is so discrete that it has been used to map the specific cortical sensory areas. It was thought at one time that the primary response was due to activity ascending to the cortex in the thalamic radiations. However, an electrode on the pial surface of the cortex samples activity to a depth of only 0.3–0.6 mm. The primary response

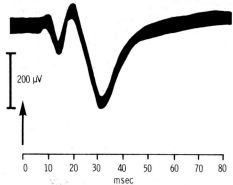

Figure 11—4. Response evoked in the contralateral sensory cortex by stimulation (at the arrow) of the sciatic nerve in a cat under barbiturate anesthesia. Upward deflection is surface-negative. (Modified from Forbes & Morrison: Cortical response to sensory stimulation under deep barbiturate narcosis. J Neurophysiol 2:112, 1939.)

is negative rather than positive when it is recorded with a microelectrode inserted in layers 2–6 of the underlying cortex, and the negative wave within the cortex is followed by a positive wave. This indicates depolarization on the dendrites and somas of the cells in the cortex, followed by hyperpolarization. The positive-negative wave sequence recorded from the surface of the cortex is due to the fact that the superficial cortical layers are positive relative to the initial negativity, then negative to the deep hyperpolarization. In unanesthetized animals the primary evoked potential is largely obscured by the spontaneous activity of the brain, but it can be demonstrated with special technics. It is somewhat more diffuse in unanesthetized animals, but still well localized compared to the diffuse secondary response.

Diffuse Secondary Response

The surface-positive diffuse secondary response is sometimes followed by a negative wave or series of waves. Unlike the primary response, the secondary response is not highly localized. It appears at the same time over most of the cortex and in many other parts of the brain. The uniform latency in different parts of the cortex and the fact that it is not affected by a circular cut through the cortical gray matter that isolates an area from all lateral connections indicates that the secondary response cannot be due to lateral spread of the primary evoked response. It therefore must be due to activity ascending from below the cortex. The pathway involved appears to be the nonspecific thalamic projection system from the midline and related thalamic nuclei.

The diffuse secondary response is present in unanesthetized animals, and in them is influenced by a variety of emotional and motivational factors. When the animal is presented with a stimulus to which it has become accustomed, the diffuse secondary response produced by it is small and inconspicuous. However, if the stimulus is followed a number of times by an elec-

tric shock, the diffuse secondary response to the same stimulus is large and is present not only in all parts of the cortex but in a variety of subcortical loci as well.

THE ELECTROENCEPHALOGRAM

The background electrical activity of the brain in unanesthetized animals was described in the 19th century, but it was first analyzed in a systematic fashion by the German psychiatrist Hans Berger, who introduced the term **electroencephalogram (EEG)** to denote the record of the variations in potential recorded from the brain. The EEG can be recorded with scalp electrodes through the unopened skull, or with electrodes on or in the brain. The term **electrocorticogram (ECoG)** is sometimes used to refer to the record obtained with electrodes on the pial surface of the cortex.

EEG records may be **bipolar** or **unipolar**. The former is the record of potential fluctuations between 2 cortical electrodes; the latter is the record of potential differences between a cortical electrode and a theoretically indifferent electrode on some part of the body distant from the cortex.

Alpha Rhythm

In an adult human who is at rest and letting his mind wander with his eyes closed, the most prominent component of the EEG is a fairly regular pattern of waves at a frequency of 8–12/sec and an amplitude of about 50 μV when recorded from the scalp. This pattern is the **alpha rhythm**. It is most marked in the parieto-occipital area, although it is sometimes ob-

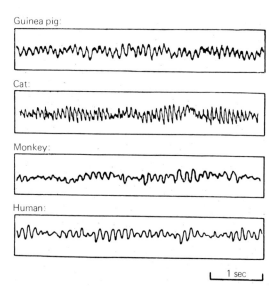

Figure 11—5. EEG records showing alpha rhythm from 4 different species. (Reproduced, with permission, from Brazier: *Electrical Activity of the Nervous System,* 2nd ed. Pitman, 1960.)

served in other locations. A similar rhythm has been observed in a wide variety of mammalian species (Fig 11–5). In the cat it is slightly more rapid than in the human, and there are other minor variations from species to species, but in all mammals the pattern is remarkably similar.

Other Rhythms

In addition to the dominant alpha rhythm, 18–30/sec patterns of lower voltage are sometimes seen over the frontal regions. This rhythm, the **beta rhythm**, may be a harmonic of the alpha. A pattern of large, regular 4–7/sec waves called the **theta rhythm** occurs in normal children and is generated in the hippocampus in experimental animals (see below). Large, slow waves with a frequency of less than 4/sec are sometimes called **delta waves**.

Variations in the EEG

In humans, the frequency of the dominant EEG rhythm at rest varies with age. In infants there is fast, beta-like activity, but the occipital rhythm is a slow 0.5–2/sec pattern. During childhood this latter rhythm speeds up, and the adult alpha pattern gradually appears during adolescence. The frequency of the alpha rhythm is decreased by a low blood glucose level, a low body temperature, a low level of adrenal glucocorticoid hormones, and a high arterial partial pressure of CO_2 (P_{CO_2}). It is increased by the reverse conditions. Forced overbreathing to lower the arterial P_{CO_2} is sometimes used clinically to bring out latent EEG abnormalities.

Alpha Block

When the eyes are opened, the alpha rhythm is replaced by fast, irregular low-voltage activity with no dominant frequency. This phenomenon is called **alpha block**. A breakup of the alpha pattern is also produced by any form of sensory stimulation (Fig 11–6) or mental concentration such as solving arithmetic problems. A common term for this replacement of the regular alpha rhythm with irregular low-voltage activity is **desynchronization**, because it represents a breaking up of the synchronized activity of neural elements responsible for the wave pattern. Because desynchronization is produced by sensory stimulation and is correlated with the aroused, alert state, it is also called the **arousal** or **alerting response**.

Sleep Patterns

When an individual in a relaxed, inattentive state becomes drowsy and falls asleep, the alpha rhythm is replaced by slower, larger waves. In deep sleep (slow wave sleep), very large, somewhat irregular delta waves at a frequency of less than 4/sec are observed. Interspersed with these waves during moderately deep sleep are bursts of alpha-like, 10–14/sec, 50 μV waves—the **sleep spindles**. However, there is a special form of sleep in which there is rapid, irregular cortical activity (REM sleep; see below). The alpha rhythm and the patterns of the drowsy and sleeping individual are **synchronized**, in contrast to the desynchronized, irregular activity seen in the alert state and REM sleep.

PHYSIOLOGIC BASIS OF THE EEG & CONSCIOUSNESS

The presence of rhythmic waves in the alpha and slow wave sleep patterns indicates a priori that neural components of some sort are discharging rhythmically, since random discharges of individual units would cancel out and no waves would be produced. The main questions to be answered are which units are discharging synchronously, and what mechanisms are responsible for desynchronization and synchronization.

Source of the EEG

EEG waves were originally thought to be the summed action potentials of cortical cells discharging in a volume conductor. However, the activity recorded in the EEG is mostly that of the most superficial layers of the cortical gray substance, and there are relatively few cell bodies in these layers. Present evidence indicates that the potential changes in the cortical EEG are due to current flow in the fluctuating dipoles formed on the dendrites of the cortical cells and the cell bodies. The dendrites of the cortical cells are a forest of similarly oriented, densely packed units in the superficial layers of the cerebral cortex (Fig 11–2). As pointed out in Chapter 4, dendrites may be conducting processes, but they generally do not produce propagated all or none spikes; rather, they are the site of nonpropagated hypopolarizing and hyperpolarizing local potential changes. As excitatory and inhibitory endings on the dendrites of each cell become active, current flows into and out of these current sinks and sources from the rest of the dendritic processes and the cell body. The cell-dendrite relationship is therefore that of a constantly shifting dipole. Current flow in this dipole would be expected to produce wave-like potential fluctuations in a volume conductor (Fig 11–7). When the sum of the dendritic activity is negative relative to the cell, the cell is hypopolarized and

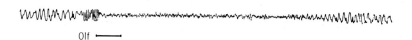

Olf ⟶

Figure 11–6. Desynchronization of the cortical EEG of a rabbit by an olfactory stimulus (indicated by the line after Olf). (Reproduced, with permission, from Green & Arduini: Hippocampal electrical activity during arousal. J Neurophysiol 17:533, 1954.)

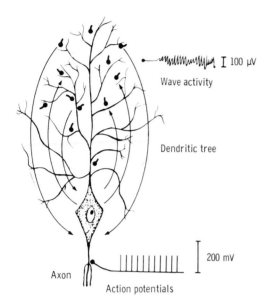

Figure 11-7. Diagrammatic comparison of the electrical responses of the axon and the dendrites of a large cortical neuron. Current flow to and from active synaptic knobs on the dendrites produces wave activity, while all or none action potentials are transmitted down the axon. (Modified and redrawn, with permission, from Bickford: Computational aspects of brain function. Institute of Radio Engineers, Medical Electronics Series [IRE, ME] 6:164, 1959.)

hyperexcitable; when it is positive, the cell is hyperpolarized and less excitable. It also seems that information can be transmitted electrotonically from one dendrite to another (see Chapter 4). The cerebellar cortex and the hippocampus are 2 other parts of the CNS where many complex, parallel dendritic processes are located subpially over a layer of cells. In both areas there is a characteristic rhythmic fluctuation in surface potential similar to that observed in the cortical EEG.

Desynchronizing Mechanisms

Desynchronization, the replacement of a rhythmic EEG pattern with irregular low-voltage activity, is produced by stimulation of the specific sensory systems up to the level of the midbrain, but stimulation above this level, stimulation of the specific sensory relay nuclei of the thalamus, or stimulation of the cortical receiving areas themselves does not have this effect. On the other hand, high-frequency stimulation of the reticular formation in the midbrain tegmentum and of the nonspecific projection nuclei of the thalamus desynchronizes the EEG and arouses a sleeping animal. Large lesions of the lateral and superior portions of the midbrain which interrupt the medial lemnisci and other ascending specific sensory systems fail to prevent the desynchronization produced by sensory stimulation, but lesions in the midbrain tegmentum which disrupt the RAS without damaging the specific systems are associated with a synchronized pattern which is unaffected by sensory stimulation

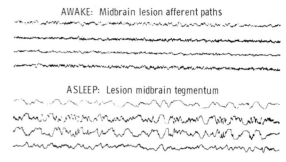

Figure 11-8. Typical EEG records of cat with lesion of lemniscal pathways *(above)* and cat with lesion of midbrain tegmentum *(below)*. (Reproduced, with permission, from Lindsley & others: Behavioral and EEG changes following chronic brain stem lesions in the cat. Electroencephalogr Clin Neurophysiol 2:483, 1950.)

(Fig 11-8). Animals with the former type of lesion are awake; those with the latter type are comatose for long periods. It therefore appears that the ascending activity responsible for desynchronization following sensory stimulation passes up the specific sensory systems to the midbrain, enters the RAS via collaterals, and continues through the thalamus and the nonspecific thalamic projection system to the cortex.

Generalized & Localized Cortical Arousal

There is some evidence for localization of function within the RAS. The hypothesis has been advanced that the lower part of the reticular system is responsible for relatively crude sleep-wakefulness changes, whereas the thalamic portions of the system mediate shifting, localized alerting of the various parts of the cortex in response to the panorama of highly specific stimuli demanding attention in any active individual. The ways in which selected parts of the brain can be alerted under certain conditions, and the relationship of these responses to conditioned learning, are discussed in Chapter 16.

Effect of RAS Stimulation on Cortical Neurons

It is not known how impulses ascending in the RAS break up synchronized cortical activity. Stimulation of the RAS inhibits burst activity, the recruiting response, and the cortical waves produced by the application of strychnine to certain parts of the brain. RAS stimulation arouses and alerts the animal, and, a priori, one might expect it to produce a heightened rather than a depressed excitability of cortical neurons. However, some of the neurons in the cortical sensory projection areas fire randomly during sleep whereas they discharge only in response to specific stimuli when the animal is awake. It is possible that RAS activity abolishes this random firing by producing some degree of cortical inhibition, leaving these neurons free to respond only to specific sensory signals. The net effect of RAS activity, therefore, might be an increase in the "signal/noise ratio" at the expense of a slight decrease in absolute excitability.

Arousal Following Cortical Stimulation

Electrical stimulation of certain portions of the cerebral cortex causes increased reticular activity and EEG arousal. The most effective cortical loci in the monkey are the superior temporal gyrus and the orbital surface of the frontal lobe. Stimulation of these regions wakes a sleeping animal but causes no movements and has few visible effects in the conscious animal. Stimulation of other cortical areas, even with strong currents, does not produce electrical or behavioral arousal. These observations indicate that a system of **corticofugal fibers** feeds into the reticular formation, providing a pathway by which intracortical events can initiate arousal. The system may be responsible for the alerting responses to emotions and related psychic phenomena which occur in the absence of any apparent external stimulus.

Alerting Effects of Epinephrine & Related Compounds

An interesting pharmacologic effect on the RAS is the arousal response produced by agents that mimic the action of the sympathetic nervous system. Epinephrine, norepinephrine, and amphetamine produce EEG arousal and behavioral alerting by lowering the threshold of reticular neurons in the brain stem. Epinephrine and norepinephrine secreted from the adrenal medulla in the stressed individual have the same effect. Therefore, one of the effects of the mass adrenergic discharge in emergency situations (see Chapter 13) is reinforcement of the alert, attentive state necessary for effective action.

It was originally thought that the alerting effect was due to a direct action of pressor agents on the neurons in the midbrain, but it has been demonstrated that any increase in blood pressure increases the excitability of the reticular formation. Apparently there are blood pressure-sensitive neurons in the midbrain because pressor agents produce EEG arousal in animals in which the brain has been transected at the top of the pons, but not in animals in which transection has been carried out at higher levels.

Clinical Correlates

Patients with tumors or other lesions that interrupt the RAS are generally comatose. This system is especially vulnerable at the top of the midbrain and in the posterior hypothalamus, where it is pushed medially by other fiber systems. Relatively small lesions in this location may cause prolonged coma while producing very few other symptoms. In animals it has been demonstrated that concussion depresses activity in the RAS and produces a sleep pattern in the EEG which persists as long as the unconsciousness lasts.

The RAS & General Anesthesia

The ability of general anesthetics to produce unconsciousness appears to be due, at least in part, to their action in depressing conduction in the RAS. The effect of ether on the response of the reticular formation and the medial lemnisci to a sensory stimulus is

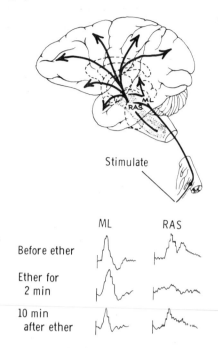

Stimulate

	ML	RAS
Before ether		
Ether for 2 min		
10 min after ether		

Figure 11–9. Effect of ether anesthesia on lemniscal (ML) and reticular (RAS) response to stimulation of the sciatic nerve. (Redrawn and reproduced, with permission, from French & King: Mechanisms involved in the anesthetic state. Surgery 38:228, 1955.)

shown in Fig 11–9. Similar blocking effects are produced by anesthetic doses of barbiturates. These effects may be simply a manifestation of general synaptic depression by these drugs. There are hundreds of synapses in the reticular pathways, whereas the specific systems have only 2–4. At each synapse, the EPSPs must build up until the firing level of the postsynaptic neurons is reached (see Chapter 4). Any agent which has a moderate depressant effect on this process will block conduction in multisynaptic paths before blocking it in those with only a few synapses.

Synchronizing Mechanisms

The wave pattern of the alpha rhythm indicates that the activity of many of the dendritic units is synchronized. Two factors contribute to this synchronization: the synchronizing effect on each unit of activity in neighboring parallel fibers, and rhythmic discharge of impulses from the thalamus.

If 2 nerve fibers are placed side by side in a volume conductor, depolarization of one of them rarely if ever causes a propagated discharge in the other but does influence its excitability. This is because external current flow into the area of depolarization in the active fiber hyperpolarizes the membrane of the neighboring fiber at 2 points and partially depolarizes it at another. Current flow in the opposite direction creates areas of positivity in fibers adjacent to sites where inhibitory endings are active (Fig 11–10). In a large population of similarly oriented neural processes this

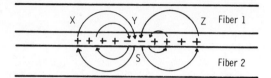

Figure 11—10. Effect of activity in one nerve fiber on the activity of a neighboring fiber in a volume conductor. Current flows into the area of depolarization (S) on fiber 2 from the surrounding membrane. At X and Z on the membrane of fiber 1, positive charges pile up, hyperpolarizing the membrane; at Y, positive charges are pulled off, partly depolarizing it.

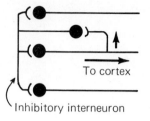

Figure 11—12. Postulated circuit in thalamus which generates rhythmic discharge to cortex. Arrows indicate direction of action potentials when neuron in center discharges.

formation of current sinks and sources in neighboring fibers tends to synchronize current flow.

The dendritic potentials of the cerebral cortex are also influenced by projections from the thalamus. A circular cut around a piece of cortex does not alter its synchronized activity if the blood supply is intact, but the rhythmicity is markedly decreased if the deep connections of the cortical "button" are severed. Large lesions of the thalamus disrupt the EEG synchrony on the side of the lesion. Stimulation of thalamic nuclei at a frequency of about 8/sec produces a characteristic 8/sec response throughout most of the ipsilateral cortex. Because the amplitude of this response waxes and wanes, it is called the **recruiting response** (Fig 11—11). The recruiting response has many similarities to the alpha rhythm and to **burst activity**, the occurrence of short trains of alpha-like waves superimposed on slower rhythms. The records of burst activity such as sleep spindles are essentially identical when recorded simultaneously from the cortex and the thalamus. These observations point to activity projected from the thalamus or reverberating activity between the thalamus and the cortex as being of importance in the genesis of the synchronized EEG rhythm. A current theory holds that synchrony is produced by a thalamic circuit which includes a pathway for **recurrent collateral inhibition**. The proposed pathway is shown in Fig 11—12. Each time the central neuron discharges, it activates via a collateral branch an inhibitory interneuron which produces IPSPs in the discharging neuron and its neighbors. The thalamic neurons are also postulated to be hyperexcitable after a period of inhibition and to discharge spontaneously during the rebound (**postinhibitory rebound excitation**). Therefore, they discharge rhythmically.

It should be noted that slow wave sleep is not solely a passive phenomenon that occurs when sensory stimuli are withdrawn; the synchronizing mechanisms

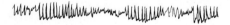

Figure 11—11. Recruiting response in cortex produced by 8/sec stimulation of intralaminar thalamic region. (Based on recordings of Morrison & Dempsey: A study of thalamo-cortical relations. Am J Physiol 135:281, 1942.)

are active. Synchrony is augmented by activation of the brain stem (see below). It is also worth noting that high-frequency stimulation of the thalamic structures produces desynchrony, whereas low-frequency (8/sec) stimulation produces synchrony. These observations are not necessarily inconsistent; the important point is that low-frequency stimulation produces one response whereas high-frequency stimulation produces another.

The relation of these observations, if any, to the production of **electrosleep** or **electric anesthesia** is not known. These terms refer to the unconscious state produced in some humans by the application of small amounts of current to the head in the form of pulses at a frequency of 20—40 Hz. However, sleep and insensibility to pain are not produced by the current in all individuals.

Clinical Uses of the EEG

The EEG is sometimes of value in localizing pathologic processes. When a collection of fluid overlies a portion of the cortex, activity over this area may be damped. This fact may aid in diagnosing and localizing conditions such as subdural hematomas. Lesions in the cortex cause local formation of irregular or slow waves which can be picked up in the EEG leads. Epileptogenic foci sometimes generate high-voltage waves which can be localized.

The waves recorded from corresponding anatomic loci on the 2 hemispheres are normally remarkably similar in timing and shape. This is presumably due to a central subcortical "pacemaker" that keeps the activity of both hemispheres in phase. A lesion in one hemisphere distorts the pattern; consequently, if records from homologous points on the 2 hemispheres are out of phase with each other, focal cortical damage is indicated.

In epileptics there are characteristic EEG patterns during seizures; between attacks, however, abnormalities are often difficult to demonstrate. **Grand mal** seizures, epileptic attacks in which an aura precedes a generalized convulsion with tonic muscular contraction and clonic jerks, have a characteristic EEG pattern. There is fast activity during the tonic phase. Slow waves, each preceded by a spike, occur at the time of each clonic jerk. For a while after the attack, slow waves are present. Similar changes are seen in experimental animals during convulsions produced by elec-

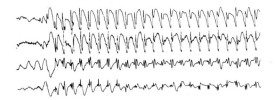

Figure 11–13. Petit mal epilepsy. Record of 4 cortical EEG leads from a 6-year-old boy who during the recording had one of his "blank spells" in which he was transiently unaware of his surroundings and blinked his eyelids. (Reproduced, with permission, from Chusid: *Correlative Neuroanatomy & Functional Neurology,* 16th ed. Lange, 1976.)

tric shocks. **Petit mal** epileptic attacks, seizures characterized by a momentary loss of responsiveness, are associated with 3/sec doublets, each consisting of a typical spike and rounded wave (Fig 11–13). **Psychomotor seizures,** attacks in which emotional lability and stereotyped behavior are seen due to discharge from a temporal lobe focus, are not associated with any typical EEG changes. During the various types of diencephalic seizures that originate in the brain stem, there are also no characteristic EEG abnormalities.

SLEEP

Sleep Stages

There are 2 different kinds of sleep: **rapid eye movement (REM) sleep** and **non-REM (NREM)** or **slow wave sleep.** NREM sleep is divided into 4 stages. As a person falls asleep, he first enters stage 1, which is characterized by low amplitude, fast frequency EEG activity (Fig 11–14). Stage 2 is marked by the appearance of sleep spindles (see above). In stage 3, the pattern is one of slower frequency and increased amplitude of the EEG waves. Maximum slowing with large waves is seen in stage 4. Thus, the characteristic of deep sleep is a pattern of synchronized slow waves.

REM Sleep

The high-amplitude slow waves seen in the EEG during sleep are sometimes replaced by rapid, low-voltage, irregular EEG activity that resembles that seen in alert animals and humans. However, sleep is not interrupted; indeed, the threshold for arousal by sensory stimuli and by stimulation of the reticular formation is elevated. The condition has been called **paradoxical sleep.** There are rapid, roving movements of

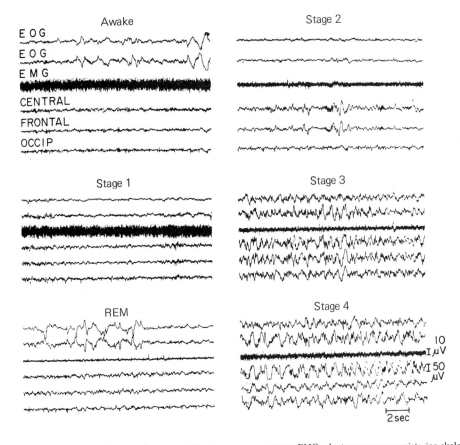

Figure 11–14. Sleep stages. EOG, electrooculogram registering eye movements; EMG, electromyogram registering skeletal muscle activity; central, frontal, occip, 3 EEG leads. Note the low muscle tone with extensive eye movements in REM. (Reproduced, with permission, from Kales & others: Sleep and dreams: Recent research on clinical aspects. Ann Intern Med 68:1078, 1968.)

the eyes during paradoxical sleep, and for this reason it is also called REM sleep. There are no such movements in slow-wave sleep, and consequently it is often called NREM sleep. REM sleep is found in all species of mammals that have been studied and in birds, but it probably does not occur in other animals. Humans aroused at a time when they show the low-voltage EEG activity generally report that they were dreaming, whereas individuals wakened from spindle sleep do not. This observation and other evidence indicate that REM sleep and dreaming are closely associated. During REM sleep, there is a marked reduction in skeletal muscle tone despite the rapid eye movements. The teeth grinding (**bruxism**) that occurs in some individuals is also associated with dreaming.

If humans are awakened every time they show REM sleep, they become somewhat anxious and irritable. If they are then permitted to sleep without interruption, they show a great deal more than the normal amount of paradoxical sleep for a few nights. The same "rebound" effect is seen in animals treated the same way. These observations have led some investigators to conclude that dreaming is necessary to maintain mental health. However, it is now established that prolonged REM deprivation does not have any adverse psychologic effects.

Distribution of Stages

In a typical night of sleep, a young adult passes through stages 1 and 2 and spends 70–100 minutes in stages 3 and 4. Sleep then lightens, and a REM period follows. This cycle is repeated at intervals of about 90 minutes throughout the night (Fig 11–15). The cycles are similar, although there is less stage 3 and 4 sleep and more REM sleep toward morning. Thus, there are 4–6 REM periods per night. At all ages, REM sleep constitutes about 25% of total sleep time. Children have more stage 3 and 4 sleep than young adults, and old people have much less.

Genesis of Slow Wave Sleep

Slow wave sleep is produced in part by the absence of desynchronizing activity transmitted via the ascending reticular system. However, the synchronizing activity of the thalamus is apparently influenced by ascending activity from the pons and hindbrain, since stimulation in the central portion of the hindbrain at slow rates produces synchrony and sleep and midpontine transection of the brain stem produces a state in which the cortex is desynchronized. Stimulation of afferents from mechanoreceptors in the skin at rates of 10/sec or less also produces sleep in animals, apparently via the brain stem, and it is of course common knowledge that regularly repeated monotonous stimuli put humans to sleep. Stimulation of the basal forebrain produces sleep, probably via a descending pathway that affects the centers in the brain stem that are concerned with sleep.

The mechanism by which the hindbrain area generates synchrony is unknown. However, there is evidence that discharge of serotonin-secreting neurons is

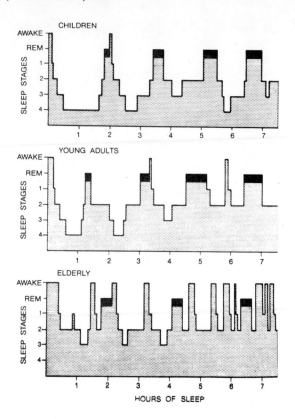

Figure 11–15. Normal sleep cycles at various ages. REM sleep is indicated by the dark areas. (Reproduced, with permission, from Kales & Kales: Sleep disorders. N Engl J Med 290:487, 1974.)

involved in the production of slow wave sleep, and the serotoninergic neurons that project to the limbic system and other rostral areas have their cell bodies in the raphe nuclei located in the hindbrain. The role of serotonin as a synaptic mediator in the CNS is discussed in Chapter 15. Parachlorophenylalanine, a drug which depletes brain serotonin, causes insomnia in cats, and this effect is overcome by administration of 5-hydroxytryptophan, which restores the serotonin content of the neurons to normal.

Genesis of REM Sleep

REM sleep appears to be initiated from nuclei in the pons. Phasic spike discharges from this region herald its onset, and destruction of the medial portion of the oral reticular nucleus of the pons abolishes REM sleep without usually affecting slow wave sleep or arousal. It is not known what initiates the discharge from the pons or how this discharge brings about the various phenomena associated with REM sleep. There is some evidence that an adrenergic mechanism in the brain is involved, since REM sleep is suppressed by brain stem lesions which deplete the forebrain of norepinephrine, presumably by interrupting ascending adrenergic fibers. However, drugs which inhibit monoamine oxidase increase brain norepinephrine and decrease REM sleep. Barbiturates also decrease the amount of REM sleep.

Sleep Disorders

Sleepwalking (**somnambulism**) and bed-wetting (**nocturnal enuresis**) have been shown to occur during slow wave sleep or, more specifically, during arousal from slow wave sleep. They are not associated with REM sleep. Episodes of sleepwalking are more common in children than adults and occur predominantly in males. They may last several minutes. Somnambulists walk with their eyes open and avoid obstacles, but when awakened they cannot recall the episodes.

Narcolepsy is a not uncommon disease of unknown cause in which there is an eventually irresistible urge to sleep during daytime activities. In some cases, it has been shown to start with the sudden onset of REM sleep. REM sleep almost never occurs without previous slow wave sleep in normal individuals.

MODULATION OF SENSORY INPUT

The first evidence that the brain regulates the generation of sensory impulses or their transmission in the specific sensory systems was the observation that stimulation of the bulbar reticular formation inhibited transmission at the first synapse in the lemniscal and spinothalamic systems and the trigeminal nuclei. Inhibitory effects on transmission in the cochlear nucleus have also been observed. It has been claimed that some of the inhibitory effects in the auditory system are due to contraction of the stapedius and tensor tympani muscles (see Chapter 9). However, efferent fibers in the auditory nerve pass all the way to the cochlea, and stimulation of these efferent fibers inhibits the initiation of impulses in the organ of Corti. There are efferent fibers in the optic nerve which when stimulated either inhibit or augment retinal activity. These observations establish the existence of brain mechanisms that can turn up or down the volume of afferent input by effects on the specific sensory pathways or the

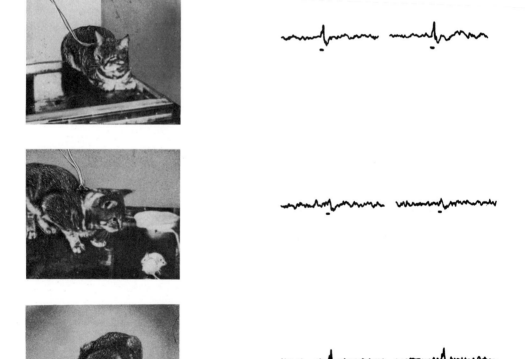

Figure 11–16. Changes in response of cochlear nucleus to repeated click stimuli (at dashes) before *(top)*, during *(middle)*, and after *(bottom)* attention is fixed on mice in a bell jar. (Reproduced, with permission, from Hernandéz-Péon, Scherrer, & Jouvet: Modification of electrical activity in cochlear nucleus during "attention." Science 123:331, 1956.)

sense organs themselves. Some of these mechanisms are reticular, but others are not. Stimulation of the sensory cortex produces presynaptic inhibition at synaptic junctions in the gracile and cuneate nuclei. There are other inhibitory mechanisms which affect transmission in the dorsal horns, the specific thalamic nuclei, and in the cortex itself.

Some of these modulating mechanisms are brought into play when the individual's attention is focused on a particular object. In the experiment illustrated in Fig 11–16, electrodes were implanted in the cochlear nucleus of a cat. After the animal recovered, the electrical activity of the cochlear nucleus was recorded while a clicker was sounded at regular intervals. While the cat sat quietly in its cage, a spike was observed with each click. However, when the animal's attention was focused on a pair of mice placed in front of it, the click response in the cochlear nucleus practically disappeared. It returned when the mice were removed, but disappeared again when the cat's atten-

tion was attracted by the smell of fish. These observations indicate that—contrary to some theories—part of the narrowing of the field of awareness during focused attention is due to "turning off" some of the incoming stimuli before they reach the cerebral cortex.

Another example of central control of sensory input is the regulatory effect of brain centers on muscle spindle sensitivity. The effect of changes in the rate of gamma efferent discharge on the sensitivity of the spindles is described in Chapter 6. The gamma efferent neurons are subjected to both facilitatory and inhibitory influences via descending tracts in the lateral funiculus of the spinal cord. Stimulation of one part of the brain stem reticular formation facilitates gamma efferent discharge, whereas stimulation of another portion inhibits it. There are also inhibitory centers in the cerebellum, basal ganglia, and motor cortex. Their function in the regulation of body posture is discussed in the next chapter.

12...
Control of Posture & Movement

Somatic motor activity depends ultimately upon the pattern and rate of discharge of the spinal motor neurons and homologous neurons in the motor nuclei of the cranial nerves. These neurons, the final common paths to skeletal muscle, are bombarded by impulses from an immense array of pathways. There are many inputs to each spinal motor neuron from the same spinal segment (see Chapter 6). Numerous suprasegmental inputs also converge on these cells, in part via interneurons and in part via the neurons of the gamma efferent system to the muscle spindles and back through the Ia afferent fibers to the spinal cord. It is the integrated activity of these multiple inputs from spinal, medullary, midbrain, and cortical levels that regulates the posture of the body and makes coordinated movement possible.

The inputs converging on the motor neurons subserve 3 semidistinct functions: they bring about skilled, voluntary activity; they adjust body posture to provide a stable background for movement; and they coordinate the action of the various muscles to make movements smooth and precise. Current evidence indicates that patterns of voluntary activity are planned within the brain and the commands are sent to the muscles via the **pyramidal** and **extrapyramidal systems.** The first of these is concerned with skilled, fine movement; the second with grosser movements and posture. The **cerebellum** and its connections are concerned with coordinating and smoothing movement. There is also some evidence that portions of the extrapyramidal system, the basal ganglia, are concerned with the generation of slow, steady movements (ramp movements) whereas the cerebellum generates rapid, ballistic movements (saccadic movements).

Encephalization

In species in which the cerebral cortex is highly developed, the process of **encephalization**, ie, the relatively greater role of the cerebral cortex in various functions, is an important phenomenon. For this reason the effects of cortical ablation in primates are generally more severe and sometimes quite different from those in cats, dogs, and other laboratory animals. Because this chapter is concerned primarily with motor function in humans, pathologic and clinical observations in humans and experiments in laboratory primates are emphasized.

Upper & Lower Motor Neurons

The motor system is commonly divided into **upper** and **lower motor neurons.** Lesions of the lower motor neurons—the spinal and cranial motor neurons that directly innervate the muscles—are associated with flaccid paralysis, muscular atrophy, and absence of reflex responses. The syndrome of spastic paralysis and hyperactive stretch reflexes in the absence of muscle atrophy is said to be due to destruction of the "upper motor neurons," the neurons in the brain and spinal cord which activate the motor neurons. However, there are 3 types of "upper motor neurons" to consider. Lesions in the extrapyramidal posture-regulating pathways do cause spastic paralysis, but lesions limited to the pyramidal tracts produce weakness **(paresis)** rather than paralysis, and the affected musculature is generally hypotonic, whereas cerebellar lesions produce incoordination. The unmodified term upper motor neuron is therefore confusing and should not be used.

PYRAMIDAL SYSTEM

ANATOMY

Tracts

The nerve fibers which form the pyramids in the medulla and hence are called the pyramidal system descend in the internal capsule from the cerebral cortex. About 80% of them cross the midline in the pyramidal decussation to form the **lateral corticospinal tract;** the remainder descend as the **anterior corticospinal tract,** decussating just before their termination (Fig 12–1). Additional uncrossed corticospinal fibers may exist. In most animals, the corticospinal axons end on interneurons rather than motor neurons. In humans, however, at least 10% of the axons make direct synaptic connections with the motor neurons. Ninety percent of the fibers in the pyramidal system are small, and 50% are unmyelinated.

Cortical Motor Areas

The cortical areas from which the pyramidal

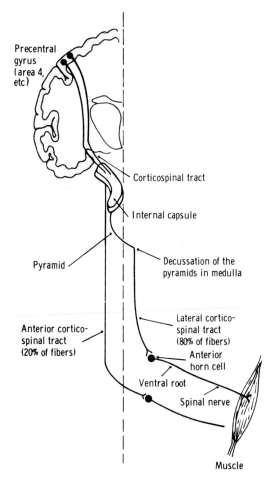

Figure 12–1. The corticospinal tracts.

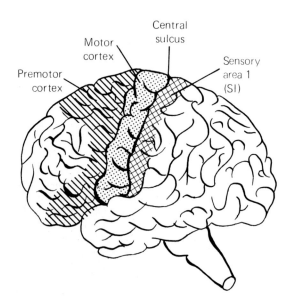

Figure 12–2. Diagram showing classical cortical motor areas.

system originates are generally held to be those where stimulation produces prompt discrete movement. There are 4 such areas in the cortex. The best known is the **motor cortex** in the precentral gyrus (Fig 12–2). However, there is a **supplementary motor area** of unknown function on and above the superior bank of the cingulate sulcus on the medial side of the hemisphere (Fig 12–3). Motor responses are also produced by stimulation of somatic sensory area I in the postcentral gyrus and by stimulation of somatic sensory area II in the wall of the sylvian fissure (see Chapter 7). It is probable that all of these areas contribute fibers to the pyramidal system and to the extrapyramidal system as well. About 60% of the pyramidal fibers arise from the precentral gyrus, but only 2% come from the large Betz cells in area 4.

By means of stimulation experiments in patients undergoing craniotomy under local anesthesia, it has been possible to outline most of the motor projection from the precentral gyrus (Fig 12–4). The various parts of the body are represented in the precentral gyrus, with the feet at the top of the gyrus and the face at the bottom. The facial area is represented bilaterally, but the rest of the representation is unilateral, the cortical motor area controlling the musculature on the opposite side of the body. The cortical representation of each body part is proportionate in size to the skill with which the part is used in fine, voluntary movement. The muscles involved in speech and hand movements are especially well represented in the cortex; use of the pharynx, lips, and tongue to form words, and the fingers and opposable thumbs to manipulate the environment are activities in which humans are especially skilled.

The conditions under which these human studies were performed precluded stimulation of the banks of the sulci and other inaccessible areas. In monkeys, meticulous study has shown that the hand area is not interposed between the trunk and face areas (Fig 12–4). Instead, there is a regular representation of the body, with the axial musculature and the proximal portions of the limbs represented along the anterior edge of the precentral gyrus and the distal part of the limbs along the posterior edge. The cells in the cortical motor areas are arranged in columns. The cells in each column receive fairly extensive sensory input from the peripheral area in which they produce movement.

Premotor Cortex

Brodmann's area 6, the region anterior to the precentral gyrus, has traditionally been called the **premotor cortex** or **premotor area** (Fig 12–2). Under certain conditions, stimulation in this region produces **adversive movements**, ie, gross rotation of the eyes, head, and trunk to the opposite side. These movements may be due to stimulation of extrapyramidal pathways, but they may also be due to intracortical spread of the stimuli to the pyramidal system. On this basis the existence of the premotor area as a separate entity has been questioned.

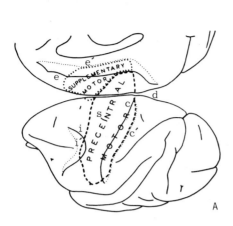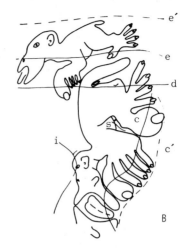

Figure 12–3. Motor "simunculi," showing the cortical localization of motor function in the monkey. *B* is an enlarged view of *A*, the various lines representing the sulci and medial edge of the hemisphere as indicated in *A*. (See Fig 12–4.) c = central sulcus; c' = bottom of central sulcus; d = medial edge of hemisphere; e = sulcus cinguli; e' = bottom of sulcus cinguli; i = inferior precentral sulcus; i' = bottom of inferior precentral sulcus; s = superior precentral sulcus. (Reproduced, with permission, from Woolsey & others: Patterns of localization in pre-central and "supplementary" motor areas and their relation to the concept of a premotor area. Res Publ Assoc Res Nerv Ment Dis 30:238, 1950.)

Other Areas

Stimulation of the frontal cortex anterior to and below area 6 causes eye movements in primates. The most common response is movement of both eyes in the same direction (**conjugate deviation**), but pupillary dilatation and nystagmus have also been observed. It is probable that this **frontal eye field** is a center concerned with integration of eye movements, but the details of the way it functions are not known. Stimulation of the occipital lobe near the visual cortex also causes conjugate deviation of the eyes to the opposite side. Stimulation of an area adjacent to the auditory cortex causes movement of the ears.

FUNCTION

Role in Movement

The pyramidal system appears to be concerned with skilled, fine movement. This does not mean that movement—even skilled movement—is impossible without it. Nonmammalian vertebrates have essentially no pyramidal system, but they move with great agility nonetheless. Cats and dogs stand, walk, run, and even eat if food is presented to them after complete destruction of the pyramidal system.

In primates it is difficult to produce selective disruption of pyramidal function, and this fact is responsible for much of the confusion about the role of the pyramidal system in humans. Even the most circumscribed lesions in the cortical motor area destroy cells concerned with extrapyramidal and cerebellar functions. Careful surgical section of the pyramids in the medulla is probably the most selective experimental approach, but even this procedure damages other fibers.

After section of one pyramid in monkeys, the limbs on the opposite side of the body hang limply much of the time. However, they are not paralyzed. The hopping and placing postural reactions are defective (see below), but otherwise the monkey uses his limbs to maintain his posture and to right himself in

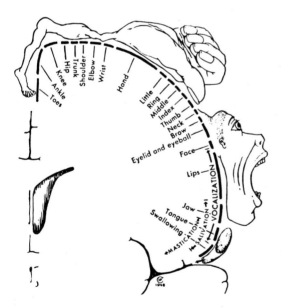

Figure 12–4. Motor homunculus. The figure represents, on a coronal section of the precentral gyrus, the location of the cortical representation of the various parts. The size of the various parts is proportionate to the amount of cortical area devoted to them. (Reproduced, with permission, from Penfield & Rasmussen: *The Cerebral Cortex of Man: A Clinical Study of Localization of Function.* Macmillan, 1950.)

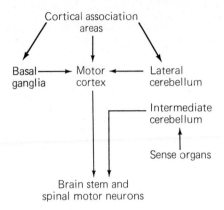

Figure 12—5. Role of the motor cortex and other structures in the control of movement.

the normal fashion. Furthermore, if use of the normal arm is prevented, he will occasionally reach for food and other objects with the affected arm, especially when motivation is strong. The motions lack precision; there is a loss of accuracy in the use of the digits, and a particular inability to maneuver objects into the palm of the hand, so that the grasp is clumsy. The main defects produced by destruction of the pyramidal system are therefore weakness and clumsiness.

What, then, is the role of the precentral motor cortex in skilled movement? It appears reasonable, on the basis of present information, to hypothesize that ideas or commands for fine movements arise in the association areas of the cortex (Fig 12—5). It also seems probable that movement patterns are generated in structures such as the basal ganglia and the cerebellum; that the patterns are modulated in the cortex in terms of the somatosensory input provided by afferents from the periphery; and that the pyramidal system is a final common path for these patterns to the spinal motor neurons. The fact that movements (such as those of the fingers) which require the most somatosensory input are most compromised by pyramidal lesions supports this hypothesis.

Effects on Stretch Reflexes

Section of the pyramids in monkeys produces prolonged hypotonia and flaccidity rather than spasticity. The anatomic arrangements in humans are such that disease processes rarely, if ever, damage the pyramidal system anywhere along its course without also destroying extrapyramidal posture-regulating pathways. When spasticity is present, it is probably due to damage to these latter pathways rather than to the pyramidal system itself.

Damage to the pyramidal tract in humans produces the **Babinski sign**: dorsiflexion of the great toe and fanning of the other toes when the lateral aspect of the sole of the foot is scratched. In normal individuals, the response to this stimulation is a plantar flexion of all the toes. The Babinski sign is valuable for the localization of disease processes, but its physiologic significance is unknown.

Relation of Movement to Perception

If the apparent position of objects in the visual field is displaced by looking at them through prisms, an individual at first has trouble reaching for them. He gradually corrects the misreaching, but correction is not simply a result of recognizing the error and correcting it. The correction and that of other experimentally produced visual and auditory displacements have been shown to be independent of their recognition and dependent on the active movements made by the individual. Without movements no correction occurs, and passive movements fail to provide the necessary information input to the perceptual apparatus; only active movements by the subject will suffice.

There is other evidence of the close connection between sensory input and motor output. If a limb is deafferented by section of the dorsal roots of the spinal nerves that supply it, it is severely paralyzed. Indeed, the paralysis is more severe than that which follows section of the pyramids. This illustrates the importance of reflexes and sensory input in the regulation of movement. However, the paralysis does not last, and motor function gradually returns. After a period of time, the deafferented animal can move its limb relatively well even when visual and other external cues are eliminated. Thus, there must be, in addition to sensory input, a central programming mechanism of some sort that can be made to work independently of peripheral sensation.

EXTRAPYRAMIDAL MECHANISMS

By definition, the extrapyramidal system is made up of those areas in the CNS other than the pyramidal and cerebellar systems that are concerned with movement. It includes a whole series of nuclei and portions of many structures, including the cerebral cortex, the basal ganglia, the midbrain, the medulla, and the spinal cord. It is concerned with the programming and initiation of movement and with posture.

Integration

The extrapyramidal mechanisms concerned with posture are integrated at various levels all the way from the spinal cord to the cerebral cortex. At the spinal cord level, afferent impulses produce simple reflex responses. At higher levels in the nervous system, neural connections of increasing complexity mediate increasingly complicated motor responses. This principle of levels of motor integration is illustrated in Table 12—1. In the intact animal, the individual motor responses are fitted into or "submerged" in the total pattern of motor activity. When the neural axis is transected, the activities integrated below the section are cut off or **released** from the "control of higher

Table 12—1. Summary of levels involved in various neural functions.*

Functions	Preparation						Level of Integration
	Normal	Decorticate	Midbrain	Hindbrain (Decerebrate)	Spinal	Decerebellate	
Initiative, memory, etc	+	0	0	0	0	+	Cerebral cortex required
Conditioned reflexes	+	+†	0	0	0	+	Cerebral cortex required
Emotional responses	+	++	0	0	0	+	Hypothalamus, limbic system
Locomotor reflexes	+	++	+	0	0	Incoordinate	Midbrain, thalamus
Righting reflexes	+	+	++	0	0	Incoordinate	Midbrain
Antigravity reflexes	+	+	+	++	0	Incoordinate	Medulla
Respiration	+	+	+	+	0	+	Lower medulla
Spinal reflexes‡	+	+	+	+	++	+	Spinal cord

Legend: 0 = absent; + = present; ++ = accentuated.
*Modified from Cobb: *Foundations of Neuropsychiatry,* 6th ed. Williams & Wilkins, 1958.
†Conditioned reflexes can be established in decorticate animals but special technics are required.
‡Other than stretch reflexes.

brain centers," and often appear to be accentuated. Release of this type, long a cardinal principle in neurology, may in some situations be due to removal of an inhibitory control by higher neural centers. A more important cause of the apparent hyperactivity is loss of differentiation of the reaction, so that it no longer fits into the broader pattern of motor activity. An additional factor may be denervation hypersensitivity of the centers below the transection, but the role of this component remains to be determined.

Postural Control

It is impossible to separate postural adjustments from voluntary movement in any rigid way, but it is possible to differentiate a series of postural reflexes (Table 12—2) that not only maintain the body in an upright, balanced position but also provide the constant adjustments necessary to maintain a stable postural background for voluntary activity. These adjustments include maintained **static** reflexes and dynamic, short-term **phasic** reflexes. The former involve sus-

Table 12—2. Principal postural reflexes.

Reflex	Stimulus	Response	Receptor	Integrated In
Stretch reflexes	Stretch	Contraction of muscle	Muscle spindles	Spinal cord, medulla
Positive supporting (magnet) reaction	Contact with sole or palm	Foot extended to support body	Proprioceptors in distal flexors	Spinal cord
Negative supporting reaction	Stretch	Release of positive supporting reaction	Proprioceptors in extensors	Spinal cord
Tonic labyrinthine reflexes	Gravity	Extensor rigidity	Otolithic organs	Medulla
Tonic neck reflexes	Head turned: (1) To side (2) Up (3) Down	Change in pattern of rigidity (1) Extension of limbs on side to which head is turned (2) Hind legs flex (3) Forelegs flex	Neck proprioceptors	Medulla
Labyrinthine righting reflexes	Gravity	Head kept level	Otolithic organs	Midbrain
Neck righting reflexes	Stretch of neck muscles	Righting of thorax and shoulders, then pelvis	Muscle spindles	Midbrain
Body on head righting reflexes	Pressure on side of body	Righting of head	Exteroceptors	Midbrain
Body on body righting reflexes	Pressure on side of body	Righting of body even when head held sideways	Exteroceptors	Midbrain
Optical righting reflexes	Visual cues	Righting of head	Eyes	Cerebral cortex
Placing reactions	Various visual, exteroceptive, and proprioceptive cues	Foot placed on supporting surface in position to support body	Various	Cerebral cortex
Hopping reactions	Lateral displacement while standing	Hops, maintaining limbs in position to support body	Muscle spindles	Cerebral cortex

tained contraction of the musculature, whereas the latter involve transient movements. Both are integrated at various levels in the CNS from the spinal cord to the cerebral cortex, and are effected largely through extrapyramidal motor pathways. A major factor in postural control is variation in the threshold of the spinal stretch reflexes caused in turn by changes in the excitability of motor neurons and, indirectly, by changes in the rate of discharge in the small motor nerve system.

SPINAL INTEGRATION

The responses of animals and humans after spinal cord transection in the cervical region illustrate the integration of reflexes at the spinal level. The individual spinal reflexes are discussed in detail in Chapter 6.

Spinal Shock

In all vertebrates, transection of the spinal cord is followed by a period of **spinal shock** during which **all spinal reflex responses are profoundly depressed. During it, the resting membrane potential of the spinal motor neurons is 2–6 mV greater than normal.** Subsequently, reflex responses return and become relatively hyperactive. The duration of spinal shock is proportionate to the degree of encephalization of motor function in the various species. In frogs it lasts for minutes, in dogs and cats it lasts for 1–2 hours, in monkeys it lasts for days, and in humans it usually lasts for a minimum of 2 weeks.

The cause of spinal shock is uncertain. Cessation of tonic bombardment of spinal neurons by excitatory impulses in descending pathways undoubtedly plays a role, but the subsequent return of reflexes and their eventual hyperactivity also need to be explained. The recovery of reflex excitability may possibly be due to the development of denervation hypersensitivity to the mediators released by the remaining spinal excitatory endings. Another possibility for which there is some evidence is the sprouting of collaterals from existing neurons with the formation of additional excitatory endings on interneurons and motor neurons.

The first reflex response to reappear as spinal shock wears off in humans is frequently a slight contraction of the leg flexors and adductors in response to a noxious stimulus. In some patients, the knee jerks come back first. The interval between cord transection and the beginning return of reflex activity is about 2 weeks in the absence of any complications, but if complications are present it is much longer. It is not known why infection, malnutrition, and other complications of cord transection inhibit spinal reflex activity.

Complications of Cord Transection

The problems in the management of paraplegic and quadriplegic humans are complex. Like all immobilized patients, they develop a negative nitrogen balance and catabolize large amounts of body protein.

The weight of the body compresses the circulation to the skin over bony prominences, so that unless the patient is moved frequently the skin breaks down at these points and **decubitus ulcers** form. The ulcers heal poorly and are prone to infection because of body protein depletion. The tissues broken down include the protein matrix of bone, and calcium is liberated in large amounts. The hypercalcemia leads to hypercalciuria, and calcium stones often form in the urinary tract. The stones and the paralysis of bladder function both cause urinary stasis, which predisposes to urinary infection. Therefore, the prognosis in patients with transected spinal cords used to be very poor, and death from septicemia, uremia, or inanition was the rule. Since World War II, however, the use of antibiotics and meticulous attention to nutrition, fluid balance, skin care, bladder function, and general nursing care have made it possible for many of these patients to survive.

Responses in Chronic Spinal Animals & Humans

Once the spinal reflexes begin to reappear after spinal shock, their threshold steadily drops. In chronically quadriplegic humans the threshold of the withdrawal reflex is especially low. Even minor noxious stimuli may cause not only prolonged withdrawal of one extremity but marked flexion-extension patterns in the other 3 limbs. Repeated flexion movements may occur for prolonged periods, and contractures of the flexor muscles develop. Stretch reflexes are also hyperactive, as are more complex reactions based on this reflex as well. For example, if a finger is placed on the sole of the foot of an animal after the spinal cord has been transected (**spinal animal**), the limb usually extends, following the examining finger. This **magnet reaction** or **positive supporting reaction** involves proprioceptive as well as tactile afferents and transforms the limb into a rigid pillar to resist gravity and support the animal. Its disappearance is also in part an active phenomenon (**negative supporting reaction**) initiated by stretch of the extensor muscles. On the basis of the positive supporting reaction, spinal cats and dogs can be made to stand, albeit awkwardly, for as long as 2–3 minutes.

Autonomic Reflexes

Reflex contractions of the full bladder and rectum occur in spinal animals and humans, although the bladder is rarely emptied completely. Hyperactive bladder reflexes can keep the bladder in a shrunken state long enough for hypertrophy and fibrosis of its wall to occur. Blood pressure is generally normal at rest, but the precise feedback regulation normally supplied by the baroreceptor reflexes is absent and wide swings in pressure are common. Bouts of sweating and blanching of the skin also occur.

The intermediolateral gray columns of the spinal cord are relatively rich in norepinephrine and serotonin. Seven days after cord section in rabbits, when the autonomic reflexes are hyperactive, the norepinephrine and serotonin content of the spinal cord below the transection is markedly reduced. These observations suggest that norepinephrine and serotonin are mediators in descending pathways which normally inhibit autonomic function.

Sexual Reflexes

Other reflex responses are present in the spinal animal, but in general they are only fragments of patterns that are integrated in the normal animal into purposeful sequences. The sexual reflexes are an example. Coordinated sexual activity depends upon a series of reflexes integrated at many neural levels, and is absent after cord transection. However, genital manipulation in the male spinal animal and human will produce erection and even ejaculation. In the female spinal dog, vaginal stimulation causes tail deviation and movement of the pelvis into the copulatory position.

Mass Reflex

In chronic spinal animals, afferent stimuli irradiate from one reflex center to another. When even a relatively minor noxious stimulus is applied to the skin, it may irradiate to autonomic centers and produce evacuation of the bladder and rectum, sweating, pallor, and blood pressure swings in addition to the withdrawal response. This distressing **mass reflex** can sometimes be used to give paraplegic patients a degree of bladder and bowel control. They can be trained to initiate urination and defecation by stroking or pinching their thighs, thus producing an intentional mild mass reflex.

MEDULLARY COMPONENTS

In experimental animals in which the hindbrain and spinal cord are isolated from the rest of the brain by transection of the brain stem at the superior border of the pons, the most prominent finding is marked spasticity of the body musculature. The operative procedure is called **decerebration**, and the resulting pattern of spasticity is called **decerebrate rigidity**. Decerebration produces no phenomenon akin to spinal shock, and the rigidity develops as soon as the brain stem is transected. Flexor and extensor muscles are both involved, but in the dog and cat the spasticity is most prominent in the extensor muscles. This produces the characteristic posture of decerebration: neck and limbs extended, back arched, and tail elevated.

Mechanism of Decerebrate Rigidity

On analysis, decerebrate rigidity is found to be due to a diffuse facilitation of stretch reflexes. The facilitation is due to 2 factors: increased general excitability of the motor neuron pool and increase in the rate of discharge in the gamma efferent neurons.

Supraspinal Regulation of Stretch Reflexes

The brain areas which facilitate and inhibit stretch reflexes are shown in Fig 12–6. Except for the

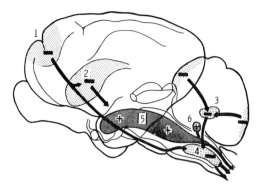

Figure 12–6. Areas in the cat brain where stimulation produces facilitation (plus signs) or inhibition (minus signs) of stretch reflexes. *1*, motor cortex; *2*, basal ganglia; *3*, cerebellum; *4*, reticular inhibitory area; *5*, reticular facilitatory area; *6*, vestibular nuclei. (Reproduced, with permission, from Lindsley, Schreiner, & Magoun: An electromyographic study of spasticity. J Neurophysiol 12:197, 1949.)

vestibular nuclei, these areas act by increasing or decreasing spindle sensitivity (Fig 12–7). The large facilitatory area in the brain stem reticular formation discharges spontaneously, possibly in response to afferent input like the reticular activating system. However, the smaller brain stem area which inhibits gamma efferent discharge does not discharge spontaneously but is driven instead by fibers from the cerebral cortex and the cerebellum. The inhibitory area in the basal ganglia may act through descending connections, as shown in Fig 12–6, or by stimulating the cortical inhibitory center. From the reticular inhibitory and facilitatory areas, impulses descend in the lateral funiculus of the spinal cord. When the brain stem is transected at the level of the top of the pons, 2 of the 3 inhibitory areas that drive the reticular inhibi-

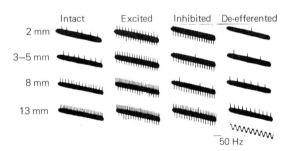

Figure 12–7. Response of single afferent fiber from muscle spindle to various degrees of muscle stretch. Figures at left indicate amount of stretch. The upward deflections are action potentials; the downward deflections are stimulus artifacts. Records were obtained before brain stimulation (first column), during stimulation of brain areas facilitating (second column) and inhibiting (third column) stretch reflexes, and after section of the motor nerve (fourth column). Reproduced, with permission, from Eldred, Granit, & Merton: Supraspinal control of muscle spindles. J Physiol [Lond] 122:498, 1953.)

tory center are removed. Discharge of the facilitatory area continues, but that of the inhibitory area is decreased. Consequently, the balance of facilitatory and inhibitory impulses converging on the gamma efferent neurons shifts toward facilitation. Gamma efferent discharge is increased, and stretch reflexes become hyperactive. The cerebellar inhibitory area is still present, and in decerebrate animals removal of the cerebellum increases the rigidity. The influence of the cerebellum is complex, however, and destruction of the cerebellum in man produces hypotonia rather than spasticity.

The vestibulospinal pathways are also facilitatory to stretch reflexes and promote rigidity. Unlike the reticular pathways, they pass primarily in the anterior funiculus of the spinal cord, and the rigidity due to increased discharge in them is not abolished by deafferentation of the muscles. This indicates that this rigidity is due to a direct action on the motor neurons rather than an effect mediated through the small motor nerve system which would, of course, be blocked by deafferentation.

Significance of Decerebrate Rigidity

Sherrington pointed out that the extensor muscles are those with which the cat and dog resist gravity; the decerebrate posture in these animals is, as he put it, "a caricature of the normal standing position." What has been uncovered by decerebration, then, are the tonic, static postural reflex mechanisms that support the animal against gravity. Additional evidence that this is the correct interpretation of the phenomenon comes from the observation that decerebration in the

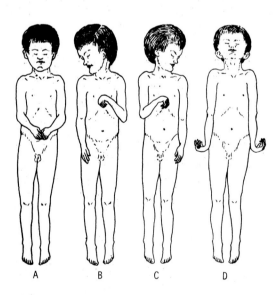

Figure 12–8. Human decorticate rigidity *(A–C)* and true decerebrate rigidity *(D).* In *A* the patient is lying supine with head unturned. In *B* and *C,* the tonic neck reflex patterns produced by turning of the head to the right or left are shown. (Reproduced, with permission, from *Textbook of Physiology,* 17th ed. Fulton JF [editor]. Saunders, 1955.)

sloth, an arboreal animal which hangs upside down from branches most of the time, causes rigidity in flexion. In humans, the pattern in true decerebrate rigidity is extensor in all 4 limbs, like that in cats and dogs. Apparently human beings are not far enough removed from their quadruped ancestors to have changed the pattern in their upper extremities even though the main antigravity muscles of the arms in the upright position are flexors. However, decerebrate rigidity is rare in disease states and the defects which produce it are usually incompatible with life. The more common pattern of extensor rigidity in the legs and moderate flexion in the arms is actually **decorticate rigidity** due to lesions of the cerebral cortex, with most of the brain stem intact (Fig 12–8).

Tonic Labyrinthine Reflexes

In the decerebrate animal the pattern of rigidity in the limbs varies with the position. No righting responses are present, and the animal stays in the position in which it is put. If the animal is placed on its back, the extension of all 4 limbs is maximal. As the animal is turned to either side, the rigidity decreases, and when it is prone the rigidity is minimal though still present. These changes in rigidity, the **tonic labyrinthine reflexes,** are initiated by the action of gravity on the otolithic organs and are effected via the vestibulospinal tracts. They are rather surprising in view of the role of rigidity in standing, and their exact physiologic significance remains obscure.

Tonic Neck Reflexes

If the head of a decerebrate animal is moved relative to the body, changes in the pattern of rigidity occur. If the head is turned to one side, the limbs on that side ("jaw limbs") become more rigidly extended while the contralateral limbs become less so. This is the position often assumed by a normal animal looking to one side. Flexion of the head causes flexion of the forelimbs and continued extension of the hindlimbs, the posture of an animal looking into a hole in the ground. Extension of the head causes flexion of the hindlimbs and extension of the forelimbs, the posture of an animal looking over an obstacle. These responses are the **tonic neck reflexes.** They are initiated by stretch of the proprioceptors in the upper part of the neck, and they can be sustained for long periods of time.

MIDBRAIN COMPONENTS

After section of the neural axis at the superior border of the midbrain (**midbrain animal**), extensor rigidity like that seen in the decerebrate animal is present only when the animal lies quietly on its back. In the decerebrate animal the rigidity, which is a static postural reflex, is prominent because there are no modifying phasic postural reflexes. Chronic midbrain preparations can rise to the standing position, walk, and right themselves. While the animals are engaged in these phasic activities, the static phenomenon of rigidity is not seen.

Righting Reflexes

All higher animals have righting reflexes that operate to maintain their normal standing position and keep their heads upright. These reflexes are a series of responses integrated for the most part in the nuclei of the midbrain.

When a midbrain animal is held by its body and tipped from side to side, the head stays level in response to the **labyrinthine righting reflexes.** The stimulus is tilting of the head, which stimulates the otolithic organs; the response is compensatory contraction of the neck muscles to keep the head level. If the animal is laid on its side, the pressure on that side of the body initiates reflex righting of the head even if the labyrinths have been destroyed. This is the **body on head righting reflex.** If the head is righted by either of these mechanisms and the body remains tilted, the neck muscles are stretched. Their contraction rights the thorax and initiates a wave of similar stretch reflexes which pass down the body, righting the abdomen and the hind quarters (**neck righting reflexes**). Pressure on the side of the body may cause body righting even if the head is prevented from righting (**body on body righting reflex**).

In cats, dogs, and primates, visual cues can initiate **optical righting reflexes** which right the animal in the absence of labyrinthine or body stimulation. Unlike the other righting reflexes, these responses depend upon an intact cerebral cortex.

Grasp Reflex

When a primate in which the brain tissue above the thalamus has been removed lies on its side, the limbs next to the supporting surface are extended. The upper limbs are flexed, and the hand on the upper side grasps firmly any object brought in contact with it (**grasp reflex**). This whole response is probably a supporting reaction that steadies the animal and aids in pulling him upright.

Other Midbrain Responses

Animals with intact midbrains show pupillary light reflexes if the optic nerves are also intact. Nystagmus, the reflex response to rotational acceleration described in Chapter 9, is also present. If a blindfolded animal is lowered rapidly, its forelegs extend and its toes spread. This response to linear acceleration is a **vestibular placing reaction** which prepares the animal to land on the floor.

CORTICAL COMPONENTS

Effects of Decortication

Removal of the cerebral cortex (**decortication**) produces little motor deficit in lower mammals. In primates the deficit is more severe, but a great deal of movement is still possible. Decorticate animals have all the reflex patterns of midbrain animals, and the responses generally are present in the immediate postoperative period whereas in midbrain preparations they take 2–3 weeks to appear. This suggests that centers between the top of the midbrain and the cerebral cortex facilitate brain stem reflexes. In addition, decorticate animals are easier to maintain than midbrain animals because temperature regulation and other visceral homeostatic mechanisms integrated in the hypothalamus (see Chapter 14) are present. The most striking defect is inability to react in terms of past experience. With certain special types of training, conditioned reflexes can be established in the absence of the cerebral cortex, but under normal laboratory conditions there is no evidence that learning or conditioning occurs.

Decorticate Rigidity

Moderate rigidity is present in the decorticate animal as a result of the loss of the cortical area that inhibits gamma efferent discharge via the reticular formation. Like the rigidity present after transection of the neural axis anywhere above the top of the midbrain, this **decorticate rigidity** is obscured by phasic postural reflexes and is only seen when the animal is at rest. Decorticate rigidity is seen on the hemiplegic side in humans after hemorrhages or thromboses in the internal capsule. Probably because of their anatomy, the small arteries in the internal capsule are especially prone to rupture or thrombotic obstruction, so this type of decorticate rigidity is common.

Suppressor Areas

The exact site of origin in the cerebral cortex of the fibers that inhibit stretch reflexes is a subject of debate. Under certain experimental conditions, stimulation of the anterior edge of the precentral gyrus is said to cause inhibition of stretch reflexes and cortically evoked movements. This region, which also projects to the basal ganglia, has been named area 4s, or the **suppressor strip.** Four other suppressor regions (Brodmann's areas 2, 8, 19, and 24) have also been described. However, the stimulation experiments on which the hypothesis of discrete suppressor areas is based have not been uniformly confirmed. Ablation of area 4s does cause spasticity in the trunk and proximal limb muscles of the contralateral side of the body, but destruction of the caudal part of area 4 produces spasticity in the distal limb muscles. Mapping experiments show that the musculature of the trunk and proximal portions of the limbs is represented in the anterior portion of the precentral gyrus, whereas that of the distal portions is represented posteriorly. It is therefore probable that the inhibitory fibers originate with the pyramidal fibers from all of the precentral motor area and that the distribution of the spasticity produced by lesions in this area depends upon the particular portion of the motor cortex destroyed.

Placing & Hopping Reactions

Two types of postural reactions are seriously disrupted by decortication, the **hopping** and **placing reactions**. The former are the hopping movements that keep the limbs in position to support the body when a standing animal is pushed laterally. The latter are the reactions that place the foot firmly on a supporting surface. They can be initiated in a blindfolded animal held suspended in the air by touching the supporting surface with any part of the foot. Similarly, when the snout or vibrissae of a suspended animal touch a table, the animal immediately places both forepaws on the table; and if one limb of a standing animal is pulled out from under it the limb is promptly replaced on the supporting surface. The vestibular placing reaction has already been mentioned. In cats, dogs, and primates, the limbs are extended to support the body when the animal is lowered toward a surface it can see. These various placing reactions are abolished on one side by unilateral decortication, but some of them reappear after subsequent removal of the other hemisphere. This casts doubt on the claim that they are entirely dependent upon an intact motor cortex, but this portion of the brain is certainly important in their regulation.

Table 12–3. The basal ganglia.

Lenticular nucleus	Caudate nucleus	Striatum (neostriatum)
	Putamen	
	Globus pallidus (pallidum)	

Subthalamic nucleus (body of Luys)
Substantia nigra
Red nucleus

BASAL GANGLIA

Anatomic Considerations

The term **basal ganglia** is generally applied to the **caudate nucleus, putamen,** and **globus pallidus**–the 3 large nuclear masses underlying the cortical mantle (Fig 12–9)–and the functionally related **subthalamic nucleus** (body of Luys), **substantia nigra,** and **red nucleus** on each side. Parts of the thalamus are intimately related to this system, but the claustrum and the amygdala probably are not properly included although they have been in some classifications. The caudate nucleus and the putamen are sometimes called the **striatum**; the putamen and the globus pallidus are sometimes called the **lenticular nucleus** (Table 12–3).

The interconnections of these nuclei are complex (Fig 12–10). On each side, the caudate nucleus projects

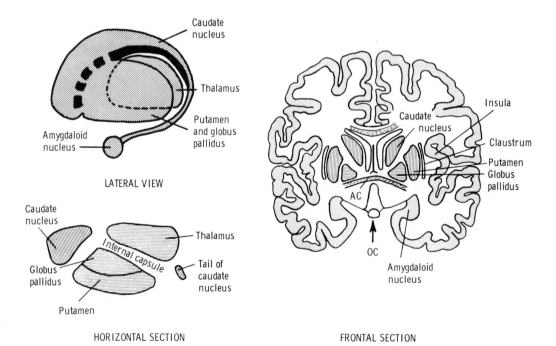

Figure 12–9. The basal ganglia. AC, anterior commissure; OC, optic chiasm.

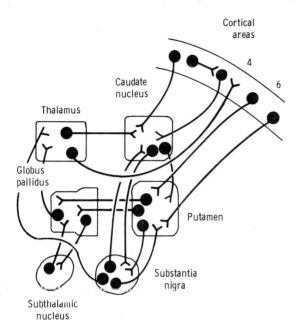

Figure 12—10. Some of the interconnections of the cerebral cortex and basal ganglia. (Modified from Carman: Anatomic basis of surgical treatment of Parkinson's disease. N Engl J Med 279:919, 1968. Courtesy of Little, Brown, Inc.)

in part to the putamen, the putamen to the globus pallidus, and the globus pallidus via the **ansa lenticularis,** the major efferent pathway from the lenticular nucleus, to the thalamus, subthalamic nuclei, red nuclei, and other structures. There is considerable evidence for a feedback circuit that projects from the motor cortex to the caudate nucleus and from there back to the cortex via the lenticular nucleus, the ansa lenticularis, and the ventrolateral nuclei of the thalamus. There is a prominent system of dopaminergic neurons that project from the substantia nigra to the striatum (nigrostriatal pathway; see Chapter 15). Cholinergic fibers also end in the striatum.

Metabolic Considerations

The metabolism of the basal ganglia is unique in a number of ways. These structures have an O_2 consumption per gram of tissue which in dogs exceeds that of the cerebral cortex (see Chapter 17). The copper content of the substantia nigra and the nearby locus ceruleus is particularly high. In Wilson's disease, a familial disorder of copper metabolism in which the plasma copper-binding protein, **ceruloplasmin,** is usually low, there is severe degeneration of the lenticular nucleus. However, the exact nature of the defect in copper metabolism in this disease is not known.

Function

The precise functions of the basal ganglia are an enigma. In birds, reptiles, and other animals in which the motor cortex is rudimentary or absent, these nuclear masses are prominent and take the place of a

motor cortex. Removal of the striatum and pallidum in decorticate animals does not produce any additional gross impairment in motor function. Stimulation studies in animals have generally produced negative results, although stimulation of the caudate nucleus inhibits stretch reflexes. This inhibition is probably mediated by activation of the cortical inhibitory areas through the thalamocortical feedback pathways. Stimulation of the globus pallidus and caudate nucleus also inhibits movements evoked by cortical stimulation. More recently, it has been shown that many neurons in the basal ganglia fire throughout slow, steady ramp movements and are silent during rapid saccadic movements. Like the motor cortex and the cerebellum, they begin to discharge before the movements begin. Thus, it appears that the basal ganglia are involved in the planning and programming of movement. The abnormalities in humans with basal ganglion disease also support this hypothesis.

Diseases of the Basal Ganglia in Humans

Disorders of movement associated with diseases of the basal ganglia in humans are of 2 general types: **hyperkinetic** and **hypokinetic.** The hyperkinetic conditions, those in which there is excessive and abnormal movement, include chorea, athetosis, and ballism. In Parkinson's disease, there are both hyperkinetic and hypokinetic features.

Hyperkinetic Disorders

Chorea is associated with degeneration of the caudate nucleus. It is characterized by rapid, involuntary "dancing" movements that may be a mixture of unrelated or conflicting cortical automatisms. **Athetosis** is due to lesions in the lenticular nucleus and is characterized by continuous slow, writhing movements that may be tonic avoiding or grasping reactions. In **ballism,** the involuntary movements are flailing, intense, and violent. They appear when the subthalamic nuclei are damaged, and a sudden onset of the movements on one side of the body **(hemiballism)** due to hemorrhage in the contralateral subthalamic nucleus is one of the most dramatic syndromes in clinical medicine.

Parkinson's Disease (Paralysis Agitans)

In the syndrome originally described by James Parkinson and named for him, there are pathologic changes in the nigrostriatal system of dopaminergic neurons. Parkinsonism was a common late complication of the type of influenza that was epidemic during World War I, and it occurs also in patients with cerebral arteriosclerosis. It is also seen as a complication of treatment with the phenothiazine group of tranquilizer drugs. These drugs block dopamine receptors. The hallmarks of parkinsonism are **akinesia** or **poverty of movement** (a hypokinetic feature) and the hyperkinetic features **rigidity** and **tremor.** The absence of motor activity can be quite striking. There is difficulty in initiating voluntary movements, and there is also a decrease in **associated movements,** the normal, unconscious movements such as swinging of the arms during walking, the panorama of facial expressions related to the emotional content of thought and speech, and the multiple "fidgety" actions and gestures that occur in all of us. The rigidity is different from spasticity because there is increased motor neuron discharge to both the agonist and antagonist muscles. Passive motion of an extremity meets with a plastic, dead-feeling resistance that has been likened to bending a lead pipe and is therefore called **lead-pipe rigidity**. Sometimes there is a series of "catches" during passive motion (**cogwheel rigidity**), but the sudden loss of resistance seen in a spastic extremity is absent. The tremor, which is present at rest and disappears with activity, is due to regular, alternating, 8/sec contractions of antagonistic muscles.

It has been difficult to reproduce parkinsonism by means of lesions in laboratory animals. An interesting feature of the syndrome in humans is the fact that even though it is due to lesions in parts of the basal ganglia, further destruction of these nuclei and other motor systems sometimes brings about clinical improvement. Ablation of the motor cortex, section of the cerebral peduncles, posterolateral spinal cordotomy, destruction of the medial part of the globus pallidus, interruption of the ansa lenticularis, and lesions of the ventrolateral nucleus of the thalamus produced by electrocoagulation or the injection of alcohol (chemopallidectomy, etc) have all been used to diminish the rigidity and the tremor. These treatments have been superseded by the use of L-dopa, which produces dramatic improvement in many patients. Dopamine appears to exert an inhibitory effect on striatal neurons, whereas acetylcholine is excitatory. Indeed, treatment with a drug that inhibits acetylcholinesterase produces tremor and rigidity in rats. Increasing the dopamine supply with L-dopa or decreasing the cholinergic influence with anticholinergic therapy restores the balance between the 2 systems in patients with Parkinson's disease (see Chapter 15).

Conclusion

The experimental and clinical data described above suggest that the basal ganglia function in some way in the programming of movement, in part by preventing oscillation and afterdischarge in motor systems. Except for these necessarily vague speculations, however, the functions of the basal ganglia remain unclear.

CEREBELLUM

The cerebellum is concerned primarily with the coordination, adjustment, and smoothing out of movement. It receives information from the motor areas of the cerebral cortex and afferent impulses from proprio-

ceptors, cutaneous tactile receptors, auditory receptors, visual receptors, and even visceral receptors. However, the exact way in which it functions in producing its effects on movement is unsettled.

ANATOMIC & FUNCTIONAL ORGANIZATION

Orientation

The cerebellum sits astride the main sensory and motor systems in the brain stem (Fig 12–11). It is connected to the brain stem on each side by a **superior peduncle** (brachium conjunctivum), **middle peduncle** (brachium pontis), and **inferior peduncle** (restiform body). The medial **vermis** and lateral **cerebellar hemispheres** are more extensively folded and fissured than the cerebral cortex; the cerebellum weighs only 10% as much as the cerebral cortex, but its surface area is about 75% of that of the cerebral cortex. There are 10 primary lobules in the vermis, numbered I–X from superior to inferior. These lobules are identified by name and number in Fig 12–12. Folia I–V and the corresponding portions of the hemispheres are sometimes called the **anterior lobe** of the cerebellum.

Afferent and Efferent Connections

The cerebellum has an external **cerebellar cortex** separated by white matter from deep **cerebellar nuclei**. Its afferent input goes to the cortex and, via collaterals, to the deep nuclei. The cortex projects to the deep nuclei, and the deep nuclei project on each side to the red nucleus, the ventrolateral nucleus of the thalamus, the vestibular nuclei, and the reticular formation.

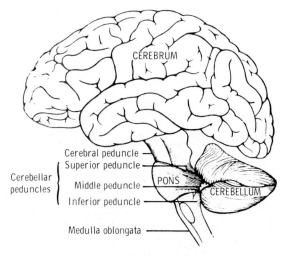

Figure 12–11. Diagrammatic representation of the principal parts of the brain. The parts are distorted to show the cerebellar peduncles and the way the cerebellum, pons, and middle peduncle form a napkin ring around the brain stem. (Reproduced, with permission, from: *Gray's Anatomy of the Human Body,* 27th ed. Goss CM [editor]. Lea & Febiger, 1959.)

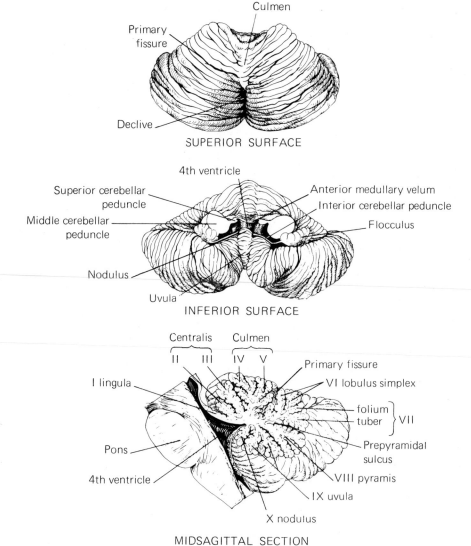

Figure 12—12. Superior and inferior views and sagittal section of the human cerebellum. The 10 principal lobules are identified by name and by number (I–X) on the basis of the comparative studies of the mammalian cerebellum by Larsell: The cerebellum of the cat and monkey. J Comp Neurol 99:135, 1953. (Modified from Chusid: *Correlative Neuroanatomy & Functional Neurology,* 16th ed. Lange, 1976.)

The afferent pathways to the cerebellum are summarized in Table 12–4. They transmit proprioceptive and sensory information from all parts of the body. One portion of the proprioceptive input is relayed via the inferior olive, and the olivocerebellar fibers form the excitatory climbing fiber input (see below). In addition, information is relayed to the cerebellum from all the motor areas in the cerebral cortex via the pontine nuclei.

The cerebellar cortex contains 3 layers (Fig 12–13): an external molecular layer, a Purkinje cell layer which is only 1 cell thick, and an internal granular layer. The Purkinje cells are among the biggest neurons in the body. They have very extensive den-

dritic arbors that extend throughout the molecular layer. Their axons, which are the only output from the cerebellar cortex, pass to the deep nuclei: the fastigial, globose, emboliform, and dentate nuclei. The **fastigial nucleus** receives axons from the vermis; the **globose** and **emboliform nuclei** and the **dentate nuclei** receive axons from the lateral portions of the hemispheres. The cerebellar cortex also contains **granule cells,** which receive input from the mossy fibers (see below) and innervate the Purkinje cells. The granule cells have their cell bodies in the granular layer. Each sends an axon to the molecular layer where the axon bifurcates to form a T. The branches of the T are straight and run long distances. Consequently, they are called **parallel**

Table 12—4. Function and major terminations of the principal afferent systems to the cerebellum.*

Afferent Tracts	Transmits	Distribution	Peduncle by Which Enters Cerebellum
Dorsal spinocerebellar	Proprioceptive and exteroceptive impulses from body	Folia I—VI, pyramis and para-median lobule	Inferior
Ventral spinocerebellar	Proprioceptive and exteroceptive impulses from body	Folia I—VI, pyramis and para-median lobule	Superior
Cuneocerebellar	Proprioceptive impulses, especially from head and neck	Folia I—VI, pyramis and para-median lobule	Inferior
Tectocerebellar	Auditory and visual impulses via inferior and superior colliculi	Folium, tuber, ansiform lobule	Superior
Vestibulocerebellar	Vestibular impulses from labyrinths direct and via vestibular nuclei	Principally flocculonodular lobe	Inferior
Pontocerebellar	Impulses from motor and other parts of cerebral cortex via pontine nuclei	All cerebellar cortex except flocculonodular lobe	Middle
Olivocerebellar	Proprioceptive input from whole body via relay in inferior olive	All cerebellar cortex and deep nuclei	Inferior

*Several other pathways transmit impulses from nuclei in the brain stem to the cerebellar cortex and to the deep nuclei.

fibers. The dendritic trees of the Purkinje cells are markedly flattened (Fig 12—13) and oriented at right angles to the parallel fibers. The parallel fibers thus make synaptic contact with the dendrites of many Purkinje cells, and the parallel fibers and Purkinje dendritic trees form a grid of remarkably regular proportions.

The other 3 types of neurons in the cerebellar cortex are in effect inhibitory interneurons. The **basket cells** (Fig 12—13) are located in the molecular layer.

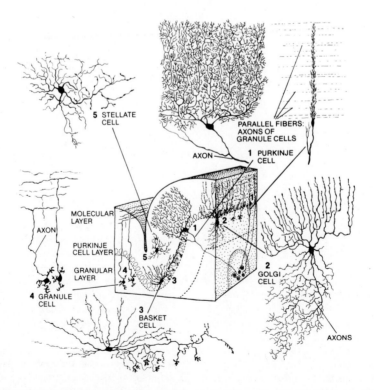

Figure 12—13. Location and structure of neurons in the cerebellar cortex. (Reproduced, with permission, from Kuffler & Nicholls: *From Neuron to Brain.* Sinauer Associates, 1976.)

They receive input from the parallel fibers, and each projects to many Purkinje cells. Their axons form a basket around the cell body and axon hillock of each Purkinje cell they innervate. The **stellate cells** are similar to the basket cells but more superficial in location. The **Golgi cells** are located in the granular layer. Their dendrites, which project into the molecular layer, receive input from the parallel fibers and their cell bodies receive input via collaterals from the incoming climbing fibers (see below) and the Purkinje cells. Their axons project to the dendrites of the granule cells.

There are 2 main sources of input to the cerebellar cortex: **climbing fibers** and **mossy fibers.** The climbing fibers come from the inferior olivary nuclei, and each projects to the primary dendrites of the Purkinje cell, around which it entwines like a climbing plant. The mossy fibers constitute most of the other incoming fibers. They end on the dendrites of granule cells in complex synaptic junctions called **glomeruli.** The glomeruli also contain the inhibitory endings of the Golgi cells mentioned above.

The fundamental circuits of the cerebellar cortex are thus relatively simple (Fig 12–14). Climbing fiber inputs exert a strong excitatory effect on single Purkinje cells, while mossy fiber inputs exert a weak excitatory effect on many Purkinje cells via the granule cells. The basket and stellate cells are also excited by granule cells via the parallel fibers, and their output inhibits Purkinje cell discharge. Golgi cells are excited by the mossy fiber collaterals, Purkinje cell collaterals,

and parallel fibers, and they inhibit transmission from mossy fibers to granule cells.

The output of the Purkinje cells is in turn inhibitory to the deep cerebellar nuclei. These nuclei also receive excitatory inputs via collaterals from the mossy and climbing fibers, and they may also receive other excitatory inputs. It is interesting, in view of their inhibitory Purkinje cell input, that the output of the deep cerebellar nuclei to the brain stem and thalamus is always excitatory. Thus, the entire cerebellar circuitry seems to be concerned solely with modulating, or possibly with timing, the excitatory output of the deep cerebellar nuclei to the brain stem and thalamus.

PHYSIOLOGY

Flocculonodular Lobe

The phylogenetically oldest part of the cerebellum, the **flocculonodular lobe,** consists of the central **nodule** and lateral **flocculus** on either side. Its connections are essentially all vestibular. Animals in which it has been destroyed walk in a staggering fashion on a broad base. They tend to fall and are reluctant to move without support. Similar defects are seen in children as the earliest signs of a midline cerebellar tumor called a medulloblastoma. This malignant tumor arises from cell rests in the nodule and early in its course produces damage that is generally localized to the flocculonodular lobe.

Motion Sickness

Selective ablation of the flocculonodular lobe in dogs abolishes the syndrome of **motion sickness,** whereas extensive lesions in other parts of the cerebellum and the rest of the brain fail to affect it. This "disease," an ubiquitous if minor complication of modern travel, is a consequence of excessive and repetitive labyrinthine stimulation due to the motion of a vehicle. In humans, it can of course be controlled by a number of antiemetic tranquilizing drugs without recourse to surgery.

Uvula & Paraflocculus

According to some authors, the uvula and paraflocculus are part of the cerebellar area coordinating movement. Although the uvula is a constant anatomic feature throughout the phylogenetic scale, the paraflocculus is variable in size. It is rudimentary or absent in humans and most terrestrial animals, but it is large in aquatic diving mammals. It may play some role in the extensive reflex adjustments necessary for diving.

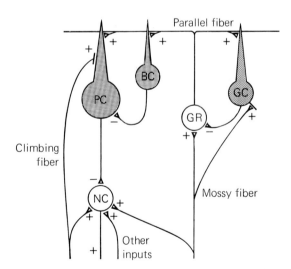

Figure 12–14. Diagram of neural connections in the cerebellum. Shaded neurons are inhibitory and + and − signs indicate whether endings are excitatory or inhibitory. BC, basket cell; GC, Golgi cell; GR, granule cell; NC, nuclear cell; PC, Purkinje cell. The connections of the stellate cells are similar to those of the basket cells, except that they end for the most part on Purkinje cell dendrites. (Modified from Eccles, Itoh, and Szentagóthai: *The Cerebellum as a Neuronal Machine.* Springer, 1967.)

Folium, Tuber, & Ansiform Lobules

Auditory and visual stimuli evoke electrical responses in the folium, tuber, and ansiform lobules, and often in the adjoining portion of the lobulus simplex. The size of this portion of the cerebellum parallels the growth of the cerebral cortex. It is very large in

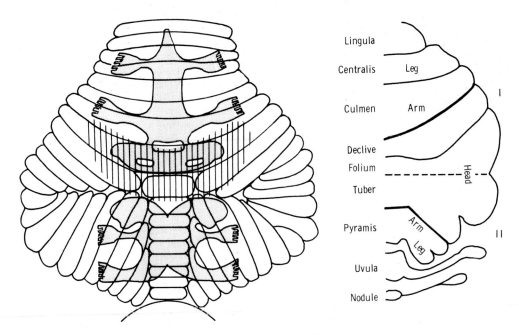

Figure 12–15. *Left:* Cerebellar homunculi. Proprioceptive and tactile stimuli are projected as shown in the figure above and the split figure below. The striped area represents the region from which evoked responses to auditory and visual stimuli are observed. (Redrawn and reproduced, with permission, from Snider: The cerebellum. Scientific American 199:84 [Aug], 1958. Copyright © 1958 by Scientific American, Inc. All rights reserved.) *Right:* Projection of the body on the cerebellum. Areas I and II (above and below the dashed line) are the 2 areas where auditory and visual stimuli are projected. (Redrawn and reproduced, with permission, from Hampson & others: Cerebro-cerebellar projections and the somatotopic localization of motor function in the cerebellum. Res Publ Assoc Res Nerv Ment Dis 30:299, 1950.)

primates, and the ansiform lobules make up a large part of the cerebellar hemispheres in man. The auditory and visual impulses reach the cerebellum via the tectocerebellar tract from the inferior and superior colliculi. Each stimulus causes a response in 2 areas: one in the tuber (area II in Fig 12–15) and another in the folium and adjacent areas (area I in Fig 12–15). The significance of this elaborate projection is far from clear. Stimulation of the region produces turning of the head and eyes to the ipsilateral side. Localized lesions of the region generally have little effect, although it has been reported that monkeys with such lesions crash into walls while running in spite of excellent vision and good coordination. Purkinje cells in folia VI and VII discharge in advance of eye movements, and the rate of discharge is inversely proportionate to the magnitude of the eye movement (Fig 12–16).

Folia I–VI, Pyramis, & Paramedian Lobules

The portions of the cerebellum that may be most concerned with the adjustment of posture and movement are folia I–VI of the vermis and their associated areas in the hemispheres, plus the pyramis and the paramedian lobules. These areas receive impulses from the motor cortex via the pons. They also receive proprioceptive input from the entire body, as well as tactile and other sensory impulses. In both the superior (folia I–VI) and inferior (paramedian) areas, there is a point-

for-point projection of peripheral sensory receptors, so that homunculi can be plotted on the cerebellar surface (Fig 12–15).

Effects on Stretch Reflexes

Stimulation of the cerebellar areas that receive proprioceptive input sometimes inhibits and sometimes facilitates movements evoked by stimulation of the cerebral cortex. In resting animals, cerebellar stimulation leads to changes in muscle tone through variations in the rate of gamma efferent discharge. Stretch reflexes are usually inhibited, especially if the site of stimulation is near the midline. However, more lateral stimuli may augment spasticity, and the response also varies with the parameters of stimulation. Lesions in folia I–VI and the paramedian areas in experimental animals cause spasticity localized to the part of the body that is represented in the part of the cerebellum destroyed. However, hypotonia is characteristic of cerebellar destruction in humans.

Effects on Movement

Except for the changes in stretch reflexes, animals with cerebellar lesions show no abnormalities as long as they are at rest. However, pronounced abnormalities are apparent when they move. There is no paralysis and no sensory deficit, but all movements are characterized by a marked **ataxia**, a defect defined as incoordination due to errors in the rate, range, force, and

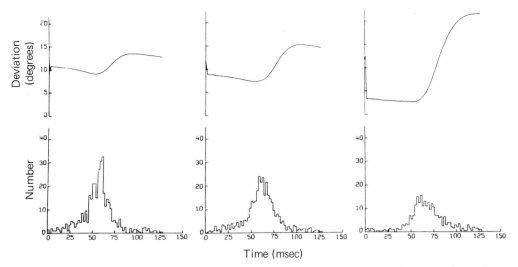

Figure 12–16. Relation between eye movement and discharge of a Purkinje cell. Deviation of the eyes of a monkey recorded in degrees on the top and the number of spikes per 2 msec from the Purkinje cell at the bottom. Note that the larger the saccadic eye movement, the smaller the number of spikes in the Purkinje cell before the movement started. (Reproduced, with permission, from Llinás R: Motor aspects of cerebellar control. Physiologist 17:19, 1974.)

direction of movement. With circumscribed lesions, the ataxia may be localized to one part of the body. If only the cortex of the cerebellum is involved, the movement abnormalities gradually disappear as **compensation** occurs. Lesions of the cerebellar nuclei produce more generalized defects, and the abnormalities are permanent.

Defects Produced by Cerebellar Lesions in Humans

The signs of cerebellar deficit in humans provide additional illustrations of the importance of the cerebellar mechanisms in the control of movement. The defects may be localized if the pathologic process is localized. Compensation for the effects of cortical lesions occurs, but compensation for the effects of lesions in the cerebellar nuclei does not occur. For this reason, care should be taken to avoid damaging the nuclei when surgical removal of parts of the cerebellum is necessary.

The hypotonia and the early symptoms of relatively selective destruction of the flocculonodular lobe have been mentioned above. The common denominator of most cerebellar signs is inappropriate rate, range, force, and direction of movement. Ataxia is manifest not only in the wide-based, unsteady, "drunken" gait of patients but also in defects of the skilled movements involved in the production of speech, so that slurred or **scanning speech** results. Other voluntary movements are also highly abnormal. For example, if the patient attempts to touch an object with his finger his motion toward the object overshoots to one side or the other. This **dysmetria** or **past-pointing** promptly initiates a gross corrective action, but the correction overshoots to the other side. Consequently, the finger oscillates back and forth, and the farther it travels the greater the excursions become. This oscillation is the

intention tremor of cerebellar disease. Unlike the resting tremor of parkinsonism, it is absent at rest; however, it appears whenever the patient attempts to perform some voluntary action. Another characteristic of cerebellar disease is inability to "put on the brakes," to stop movement promptly. For example, if a normal subject flexes his forearm against resistance and the resistance is suddenly released, movement of the limb is quickly checked. The patient with cerebellar disease cannot brake the movement, and the released forearm flies backward in a wide arc. This abnormal response is known as the **rebound phenomenon**, and similar impairment is detectable in other motor activities. This is one of the important reasons these patients show **adiadochokinesia**, the inability to perform rapidly alternating opposite movements such as repeated pronation and supination of the hands. Finally, patients with cerebellar disease have difficulty performing actions that involve simultaneous motion at more than one joint. They dissect such movements and carry them out one joint at a time, a phenomenon known as **decomposition of movement**.

Nature of Cerebellar Control

Movement depends not only on the coordinated activity of the muscles primarily responsible for the movement (**agonists** or **protagonists**) but also on that of **antagonistic** muscles, **synergistic** muscles, and muscles that anchor various parts of the body to form a base for movement (**fixation** muscles). Phasic reflex responses as well as skilled voluntary motion require a delicately adjusted interaction of all these muscles. Organizing this "cooperation in movement" has generally been regarded to be the function of the cerebellum.

In general terms, the motor cortex projects to the

cerebellum and the cerebellum in turn projects to the cerebral cortex via the ventrolateral nucleus of the thalamus. The basal ganglia, the cerebral cortex, and the cerebellum project to the skeletal muscles via the motor neurons of the spinal cord and the brain stem (Fig 12–5). The cerebral cortex and the cerebellum receive input from the sense organs. It now appears that the cerebellum functions in the regulation of movement both before and during movement. The lateral portions of the cerebellar cortex appear to be involved in the generation of rapid, ballistic movements (saccadic movements) and these movements, unlike slow ramp movements, are not subject to feedback control. Instead, the Purkinje cells discharge before the movement starts (Fig 12–16). Thus, the function of part of the cerebellar cortex may be to convert the energies needed for different movements into the requisite different durations of action potential trains to the motor neurons. This interesting concept—that the cerebellar cortex functions as a clock preprogramming the duration of fast movements—should stimulate additional research into the problem of how the cerebellum exerts its effects on movement.

The intermediate portion of the cerebellar cortex receives a massive input from proprioceptors throughout the body and appears to regulate movement that is under way. Thus, it functions as a feedback, stabilizing comparator circuit that, by continuous comparison of the motor program to the actual performance, adjusts motion so that it is smooth and precise (Fig 12–5).

The relation of the electrical events in the cerebellum to its function in motor control is another interesting problem. The cerebellar cortex has a basic, 150–300/sec, 200 μV electrical rhythm and, superimposed on this, a 1000–2000/sec component of smaller amplitude. The frequency of the basic rhythm is thus more than 10 times as great as that of the similarly recorded cerebral cortical EEG, and the amplitude is considerably less. Incoming stimuli generally alter the amplitude of the cerebellar rhythm, like a broadcast signal modulating a carrier frequency in radio transmission. However, the significance of these electrical phenomena in terms of cerebellar function is not known.

13...
Efferent Pathways to Visceral Effectors

The autonomic nervous system, like the somatic nervous system, is organized on the basis of the reflex arc. Impulses initiated in visceral receptors are relayed via afferent autonomic pathways to the CNS, integrated within it at various levels, and transmitted via efferent pathways to visceral effectors. This organization deserves emphasis because the functionally important afferent components have often been ignored. The visceral receptors and afferent pathways have been considered in Chapters 5 and 7, and the major autonomic effector, smooth muscle, in Chapter 3. The efferent pathways to the viscera are the subject of this chapter. Autonomic integration in the CNS is considered in Chapter 14.

ANATOMIC ORGANIZATION OF AUTONOMIC OUTFLOW

The peripheral motor portions of the autonomic nervous system are made up of **preganglionic and post-** ganglionic neurons (Figs 13–1 and 13–2). The cell bodies of the preganglionic neurons are located in the visceral efferent (lateral gray) column of the spinal cord or the homologous motor nuclei of the cranial nerves. Their axons are mostly myelinated, relatively slow-conducting B fibers. The axons synapse on the cell bodies of postganglionic neurons which are located in all cases outside the CNS. Each preganglionic axon diverges to an average of 8–9 postganglionic neurons. In this way, autonomic output is diffused. The axons of the postganglionic neurons, mostly unmyelinated C fibers, end on the visceral effectors.

Anatomically, the autonomic outflow is divided into 2 components: the **sympathetic** and **parasympathetic** divisions of the autonomic nervous system.

Sympathetic Division

The axons of the sympathetic preganglionic neurons leave the spinal cord with the ventral roots of the first thoracic to the third or fourth lumbar spinal nerves. They pass via the **white rami communicantes** to

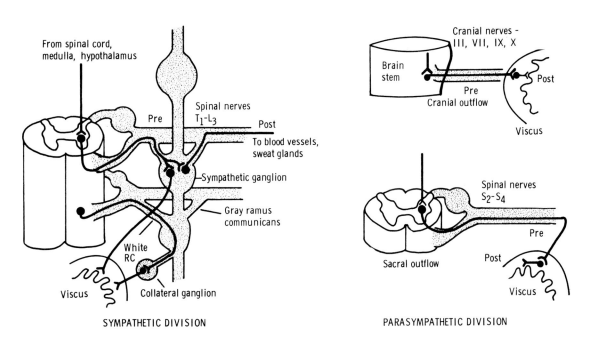

SYMPATHETIC DIVISION

PARASYMPATHETIC DIVISION

Figure 13–1. Autonomic nervous system. Pre, preganglionic neuron; Post, postganglionic neuron; RC, ramus communicans.

the **paravertebral sympathetic ganglion chain,** where most of them end on the cell bodies of the postganglionic neurons. The axons of some of the postganglionic neurons pass to the viscera in the various sympathetic nerves. Others reenter the spinal nerves via the **gray rami communicantes** from the chain ganglia and are distributed to autonomic effectors in the areas supplied by these spinal nerves. The postganglionic sympathetic nerves to the head originate in the **superior, middle,** and **stellate** ganglia in the cranial extension of

the sympathetic ganglion chain and travel to the effectors with the blood vessels. Some preganglionic neurons pass through the paravertebral ganglion chain and end on postganglionic neurons located in **collateral ganglia** close to the viscera. The myometrium of the uterus, unlike the rest of the organ, is innervated by a special system of **short adrenergic neurons** (not shown in Fig 13–2) with cell bodies in the uterus, and the preganglionic fibers to these postganglionic neurons presumably go all the way to the uterus.

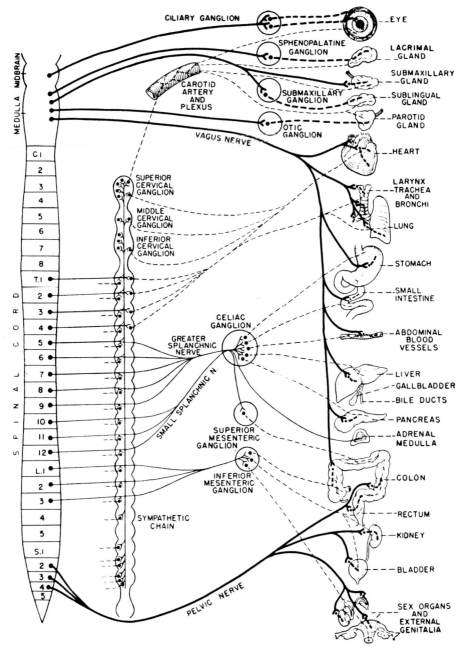

Figure 13–2. Diagram of the efferent autonomic pathways. Preganglionic neurons are shown as solid lines, postganglionic neurons as dashed lines. The heavy lines are parasympathetic fibers; the light lines are sympathetic. (Reproduced, with permission, from Youmans: *Fundamentals of Human Physiology,* 2nd ed. Year Book, 1962.)

Parasympathetic Division

The **cranial outflow** of the parasympathetic division supplies the visceral structures in the head via the oculomotor, facial, and glossopharyngeal nerves, and those in the thorax and upper abdomen via the vagus nerves. The **sacral outflow** supplies the pelvic viscera via the pelvic branches of the second to fourth sacral spinal nerves. The preganglionic fibers in both outflows end on short postganglionic neurons located on or near the visceral structures (Fig 13–2).

CHEMICAL TRANSMISSION AT AUTONOMIC JUNCTIONS

Transmission at the synaptic junctions between pre- and postganglionic neurons and between the postganglionic neurons and the autonomic effectors is chemically mediated. The principal transmitter agents involved are **acetylcholine** and **norepinephrine**.

Acetylcholine

The mediator liberated at all preganglionic endings and at anatomically parasympathetic postganglionic endings is acetylcholine. The biosynthesis and metabolism of this transmitter and its mechanism of action are described in detail in Chapter 4. It is stored in clear vesicles in the synaptic terminals of cholinergic neurons. It is released from the terminals by the nerve impulses. The secreted acetylcholine is in turn hydrolyzed. The enzyme responsible for the hydrolysis is acetylcholinesterase, and choline acetyltransferase catalyzes the synthesis of acetylcholine from choline and active acetate. There are a number of esterases in the body, including a pseudocholinesterase in plasma that is capable of hydrolyzing acetylcholine, but only acetylcholinesterase is found in high concentration in cholinergic nerve endings.

Although the same transmitter is released by preganglionic and by postganglionic cholinergic neurons, the properties of the receptors on which the acetylcholine acts are different in the 2 locations. Muscarine, the alkaloid responsible for the toxicity of toadstools, has little effect on autonomic ganglia but mimics the stimulatory action of acetylcholine on smooth muscle and glands. These actions of acetylcholine are therefore called **muscarinic actions**, and the receptors involved are **muscarinic receptors**. Muscarinic receptors are blocked by the drug atropine, and there is evidence that the effects of stimulating muscarinic receptors are mediated via intracellular liberation of cyclic GMP. In sympathetic ganglia, small amounts of acetylcholine stimulate postganglionic neurons and large amounts block transmission of impulses from pre- to postganglionic neurons. These actions are unaffected by atropine but mimicked by nicotine. Consequently, these actions of acetylcholine are **nicotinic actions** and the receptors are **nicotinic receptors**. The receptors in the motor end plates of skeletal muscle are

also nicotinic but are not identical to those in sympathetic ganglia since they respond differently to certain drugs.

Norepinephrine

The chemical transmitter at most sympathetic postganglionic endings is norepinephrine (levarterenol). It is stored in synaptic knobs of adrenergic neurons in characteristic vesicles that have a dense core (granulated vesicles). Norepinephrine and its methyl derivative, epinephrine, are secreted by the adrenal medulla, but epinephrine is not normally a mediator at postganglionic sympathetic endings.

The endings of sympathetic postganglionic neurons in smooth muscle are discussed in Chapter 4; each neuron has multiple varicosities along its course, and each of these varicosities appears to be a site at which norepinephrine is liberated. There are also norepinephrine-secreting, dopamine-secreting, and epinephrine-secreting neurons in the brain (see discussion in Chapter 15).

Biosynthesis & Release of Catecholamines

The principal **catecholamines** found in the body—norepinephrine, epinephrine, and dopamine—are formed by hydroxylation and decarboxylation of the amino acids phenylalanine and tyrosine (Fig 13–3). Phenylalanine hydroxylase is found in the liver. Tyrosine is transported into adrenergic nerve endings by a concentrating mechanism. It is converted to dopa and then to dopamine in the cytoplasm of the neurons by tyrosine hydroxylase and aromatic L-amino acid decarboxylase (dopa decarboxylase). The dopamine then enters the granulated vesicles, within which it is converted to norepinephrine by dopamine β-hydroxylase. L-Dopa is the isomer involved, and it is the L isomer of norepinephrine that is produced. The rate-limiting step in synthesis is the conversion of tyrosine to dopa. Tyrosine hydroxylase, which catalyzes this step, is subject to feedback inhibition by dopamine and norepinephrine, thus providing internal control of the synthetic process. The cofactor for tyrosine hydroxylase is tetrahydrobiopterin, which is converted to dihydrobiopterin when tyrosine is converted to dopa.

Synthesis of catecholamines in adrenal medullary cells is presumably similar to synthesis in neurons; however, unlike the postganglionic adrenergic endings, some of the granules in the adrenal medullary cells also contain the enzyme phenylethanolamine-N-methyltransferase (PNMT). This enzyme catalyzes the conversion of norepinephrine to epinephrine. In the granulated vesicles, norepinephrine and epinephrine are bound to ATP and a binding protein called chromogranin. The amines are held in the granulated vesicles by an active transport system, and the action of this transport system is inhibited by the drug reserpine.

Catecholamines are released from autonomic neurons and adrenal medullary cells by exocytosis (see Chapter 1). ATP, chromogranin, and dopamine β-hydroxylase are therefore released with norepinephrine and epinephrine in the same proportions as they exist

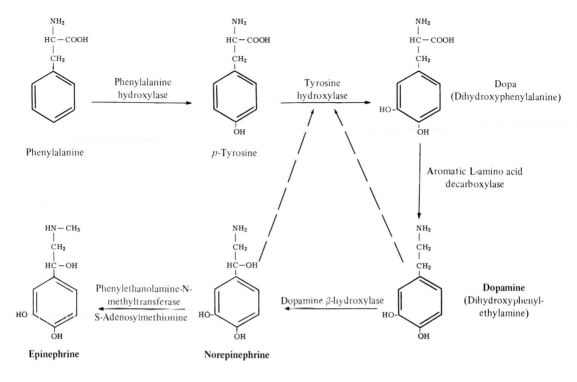

Figure 13—3. Biosynthesis of catecholamines.

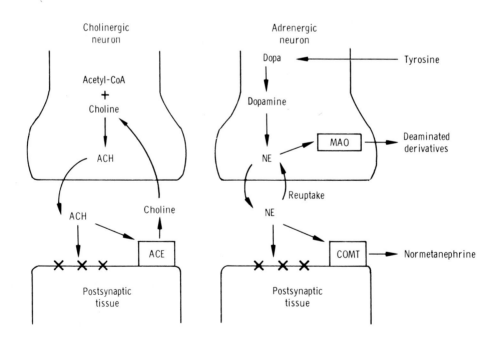

Figure 13—4. Comparison of the biochemical events at cholinergic endings with those at adrenergic endings. ACH, acetylcholine; ACE, acetylcholinesterase; NE, norepinephrine; X, receptor. Note that monoamine oxidase (MAO) is intracellular, so that some norepinephrine is being constantly deaminated in adrenergic endings. Catechol-O-methyltransferase (COMT) acts on norepinephrine after it is secreted.

in the granulated vesicles. Circulating levels of dopamine β-hydroxylase were originally thought to be a good index of sympathetic activity. However, the half-life of circulating dopamine β-hydroxylase is much longer than that of the catecholamines, and circulating levels are affected by genetic and other factors in addition to the rate of sympathetic activity.

Some of the norepinephrine in nerve endings is manufactured there, but some of it is also norepinephrine that has been secreted and then taken up again into the adrenergic neurons. An active **reuptake mechanism** is characteristic of adrenergic neurons. Circulating norepinephrine and epinephrine are also picked up in small amounts by adrenergic neurons in the autonomic nervous system. In this regard, adrenergic neurons differ from cholinergic neurons. Acetylcholine is not taken up to any appreciable degree, but the choline formed by the action of acetylcholinesterase is actively taken up and recycled (Fig 13–4).

The pathways involved in the metabolism of phenylalanine are of considerable clinical importance because they are the site of several **inborn errors of metabolism**, diseases caused by congenital absence of various specific enzymes. Each of these diseases is believed to be due to inheritance from both parents of a particular mutant gene which fails to perform its normal function of initiating the synthesis of a particular enzyme or enzyme subunit. **Phenylpyruvic oligophrenia**, a disorder characterized by severe mental deficiency and the accumulation in the blood and tissues of large amounts of phenylalanine and its keto acid derivatives, is due to congenital absence of phenylalanine hydroxylase (Fig 13–3). The mental deficiency must be secondary to the accumulation of phenylalanine derivatives; if the condition is diagnosed at birth and a low-phenylalanine diet is instituted immediately, the mental retardation is often at least partially prevented. There is evidence that high phenylalanine levels in the blood inhibit protein synthesis in the brain. There is also a deficiency of brain catecholamines and serotonin (see Chapter 15) in this disease, and some investigators believe that the serotonin deficiency is a major factor in the production of the mental abnormality. Ingested tyrosine presumably makes up for the deficiency in the formation of tyrosine from phenylalanine, but it appears that the formation of catecholamines from tyrosine is inhibited, possibly because tyrosine hydroxylase is inhibited by the excess phenylalanine.

Catabolism of Catecholamines

Epinephrine and norepinephrine are metabolized to biologically inactive products by oxidation and methylation. The former reaction is catalyzed by **monoamine oxidase (MAO)** and the latter by **catechol-O-methyltransferase (COMT)** (Figs 13–4, 13–5). MAO is found in the mitochondria. It is widely distributed, being particularly plentiful in the brain, liver, and kidneys, and large amounts are found in the mitochondria of the adrenergic nerve endings. COMT is also widely distributed, with high concentrations in the

liver and kidneys, but it is not found in adrenergic nerve endings. Consequently, there are 2 different patterns of catecholamine metabolism.

Circulating epinephrine and norepinephrine are for the most part O-methylated, and measurement of the O-methylated derivatives normetanephrine and metanephrine in the urine is a good index of the rate of secretion of norepinephrine and epinephrine. The O-methylated derivatives that are not excreted are largely oxidized, and VMA (Fig 13–5) is the most plentiful catecholamine metabolite in the urine.

In the adrenergic nerve endings, on the other hand, some of the norepinephrine is being constantly converted by MAO to the physiologically inactive deaminated derivatives 3,4-dihydroxymandelic acid and its corresponding glycol (Fig 13–4). These compounds enter the circulation and may subsequently be converted to their corresponding O-methyl derivatives.

The reuptake of released norepinephrine mentioned above is a major mechanism by which norepinephrine is removed from the vicinity of autonomic endings. The hypersensitivity of the sympathetically denervated structures (see Chapter 4) is probably explained in part on this basis. After the adrenergic neurons are cut, their endings degenerate; consequently, there is no reuptake, and more of a given dose of norepinephrine is available to stimulate the receptors of the autonomic effectors.

Chemical Divisions of the Autonomic Nervous System

On the basis of the chemical mediator released, the autonomic nervous system can be divided into cholinergic and adrenergic divisions. The neurons which are cholinergic are (1) all preganglionic neurons; (2) the anatomically parasympathetic postganglionic neurons; (3) the anatomically sympathetic postganglionic neurons which innervate sweat glands; and (4) the anatomically sympathetic neurons which end on blood vessels in skeletal muscles and produce vasodilatation when stimulated (sympathetic vasodilator nerves). The remaining postganglionic sympathetic neurons are adrenergic. The adrenal medulla is essentially a sympathetic ganglion in which the postganglionic cells have lost their axons and become specialized for secretion directly into the blood stream. The cholinergic preganglionic neurons to these cells have consequently become the secretomotor nerve supply of this gland.

Transmission in Sympathetic Ganglia

The responses produced in postganglionic neurons by stimulation of their preganglionic innervation include not only a rapid depolarization **(fast EPSP)** which generates action potentials (Fig 13–6) but also a prolonged inhibitory postsynaptic potential **(slow IPSP)** and a prolonged excitatory postsynaptic potential **(slow EPSP)**. These latter 2 responses apparently modulate and regulate transmission through the sympathetic ganglia. The initial depolarization is produced by acetylcholine via a nicotinic receptor. The slow IPSP is produced by dopamine, which appears to

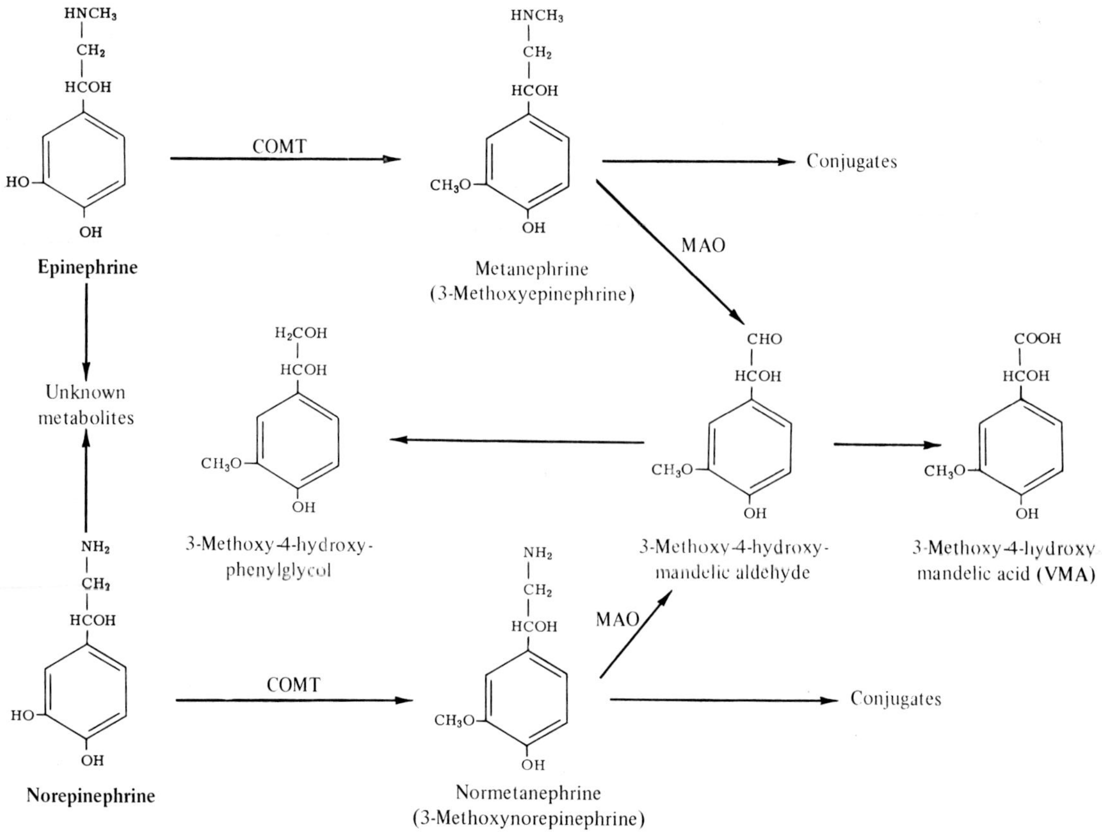

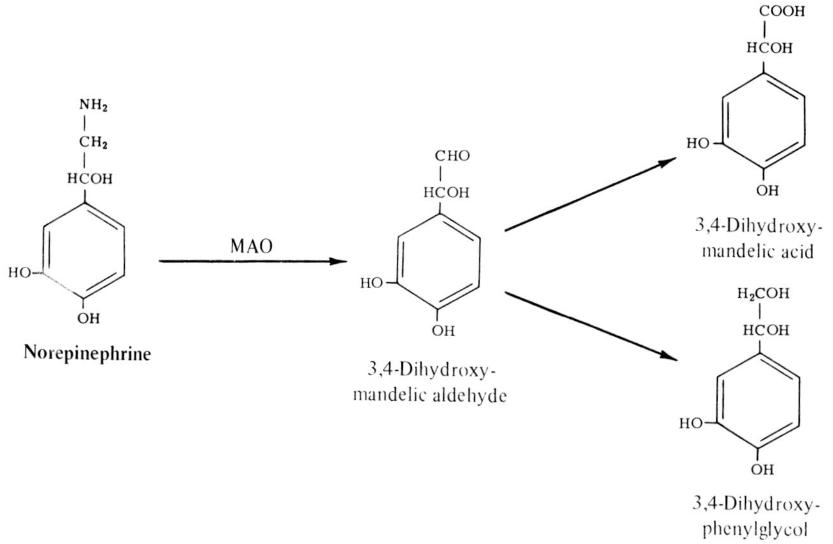

Figure 13–5. *Top:* Catabolism of circulating epinephrine and norepinephrine. The main site of catabolism is the liver. The conjugates are mostly glucuronides and sulfates. *Bottom:* Catabolism of norepinephrine in adrenergic nerve endings. The acid and the glycol enter the circulation, and may be subsequently O-methylated to VMA and 3-methoxy-4-hydroxyphenylglycol. MAO, monoamine oxidase; COMT, catechol-O-methyltransferase.

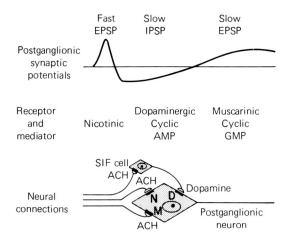

Figure 13—6. Synaptic potentials in postganglionic neurons. The neural connections are those presumed to underlie the potentials. ACH, acetylcholine; N, D, M, nicotinic, dopaminergic, and muscarinic receptors. The receptor on the SIF cell is muscarinic. (Modified from Greengard & Kebabian: Role of cyclic AMP in synaptic transmission in the mammalian peripheral nervous system. Fed Proc 33:1059, 1974.)

be secreted by an interneuron within the ganglion. The interneuron is excited by activation of a muscarinic receptor. Sympathetic ganglia are known to contain small, intensely fluorescent cells (**SIF cells**), and these cells are probably the dopaminergic interneurons. The slow EPSP is produced by acetylcholine acting on a muscarinic receptor on the membrane of the postganglionic neuron. There is evidence that the effects of activating the dopamine receptor are mediated intracellularly by cyclic AMP and that the effects of activating the muscarinic receptor are mediated via cyclic GMP.

RESPONSES OF EFFECTOR ORGANS TO AUTONOMIC NERVE IMPULSES

General Principles

The effects of stimulation of the adrenergic and cholinergic postganglionic nerve fibers to the viscera are listed in Table 13—1. The smooth muscle in the walls of the hollow viscera is generally innervated by both adrenergic and cholinergic fibers, and activity in one of these systems increases the intrinsic activity of the smooth muscle whereas activity in the other decreases it. However, there is no uniform rule about which system stimulates and which inhibits. In the case of sphincter muscles, both adrenergic and cholinergic innervations are excitatory, but one supplies the constrictor component of the sphincter and the other the dilator.

There is usually no acetylcholine in the circulating blood, and the effects of localized cholinergic discharge are generally discrete and of short duration because of the high concentration of acetylcholinesterase at cholinergic nerve endings. Norepinephrine spreads farther and has a more prolonged action than acetylcholine. Normal plasma contains about 300 pg of norepinephrine, 200 pg of dopamine, and 30 pg of epinephrine per ml. Some of this catecholamine titer is due to adrenal medullary secretion, but much of the norepinephrine is apparently liberated into the blood stream from adrenergic nerve endings.

Cholinergic Discharge

In a general way, the functions promoted by activity in the cholinergic division of the autonomic nervous system are those concerned with the vegetative aspects of day-to-day living. For example, cholinergic action favors digestion and absorption of food by increasing the activity of the intestinal musculature, increasing gastric secretion, and relaxing the pyloric sphincter. For this reason, and to contrast it with the "catabolic" adrenergic division, the cholinergic division is sometimes called the anabolic nervous system.

Adrenergic Discharge

The adrenergic division discharges as a unit in emergency situations. The effects of this discharge are of considerable value in preparing the individual to cope with the emergency, although it is important to avoid the teleologic fallacy involved in the statement that the system discharges in order to do this. For example, adrenergic discharge relaxes accommodation and dilates the pupil (letting more light into the eye), accelerates the heart beat and raises the blood pressure (providing better perfusion of the vital organs and muscles), and constricts the blood vessels of the skin (which limits bleeding if wounded). Adrenergic discharge also leads to lower thresholds in the reticular formation (reinforcing the alert, aroused state) and elevated blood glucose and free fatty acid levels (supplying more energy). On the basis of effects like these, Cannon called the emergency-induced discharge of the adrenergic nervous system the "preparation for flight or fight."

The emphasis on mass discharge in stressful situations should not obscure the fact that the adrenergic autonomic fibers also subserve other functions. For example, tonic adrenergic discharge to the arterioles maintains arterial pressure, and variations in this tonic discharge are the mechanism by which the carotid sinus feedback regulation of blood pressure is effected.

a & β Receptors

The effectors on which epinephrine and norepinephrine act can be separated into 2 categories on the basis of their different sensitivities to certain drugs. These differences are in turn due to the existence of 2 types of catecholamine receptors, the a and $β$ receptors, in the effector organs. The a receptors mediate vasoconstriction, whereas the $β$ receptors mediate such actions as increases in the cardiac rate and the strength of cardiac contraction. Beta receptors are now subdivided into 2 types: $β_1$ and $β_2$ re-

Table 13–1. Responses of effector organs to autonomic nerve impulses and circulating catecholamines.*

Effector Organs	Cholinergic Impulses Response	Receptor Type	Adrenergic Impulses Response
Eye			
Radial muscle of iris	. . .	a	Contraction (mydriasis)
Sphincter muscle of iris	Contraction (miosis)		. . .
Ciliary muscle	Contraction for near vision	β	Relaxation for far vision
Heart			
S-A node	Decrease in heart rate; vagal arrest	β†	Increase in heart rate
Atria	Decrease in contractility, and (usually) increase in conduction velocity	β†	Increase in contractility and conduction velocity
A-V node and conduction system	Decrease in conduction velocity; A-V block	β†	Increase in conduction velocity
Ventricles	. . .	β†	Increase in contractility, conduction velocity, automaticity, and rate of idiopathic pacemakers
Blood vessels			
Coronary	Dilatation	a	Constriction
		β	Dilatation
Skin and mucosa	. . .	a	Constriction
Skeletal muscle	Dilatation	a	Constriction
		β	Dilatation
Cerebral	. . .	a	Constriction (slight)
Pulmonary	. . .	a	Constriction
Abdominal viscera	. . .	a	Constriction
		β	Dilatation
Renal	. . .	a	Constriction
Salivary glands	Dilatation	a	Constriction
Lung			
Bronchial muscle	Contraction	β	Relaxation
Bronchial glands	Stimulation		Inhibition (?)
Stomach			
Motility and tone	Increase	β	Decrease (usually)
Sphincters	Relaxation (usually)	a	Contraction (usually)
Secretion	Stimulation		Inhibition (?)
Intestine			
Motility and tone	Increase	a, β	Decrease
Sphincters	Relaxation (usually)	a	Contraction (usually)
Secretion	Stimulation		Inhibition (?)
Gallbladder and ducts	Contraction		Relaxation
Urinary bladder			
Detrusor	Contraction	β	Relaxation (usually)
Trigone and sphincter	Relaxation	a	Contraction
Ureter			
Motility and tone	Increase (?)		Increase (usually)
Uterus	Variable‡	a, β	Variable‡
Male sex organs	Erection		Ejaculation
Skin			
Pilomotor muscles	. . .	a	Contraction
Sweat glands	Generalized secretion	a	Slight, localized secretion§
Spleen capsule	. . .	a	Contraction
Adrenal medulla	Secretion of epinephrine and norepinephrine		. . .
Liver	. . .	β	Glycogenolysis
Pancreas			
Acini	Secretion		. . .
Islets	Insulin secretion	a	Inhibition of insulin secretion
		β	Insulin secretion
Salivary glands	Profuse, watery secretion	a	Thick, viscous secretion
Lacrimal glands	Secretion		. . .
Nasopharyngeal glands	Secretion		. . .
Adipose tissue	. . .	β	Lipolysis
Juxtaglomerular cells	. . .	β	Renin secretion

*Modified from Goodman & Gilman: *The Pharmacological Basis of Therapeutics,* 5th ed. Macmillan, 1975.

†The β receptors of the heart have been classified as β_1 receptors and most other β receptors as β_2 receptors.

‡Depends on stage of menstrual cycle, amount of circulating estrogen and progesterone, and other factors. Responses of pregnant uterus different from those of nonpregnant.

§On palms of hands and in some other locations ("adrenergic sweating").

Table 13–2. Some drugs which affect sympathetic activity. Only the principal actions of the drugs are listed. Note that guanethidine is believed to have 2 principal actions.

Site of Action	Drugs Which Augment Sympathetic Activity	Drugs Which Depress Sympathetic Activity
Sympathetic ganglia	**Stimulate postganglionic neurons** Acetylcholine Nicotine Dimethphenylpiperazinium **Inhibit acetylcholinesterase** DFP (diisopropyl fluorophosphate) Physostigmine (eserine) Neostigmine (Prostigmin) Parathion	**Block conduction** Chlorisondamine (Ecolid) Hexamethonium (Bistrium, C-6) Mecamylamine (Inversine) Pentolinium (Ansolysen) Tetraethylammonium (Etamon, TEA) Trimethaphan (Arfonad) High concentrations of acetyl-choline, anticholinesterase drugs
Endings of postganglionic neurons	**Release norepinephrine** Tyramine Ephedrine Amphetamine	**Block norepinephrine synthesis** a-Methyl-p-tyrosine **Interfere with norepinephrine storage** Reserpine Guanethidine (Ismelin) **Prevent norepinephrine release** Bretylium tosylate (Darenthin) Guanethidine (Ismelin) **Form false transmitters** a-Methyldopa (Aldomet)
a receptors	**Stimulate a receptors** Norepinephrine (levarterenol; Levophed) Epinephrine Metaraminol (Aramine) Methoxamine (Vasoxyl) Phenylephrine (Neo-Synephrine)	**Block a receptors** Phenoxybenzamine (Dibenzyline) Phentolamine (Regitine) Ergot alkaloids
β receptors	**Stimulate β receptors** Isoproterenol (Isuprel) Epinephrine Norepinephrine	**Block β receptors** Dichloroisoproterenol Pronethalol Propranolol (Inderal)

ceptors. The β_1 receptors are the β receptors in the heart, whereas most other receptors are β_2 receptors. The effects of β receptor stimulation are brought about by activation of adenylate cyclase with a consequent increase in intracellular cyclic AMP. Evidence is available that suggests that in some locations, a receptor activation inhibits adenylate cyclase.

Autonomic Pharmacology

The junctions in the peripheral autonomic motor pathways are a logical point of attack for pharmacologic manipulation of visceral function because transmission across them is chemical. The transmitter agents are synthesized, stored in the nerve endings, and released near the neurons, muscle cells, or gland cells on which they act. They bind to receptors on these cells, thus initiating their characteristic actions, and they are then removed from the area by reuptake or metabolism. Each of these 5 steps can be stimulated or inhibited, with predictable consequences. In adrenergic endings, certain drugs also cause the formation of compounds which replace norepinephrine in the granules, and these weak or inactive "false transmitters" are released instead of norepinephrine by the action potentials reaching the endings.

Drugs with muscarinic actions include congeners of acetylcholine and drugs that inhibit acetylcholinesterase. Among the latter are diisopropyl fluorophosphate (DFP) and a number of other derivatives of the so-called nerve gases, which kill by producing massive inhibition of acetylcholinesterase. Atropine, scopolamine, and other natural and synthetic belladonna-like drugs block muscarinic receptors.

A list of some of the commonly used drugs which affect sympathetic activity and the mechanisms by which they produce their effects are summarized in Table 13–2. The drugs which block the effects of norepinephrine on visceral effectors are referred to as adrenergic blocking agents, peripheral sympathetic blocking agents, adrenolytic agents, or sympatholytic agents. Monoamine oxidase inhibitors increase the catecholamine content of the brain but do not affect circulating levels of these amines. When COMT is inhibited, there is a slight prolongation of the physiologic effects of catecholamines; but even when both MAO and COMT are inhibited, the metabolism of epinephrine and norepinephrine is still rapid. Presumably the catecholamines are being inactivated via the other pathways (Fig 13–5) that normally account for only a small portion of their metabolism.

14 ...
Neural Centers Regulating Visceral Function

The levels of autonomic integration within the CNS are arranged, like their somatic counterparts, in a hierarchy. Simple reflexes such as contraction of the full bladder are integrated in the spinal cord (see Chapter 12). The more complex reflexes that regulate respiration and blood pressure are integrated in the medulla oblongata. Those that control the pupillary responses to light and accommodation are integrated in the midbrain. The complex autonomic mechanisms that maintain the chemical constancy and temperature of the internal environment are integrated in the hypothalamus. The brain stem and diencephalic visceral regulatory centers are the subject of this chapter. The hypothalamus also functions with the limbic system as a unit that regulates emotional and instinctual behavior, and these aspects of hypothalamic function are discussed in the next chapter.

MEDULLA OBLONGATA

Control of Respiration, Heart Rate, & Blood Pressure

The medullary centers for the autonomic reflex control of the circulation, heart, and lungs are called the **vital centers** because damage to them is usually fatal. The afferent fibers to these centers originate in a number of instances in highly specialized visceral receptors. The specialized receptors include not only those of the carotid and aortic sinuses and bodies, but also receptor cells that are apparently located in the medulla itself. The motor responses are graded and delicately adjusted, and include somatic as well as visceral components. The details of the reflexes themselves are discussed in the chapters on the regulation of the circulation and respiration.

Other Medullary Autonomic Reflexes

Swallowing, coughing, sneezing, gagging, and vomiting are also reflex responses integrated in the medulla oblongata. The swallowing reflex is initiated by the voluntary act of propelling the oral contents toward the back of the pharynx. Coughing is initiated by irritation of the lining of the respiratory passages. The glottis closes and strong contraction of the respi-

ratory muscles builds up intrapulmonary pressure, whereupon the glottis suddenly opens, causing an explosive discharge of air. Sneezing is a somewhat similar response to irritation of the nasal epithelium. It is initiated by stimulation of pain fibers in the trigeminal nerves.

Vomiting

Vomiting is another example of the way visceral reflexes integrated in the medulla include coordinated and carefully timed somatic as well as visceral components. Vomiting starts with salivation and the sensation of nausea. The glottis closes, preventing aspiration of vomitus into the trachea. The breath is held in mid-inspiration. The muscles of the abdominal wall contract, and because the chest is held in a fixed position the contraction increases intra-abdominal pressure. The esophagus and gastric cardiac sphincter relax, reverse peristalsis begins, and the gastric contents are ejected.

The "vomiting center" in the reticular formation of the medulla at the level of the olivary nuclei controls these activities (Fig 14–1).

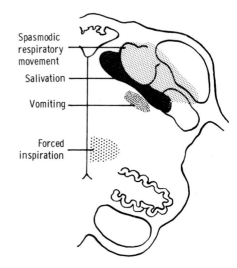

Figure 14–1. Cross-section of the medulla oblongata, showing approximate location of areas concerned with components of the vomiting reflex. (Reproduced, with permission, from: *Research in the Service of Medicine*, Vol 44. Searle & Co, 1956.)

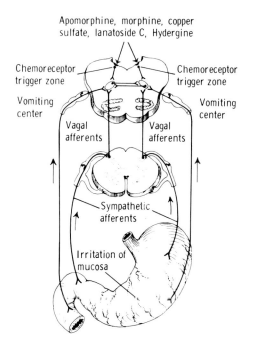

Figure 14—2. Afferent pathways for the vomiting reflex, showing the chemoreceptor trigger zone in the medulla. (Redrawn and reproduced, with permission, from: *Research in the Service of Medicine,* Vol 44. Searle & Co, 1956.)

Afferents

Irritation of the mucosa of the upper gastrointestinal tract causes vomiting. Impulses are relayed from the mucosa to the vomiting center over visceral afferent pathways in the sympathetic nerves and vagi. Other afferents presumably reach the vomiting center from the diencephalon and limbic system, because emetic responses to emotionally charged stimuli also occur. Thus, we speak of "nauseating smells" and "sickening sights."

It has been claimed that there are chemoreceptor cells in the medulla which initiate vomiting when they are stimulated by circulating chemical agents. The **chemoreceptor trigger zone** in which these cells are located (Fig 14–2) is in or near the **area postrema**, a V-shaped band of tissue on the lateral walls of the fourth ventricle near the obex. This region is known to be more permeable to many substances than the underlying medulla (see Chapter 17). Lesions of the area postrema have little effect on the vomiting response to gastrointestinal irritation but abolish the vomiting that follows injection of apomorphine and a number of other emetic drugs. Such lesions also decrease vomiting in uremia and radiation sickness, both of which may be associated with endogenous production of circulating emetic substances. A chemoreceptor mechanism stimulated by circulating toxins would explain vomiting in many clinical disorders.

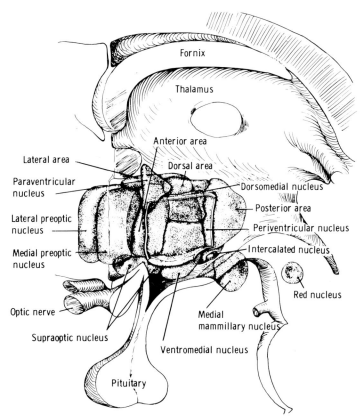

Figure 14—3. The human hypothalamus. (Redrawn from an original by Netter in Ciba Clinical Symposia. Copyright © 1956, Ciba Pharmaceutical Co. Reproduced with permission.)

HYPOTHALAMUS

ANATOMIC CONSIDERATIONS

The hypothalamus is that portion of the anterior end of the diencephalon that lies below the hypothalamic sulcus and in front of the interpeduncular nuclei. It is divided into the nuclei and nuclear areas shown in semidiagrammatic form in Fig 14–3. The supraoptic, the paraventricular, and, in some species, the ventromedial nuclei are clearly delineated, but most of the other nuclei and areas are rather ill-defined collections of small cells.

Relation to the Pituitary Gland

There are neural connections between the hypothalamus and the posterior lobe of the pituitary gland and vascular connections between the hypothalamus and the anterior lobe. The detailed anatomy of the pituitary and the adjacent ventral hypothalamus is shown in Fig 14–4. Embryologically, the posterior pituitary arises as an evagination of the floor of the third ventricle. In the adult it retains its essentially neural character. It receives an abundant supply of nerve fibers, the **hypothalamohypophysial tract**, from the supraoptic and paraventricular nuclei. Most of the supraoptic fibers end in the posterior lobe itself,

whereas many of the paraventricular fibers end in the pituitary stalk. The anterior and intermediate lobes of the pituitary arise in the embryo from Rathke's pouch, an evagination from the roof of the pharynx. Sympathetic nerve fibers reach the anterior lobe from its capsule, and parasympathetic fibers reach it from the petrosal nerves, but very few nerve fibers pass to it from the hypothalamus. However, the **portal hypophysial vessels** form a direct vascular link between the hypothalamus and the anterior pituitary. Arterial twigs from the carotid arteries and circle of Willis end in a network of fenestrated capillaries called the primary plexus on the ventral surface of the hypothalamus (Fig 14–4). Capillary loops also penetrate into the median eminence. The capillaries drain into sinusoidal vessels which carry blood down the pituitary stalk to the capillaries of the anterior pituitary. This system begins and ends in capillaries without going through the heart, and is therefore a true portal system. In birds and some mammals, including humans, there is no other anterior hypophysial arterial supply except capsular vessels and anastomotic connections from the capillaries of the posterior pituitary. In other mammals, some blood reaches the anterior lobe through a separate set of anterior hypophysial arteries; but in all vertebrates a large fraction of the anterior lobe blood supply is carried by the portal vessels. The **median eminence** is generally defined as the portion of the ventral hypothalamus from which the portal vessels arise. This region is "outside the blood-brain barrier" (see Chapter 17).

**Afferent & Efferent Connections
of the Hypothalamus**

The principal afferent and efferent neural pathways to and from the hypothalamus are listed in Table 14–1. Most of the fibers are unmyelinated. Many connect the hypothalamus to the limbic system. There are also important connections between the hypothalamus and a group of nuclei in the midbrain tegmentum. The hypothalamus thus represents, to use Nauta's term, a "nodal point" on the circuits that connect the limbic system and the "limbic midbrain area."

Norepinephrine-secreting neurons with their cell bodies in the hindbrain end in the supraoptic and paraventricular nuclei, the periventricular area, and the median eminence. A few neurons that appear to secrete epinephrine have their cell bodies in the hindbrain and end in the ventral hypothalamus. There is an intrahypothalamic system of dopamine-containing neurons which have their cell bodies in the arcuate nucleus and end on or near the capillaries that form the portal vessels in the median eminence (Fig 15–11).

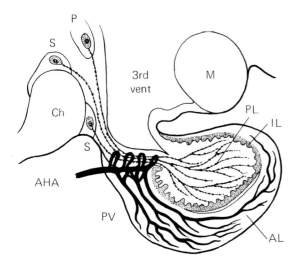

Figure 14–4. Diagram of the connections between the hypothalamus and pituitary in mammals. The capillary loops (primary plexus) in the median eminence of the hypothalamus drain into the portal hypophysial vessels. Ch, chiasm; S, supraoptic nucleus; AHA, anterior hypophysial artery; P, paraventricular nucleus; PV, portal vessels; M, mammillary body; 3rd vent, third ventricle; AL, anterior lobe; IL, intermediate lobe; PL, posterior lobe. (Based on a diagram by Ortman in: *Handbook of Physiology.* Field J, Magoun HW [editors]. Washington: The American Physiological Society, 1960. Section 1, pp 1039–1066.)

HYPOTHALAMIC FUNCTION

The major functions of the hypothalamus are summarized in Table 14–2. Some are fairly clear-cut

Table 14—1. Principal pathways to and from the hypothalamus.

Tract		Description
Medial forebrain bundle	A, E	Connects limbic lobe and midbrain via lateral hypothalamus, where fibers enter and leave it; includes direct amygdalohypothalamic fibers, which are sometimes referred to as a separate pathway.
Fornix	A	Connects hippocampus to hypothalamus, mostly mammillary bodies; some efferent fibers (?).
Stria terminalis	A	Connects amygdala to hypothalamus, especially ventromedial region.
Mammillary peduncle	A	Diverges from sensory pathways in midbrain to enter hypothalamus; may be the pathway by which sensory stimuli enter.
Ventral noradrenergic bundle	A	Noradrenergic neurons projecting from various hindbrain nuclei to ventral hypothalamus.
Dorsal noradrenergic bundle	A	Noradrenergic neurons projecting from locus ceruleus to dorsal hypothalamus.
Serotoninergic fibers	A	Serotonin-secreting fibers projecting from raphe nuclei to hypothalamus.
Epinephrinergic fibers	A	Epinephrine-secreting fibers from medulla to ventral hypothalamus.
Retinohypothalamic fibers	A	Optic nerve fibers to suprachiasmatic nuclei from optic chiasm.
Thalamohypothalamic and pallidohypothalamic fibers	A	Connections from thalamus and lenticular nucleus.
Periventricular system (including dorsal longitudinal fasciculus of Schütz)	A, E	Interconnects hypothalamus and midbrain; efferent projections to spinal cord, afferent from sensory pathways.
Mammillothalamic tract of Vicq d'Azyr	E	Connects mammillary nuclei to anterior thalamic nuclei.
Mammillotegmental tract	E	Connects hypothalamus with reticular portions of midbrain.
Hypothalamohypophysial tract (supraopticohypophysial and paraventriculohypophysial tracts)	E	Axons of neurons in supraoptic and paraventricular nuclei that end in pituitary stalk and posterior pituitary.

A = principally afferent; E = principally efferent.

Table 14—2. Summary of hypothalamic regulatory mechanisms.

Function	Afferents From	Integrating Areas
Temperature regulation	Cutaneous cold receptors; temperature-sensitive cells in hypothalamus	Anterior hypothalamus, response to heat; posterior hypothalamus, response to cold
Neuroendocrine control of:		
Catecholamines	Emotional stimuli, probably via limbic system	Dorsomedial and posterior hypothalamus
Vasopressin	Osmoreceptors, "volume receptors," others	Supraoptic and paraventricular nuclei
Oxytocin	Touch receptors in breast, uterus, genitalia	Supraoptic and paraventricular nuclei
Thyroid-stimulating hormone (TSH)	Temperature receptors, perhaps others (?)	Anterior median eminence and anterior hypothalamus
Adrenocorticotropic hormone (ACTH)	Limbic system (emotional stimuli); reticular formation ("systemic" stimuli); hypothalamic or anterior pituitary cells sensitive to circulating blood cortisol level; others (?)	Ventral hypothalamus
Follicle-stimulating hormone (FSH) and luteinizing hormone (LH)	Hypothalamic cells sensitive to estrogens; eyes, touch receptors in skin and genitalia of reflex ovulating species	Anterior hypothalamus, other areas
Prolactin	Touch receptors in breasts, other unknown receptors	Arcuate nucleus, median eminence (hypothalamus inhibits secretion)
Growth hormone	Unknown receptors	Anterior median eminence
"Appetitive" behavior		
Thirst	Osmoreceptors	Lateral superior hypothalamus
Hunger	"Glucostat" cells sensitive to rate of glucose utilization	Ventromedial satiety center, lateral hunger center, also limbic components
Sexual behavior	Cells sensitive to circulating estrogen and androgen, others	Anterior ventral hypothalamus, plus, in the male, piriform cortex
Defensive reactions		
Fear, rage	Sense organs and neocortex, paths unknown	Diffuse, in limbic system and hypothalamus
Control of various endocrine and activity rhythms	Retina via retinohypothalamic fibers	Suprachiasmatic nuclei

visceral reflexes, and others include complex behavioral and emotional reactions; but all involve a particular response to a particular stimulus. It is important to keep this pattern of stimulus-integration-response in mind in considering hypothalamic function.

RELATION OF HYPOTHALAMUS TO AUTONOMIC FUNCTION

Many years ago, Sherrington called the hypothalamus "the head ganglion of the autonomic system." Stimulation of the hypothalamus does produce autonomic responses, but there is little evidence that the hypothalamus is concerned with the regulation of visceral function per se. Rather, the autonomic responses triggered in the hypothalamus are part of more complex phenomena such as rage and other emotions.

"Parasympathetic Center"

Stimulation of the superior anterior hypothalamus occasionally causes contraction of the urinary bladder, a parasympathetic response. Largely on this basis, the statement is often made that there is a "parasympathetic center" in the anterior hypothalamus. However, bladder contraction can also be elicited by stimulation of other parts of the hypothalamus, and hypothalamic stimulation causes very few other parasympathetic responses. Thus, there is very little evidence that a localized "parasympathetic center" exists. Stimulation of the hypothalamus can cause cardiac arrhythmias, and there is reason to believe that these are due to simultaneous activation of vagal and sympathetic nerves to the heart.

Sympathetic Responses

Stimulation of various parts of the hypothalamus, especially the lateral areas, produces a rise in blood pressure, pupillary dilatation, piloerection, and other signs of diffuse adrenergic discharge. The stimuli which trigger this pattern of responses in the intact animal are not regulatory impulses from the viscera but emotional stimuli, especially rage and fear. Adrenergic responses are also triggered as part of the reactions which conserve heat (see below).

Low-voltage electrical stimulation of the mid-dorsal portion of the hypothalamus causes vasodilatation in muscle. Associated vasoconstriction in the skin and elsewhere maintains blood pressure at a fairly constant level. This observation and other evidence support the conclusion that the hypothalamus is a way station on the so-called cholinergic sympathetic vasodilator system that originates in the cerebral cortex. It may be this system which is responsible for the dilatation of muscle blood vessels that occurs at the start of exercise.

Stimulation of the dorsomedial nuclei and posterior hypothalamic areas produces increased secretion

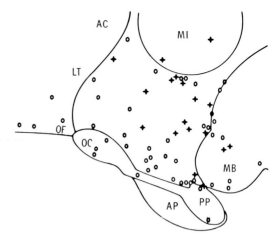

Figure 14–5. Points in the hypothalamus where low-intensity stimulation produces increased catecholamine secretion from the adrenal medulla of dogs. + = catecholamine output increased; 0 = catecholamine output unchanged. Points are projected on a midsagittal view of the hypothalamus. MI, massa intermedia; OC, optic chiasm; AP, anterior pituitary; PP, posterior pituitary; MB, mammillary body; OF, orbital surface of the frontal lobe; AC, anterior commissure; LT, lamina terminalis. (Reproduced, with permission, from Goldfien & Ganong: The adrenal medullary and adrenal cortical response to stimulation of the diencephalon. Am J Physiol 202:205, 1962.)

of epinephrine and norepinephrine from the adrenal medulla (Fig 14–5). Increased adrenal medullary secretion is one of the physical changes associated with rage and fear, and may occur when the cholinergic sympathetic vasodilator system is activated. It has been claimed that there are separate hypothalamic centers for the control of epinephrine and norepinephrine secretion. Differential secretion of one or the other of these adrenal medullary catecholamines does occur in certain physiologic situations, but the evidence for separate hypothalamic control centers is scanty and unconfirmed.

RELATION TO SLEEP

Lesions of the posterior hypothalamus cause prolonged sleep, and stimulation of the dorsal hypothalamus in conscious animals causes them to go to sleep. These observations have led to considerable speculation about the existence of "sleep centers" and "wakefulness centers" in the hypothalamus, but study of the functions of the RAS and nonspecific projection nuclei of the thalamus (see Chapter 11) has provided alternative explanations.

The posterior hypothalamic lesions that cause coma involve fibers of the RAS as they pass to the thalamus and cortex. The sleep-producing effects of posterior hypothalamic lesions are therefore probably explicable on the basis of damage to the RAS rather than destruction of a hypothetical hypothalamic "wakefulness center."

The hypothalamic loci where stimulation produces sleep are close to the nonspecific projection nuclei of the thalamus. The stimulating frequency that produces sleep is approximately 8/sec. Stimulation at greater frequencies arouses rather than depresses the animal. As noted in Chapter 11, stimulation of the thalamus, the orbital surface of the frontal lobe, and some parts of the brain stem at a frequency of 8/sec produces sleep. It therefore seems likely that the reported effects of hypothalamic stimulation are actually due to stimulation of a diffuse system, the slow frequency stimulation of which produces sleep. On the basis of these considerations, it seems unlikely that the hypothalamus plays any direct or unique role in the regulation of sleep.

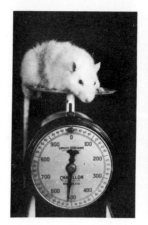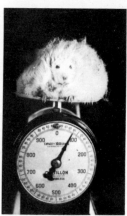

Figure 14–6. Hypothalamic obesity. The animal on the right, in which bilateral lesions have been placed in the ventromedial nuclei 4 months previously, weighs 1080 g. The control animal on the left weighs 520 g. (Reproduced, with permission, from Stevenson, in: *The Hypothalamus.* Haymaker W, Anderson E, Nauta WJH [editors]. Thomas, 1969.)

RELATION TO CYCLIC PHENOMENA

Lesions of the suprachiasmatic nuclei disrupt the circadian rhythm in the secretion of ACTH from the pituitary gland and melatonin from the pineal gland. In addition, these lesions interrupt estrous cycles and activity patterns in laboratory animals. The suprachiasmatic nuclei receive an important input from the eyes via the retinohypothalamic fibers, and it appears that they normally function to entrain various body rhythms to the 24-hour light-dark cycle. There is a prominent serotoninergic input from the raphe nuclei to the suprachiasmatic nuclei (see Chapter 15), but the exact relation of this input to the function of the latter is not known.

HUNGER

Feeding & Satiety Centers

Hypothalamic regulation of the appetite for food depends primarily upon the interaction of 2 areas: a lateral **"feeding center"** in the bed nucleus of the medial forebrain bundle at its junction with the pallidohypothalamic fibers, and a medial **"satiety center"** in the ventromedial nucleus. Stimulation of the feeding center evokes eating behavior in conscious animals, and its destruction causes severe, fatal anorexia in otherwise healthy animals. Stimulation of the ventromedial nucleus causes cessation of eating, whereas lesions in this region cause hyperphagia and, if the food supply is abundant, the syndrome of **hypothalamic obesity** (Fig 14–6). Destruction of the feeding center in rats with lesions of the satiety center causes anorexia, which indicates that the satiety center functions by inhibiting the feeding center (Fig 14–7). It appears that the feeding center is chronically active and that its activity is transiently inhibited by activity in the satiety center after the ingestion of food. However, it is not certain

that the feeding center and the satiety center simply control the desire for food. For example, rats with ventromedial lesions gain weight for a while, but their food intake then levels off. After their intake reaches a plateau, their appetite mechanism operates to maintain their new, higher weight. Thus, if they are made more obese by force feeding, their spontaneous food intake drops until their weight falls, and if they are starved their spontaneous intake increases until they regain the weight they had lost. One theory that has been advanced to explain these observations is that it is the setpoint for body weight rather than food intake per se which is regulated by the hypothalamic centers.

Afferent Mechanisms

There is considerable debate about the signals that are sensed by the satiety and feeding center to regulate food intake. The activity of the satiety center is probably governed in part by the level of glucose utilization of cells within the center. These cells have therefore been called **glucostats**. It has been postulated that when their glucose utilization is low—and consequently when the arteriovenous blood glucose difference across them is low—their activity is decreased. Under these conditions, the activity of the feeding center is unchecked, and the individual is hungry. When utilization is high, the activity of the glucostats is increased, the feeding center is inhibited, and the individual feels sated. This **glucostatic hypothesis** of appetite regulation is supported by an appreciable body of experimental data. Other factors undoubtedly affect appetite, but the glucostatic hypothesis has the merit of explaining the increased appetite in diabetes, in which the blood sugar is high but the glucose utilization of the cells is low because of the insulin deficiency. The objection has been raised that most neural tissue does not require insulin to metabolize glucose.

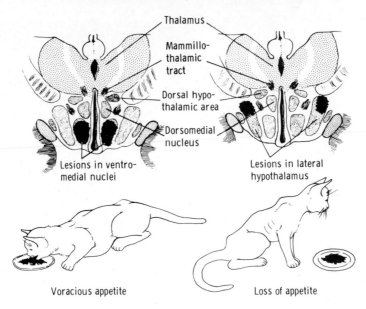

Figure 14–7. Diagrammatic summary of the effects of hypothalamic lesions on feeding. (Redrawn from an original by Netter in Ciba Clinical Symposia. Copyright © 1956, Ciba Pharmaceutical Co. Reproduced with permission.)

However, the region of the ventromedial nucleus has been shown to be different from the rest of the brain in that its rate of glucose utilization does vary with the amount of insulin in the circulation.

Relatively large amounts of radioactive glucose are taken up by cells of the ventromedial nuclei. This affinity for glucose probably explains why injections of gold thioglucose produce obesity in the mice. The ventromedial cells presumably take up the toxic gold-substituted glucose molecules, which destroy the cells and thus prevent inhibition of the lateral feeding center. Animals which have received gold thioglucose injections and have become obese have demonstrable lesions in the ventromedial nuclei.

The limbic system is also involved in the neural regulation of appetite. Lesions of the amygdaloid nuclei produce moderate hyperphagia. However, unlike animals with ventromedial hypothalamic lesions, animals with amygdaloid lesions will eat adulterated or tainted food. They are omniphagic and attempt to eat all sorts of objects (see Chapter 16). This suggests that fundamentally different mechanisms underlie the hyperphagia.

The ascending noradrenergic fibers in the ventral bundle (see Chapter 15) inhibit appetite, and discrete bilateral lesions in the bundle cause hyperphagia. However, the type of hyperphagia produced by such lesions differs from that produced by ventromedial lesions, and ventromedial lesions do not deplete hypothalamic norepinephrine. Amphetamine may exert its inhibitory effect on appetite by causing the release of norepinephrine from the terminals of the ascending noradrenergic fibers.

Other Factors Regulating Food Intake

There is some evidence that the size of body fat depots is sensed, by either neural or hormonal signals to the brain, and that appetite is controlled in this fashion (**lipostatic hypothesis**). A cold environment stimulates and a hot environment depresses appetite. Distention of the gastrointestinal tract inhibits and contractions of the empty stomach (**hunger contractions**) stimulate appetite, but denervation of the stomach and intestines does not affect the amount of food eaten. In animals with esophageal fistulas, chewing and swallowing food does cause some satiety even though the food never reaches the stomach. Especially in humans, cultural factors, environment, and past experiences relative to the sight, smell, and taste of food also affect food intake.

The net effect of all the appetite-regulating mechanisms in normal adult animals and humans is an adjustment of food intake to the point where caloric intake balances energy expenditures, with the result that body weight is maintained. In hyperthyroidism and diabetes mellitus, hunger increases as energy output increases. However, the link between energy needs and food intake is indirect, and in some situations intake is not correlated with immediate energy expenditure. For example, during growth, after exercise, and during recovery from debilitating illnesses, food intake is increased. How these long-term adjustments are brought about is not known.

THIRST

Another appetitive mechanism that is under hypothalamic control is thirst. Appropriately placed hypothalamic lesions diminish or abolish fluid intake, in some instances without any change in food intake,

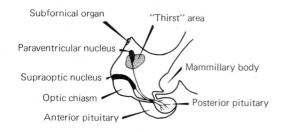

Figure 14—8. Hypothalamic areas concerned with water metabolism in dogs.

and electrical stimulation of the hypothalamus causes drinking. In the rat the area concerned with thirst is in the lateral hypothalamus posterior to the feeding center; in dogs and goats it is in the dorsal hypothalamus lateral and posterior to the paraventricular nuclei (Fig 14—8).

Drinking is increased by increased effective osmotic pressure of the plasma, by decreases in ECF volume, and by psychologic and other factors. Injection of hypertonic saline into the anterior hypothalamus causes drinking in conscious animals. This observation suggests that in the hypothalamus there are **osmoreceptors,** cells that are stimulated by an increased osmotic pressure of the body fluids to initiate thirst and drinking.

Decreases in ECF volume also stimulate thirst, and hemorrhage causes increased drinking even though there is no change in the osmolality of the plasma. The effect of ECF volume depletion on thirst is mediated in part via the renin-angiotensin system. Renin secretion is increased by hypovolemia, and there is a resultant increase in circulating angiotensin II. The angiotensin II acts on the **subfornical organ,** a specialized receptor area situated in the diencephalon (Fig 14—8), to stimulate the neural areas concerned with thirst. The subfornical area is highly permeable, and is one of the circumventricular organs located "outside the blood-brain barrier" (see Chapter 17). The link from the subfornical organ to the neural areas is apparently cholinergic. Drugs which block the action of angiotensin II do not completely block the thirst response to hypovolemia, and it appears that afferents from the thoracic venous and arterial baroreceptors are also involved.

Whenever the sensation of thirst is obtunded, either by direct damage to the diencephalon or by depressed or altered states of consciousness, patients stop drinking adequate amounts of fluid. Dehydration results if appropriate measures are not instituted to maintain water balance. If the protein intake is high, the products of protein metabolism cause an osmotic diuresis, and the amounts of water required to maintain balance are large. Most cases of hypernatremia are actually due to simple dehydration in patients with psychoses or cerebral disease who do not or cannot increase their water intake when their thirst mechanism is stimulated.

Other Factors Regulating Water Intake

A number of other well-established factors contribute to the regulation of water intake. Psychologic and social factors are important. Dryness of the pharyngeal mucous membrane causes a sensation of thirst. Patients in whom fluid intake must be restricted sometimes get appreciable relief of thirst by sucking ice chips or a wet cloth. Rats with lesions in their thirst areas will drink small amounts of water when their throats become dry even though they do not respond to dehydration per se.

Dehydrated dogs, cats, camels, and some other animals rapidly drink just enough water to make up their water deficit. They stop drinking before the water is absorbed (while their plasma is still hypertonic), so some kind of pharyngeal or gastrointestinal "metering" must be involved. In humans, this ability to drink just the right amount of water is not so well developed, and deficits are usually made up more slowly.

CONTROL OF POSTERIOR PITUITARY SECRETION

Posterior Pituitary Hormones

The 2 hormones of the posterior pituitary gland are synthesized in the cell bodies of neurons in the supraoptic and paraventricular nuclei and transported down their axons to the posterior pituitary. In all mammals studied except members of the pig family, the hormones are **oxytocin** and **arginine vasopressin.** In pigs and hippopotamuses, arginine in the vasopressin molecule is replaced by lysine to form **lysine vasopressin.** The posterior pituitaries of some African warthogs and peccaries contain a mixture of arginine and lysine vasopressin. The posterior lobe hormones are nonapeptides (considering each half cystine as a single amino acid) with a disulfide ring at one end (Fig 14—9).

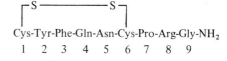

Figure 14—9. Arginine vasopressin and oxytocin. In pigs and hippopotamuses, lysine is substituted for arginine in position 8 of the vasopressin molecule.

Synthetic peptides more active than the naturally occurring substances have been produced by altering the amino acid residues.

In the posterior pituitary, oxytocin and vasopressin are stored bound to polypeptides called **neurophysins.** There is one neurophysin for oxytocin and another for vasopressin. The storage granules contain oxytocin or vasopressin, ATP, and neurophysin. Release is by exocytosis, and when the posterior lobe is stimulated, all 3 are secreted. Consequently, neurophysins are present in the peripheral blood, where they can be measured by immunoassay.

Effects of Vasopressin

Because its principal physiologic effect is the retention of water by the kidney, vasopressin is often called the antidiuretic hormone (ADH). It increases the permeability of the collecting ducts of the kidney, so that water enters the hypertonic interstitium of the renal pyramids. The urine becomes concentrated and its volume decreases. The overall effect is therefore retention of water in excess of solute; consequently, the effective osmotic pressure of the body fluids is decreased. In the absence of vasopressin, the urine is hypotonic to plasma, urine volume is increased, and there is a net water loss. Consequently, the osmolality of the body fluids rises. Vasopressin also increases the permeability of the collecting ducts to urea and decreases blood flow in the renal medulla. In addition, it increases the permeability of the bladder of toads and the skin of frogs to water.

In large doses, vasopressin elevates arterial blood pressure by an action on the smooth muscle of the arterioles. However, it is doubtful if enough endogenous vasopressin is ever secreted to exert any appreciable effect on blood pressure homeostasis. Hemorrhage is a potent stimulus to vasopressin secretion, but the blood pressure fall after hemorrhage is not significantly greater or more prolonged in the absence of the posterior pituitary than when it is present.

Circulating vasopressin is rapidly inactivated, principally in the liver and kidneys. It has a **biologic half-life** (time required for inactivation of half a given amount) of about 18 minutes in humans. Its effects on the kidney develop rapidly but are of short duration.

Mechanism of Action

Vasopressin acts by increasing intracellular cyclic adenosine-3′,5′-monophosphate (cyclic AMP) in the cells of the collecting ducts. The cyclic AMP then acts in some undefined way to increase the permeability of the renal epithelium. There is evidence that many other hormones also exert their effects by increasing cyclic AMP in their target organs.

Control of Vasopressin Secretion: Osmotic Stimuli

Vasopressin is stored in the posterior pituitary and released into the blood stream by impulses in the nerve fibers that contain the hormone. There are cell bodies of vasopressin-secreting neurons in both the

Table 14–3. Summary of stimuli affecting vasopressin secretion.

Vasopressin Secretion Increased	Vasopressin Secretion Decreased
Increased effective osmotic pressure of plasma	Decreased effective osmotic pressure of plasma
Decreased extracellular fluid volume	Increased extracellular fluid volume
Morphine, nicotine, barbiturates	Alcohol
Pain, emotion, "stress," exercise	

supraoptic and paraventricular nuclei. When the effective osmotic pressure of the plasma is increased, the rate of discharge of these neurons increases; when the effective osmotic pressure is decreased, supraoptic discharge is inhibited (Table 14–3, Fig 14–10). The changes are mediated via **osmoreceptor** cells sensitive to changes in the osmotic pressure of the plasma. These cells are located in the anterior hypothalamus. They may be the supraoptic and paraventricular neurons themselves, but they are more likely separate cells located in the perinuclear zone. It is not known if they are the same osmoreceptors that regulate water intake (see above).

Vasopressin secretion is thus controlled by a delicate feedback mechanism that operates continuously to defend the osmolality of the plasma. There is a steady, moderate level of vasopressin secretion when the plasma osmolality is normal, and the normal plasma vasopressin level is maintained at about 2 pg/ml (Fig 14–11). Whenever the effective osmotic pressure of plasma is increased, vasopressin secretion is increased; whenever plasma osmolality is decreased, vasopressin secretion is decreased. Significant changes in secretion occur when osmolality is changed as little as 2%. In this way, the osmolality of the plasma in normal individuals is maintained very close to 290 mOsm/liter.

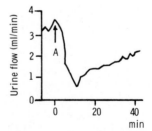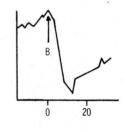

Figure 14–10. Inhibition of water diuresis in a dog by injection of 10.5 ml of 1.5% NaCl (at A) and 11 ml of 1.5% NaCl (at B) into the carotid artery. (Redrawn and reproduced, with permission, from Verney: The antidiuretic hormone and the factors which determine its release. Proc R Soc Lond [Biol] 135:25, 1947.)

Volume Effects

ECF volume also affects vasopressin secretion. Vasopressin secretion is increased when ECF volume is low and decreased when ECF volume is high (Table 14–3). There is an inverse relationship between the rate of vasopressin secretion and the rate of discharge in afferents from stretch receptors in the low and high pressure portions of the vascular system. The low pressure receptors are those in the great veins, right and left atria, and pulmonary vessels; the high pressure receptors are those in the carotid sinuses and aortic arch. The low pressure receptors monitor the fullness of the vascular system. Moderate decreases in ECF volume and, consequently, in blood volume increase vasopressin secretion without causing any change in the arterial blood pressure; it therefore appears that the low pressure receptors are the primary mediators of volume effects on vasopressin secretion. However, when the volume changes are large enough to produce changes in blood pressure, the carotid and aortic receptors also play a role. It has also been established that angiotensin II acts on the brain to increase the secretion of vasopressin.

There is a statistically significant increase in vasopressin secretion upon rising from the recumbent to the upright position (Fig 14–11) because blood pools in the legs. Hemorrhage causes a greater response. It releases much greater amounts of vasopressin than plasma hyperosmolality, and hypovolemia causes vasopressin secretion even if the plasma is hypotonic.

Other Stimuli Affecting Vasopressin Secretion

A variety of stimuli in addition to osmotic pressure changes and ECF volume aberrations increase vasopressin secretion. These include pain, surgical stress, some emotions, and a number of drugs, including morphine, nicotine, and large doses of barbiturates. Alcohol decreases vasopressin secretion.

Clinical Implications

In various clinical conditions, volume and other nonosmotic stimuli override the osmotic control of vasopressin secretion, producing water retention and a decrease in plasma osmolality. In patients with such hypersecretion, a high fluid intake can cause water intoxication. The water retention and hyponatremia seen after surgery are partly explained on this basis. Water retention occurs in addition to salt retention in patients with edema due to congestive heart failure, cirrhosis of the liver, and nephrosis. It has been argued that the water retention is due to diminished removal of vasopressin from the plasma by the liver and kidney, prolonging the half-life of the hormone. This may be a factor, but water retention does not occur unless there is abnormal posterior pituitary secretion as well. If the osmoreceptor mechanism were normal, the decreased plasma osmolality would inhibit posterior pituitary secretion and the defect would correct itself. The cause of excess vasopressin secretion in diseases of the heart, liver, and kidneys is not known with certainty, but it is probably due to abnormal activity of the "volume-sensing" mechanism described above.

An "inappropriate" hypersecretion of vasopressin is believed to be responsible for the hyponatremia which occurs with high levels of salt excretion in some patients with cerebral or pulmonary disease. In these cases of "cerebral salt wasting" and "pulmonary salt wasting," water retention is sufficient to expand ECF volume. This inhibits the secretion of aldosterone by the adrenal cortex, and salt is lost in the urine. The syndrome is different from that seen in patients with edema because the latter retain salt and usually have a high level of aldosterone secretion. Hypersecretion of vasopressin in patients with pulmonary diseases such as lung cancer may be due in part to the interruption of inhibitory impulses in vagal afferents from the stretch receptors in the atria and great veins. However, it has been demonstrated that some lung tumors and other malignancies can secrete a substance with antidiuretic activity.

Diabetes insipidus is the syndrome that results when vasopressin deficiency develops due to disease processes in the supraoptic and paraventricular nuclei, the hypothalamohypophysial tract, or the posterior pituitary gland. It also develops after surgical removal of the posterior lobe of the pituitary. It may be temporary if only the distal ends of the supraoptic and paraventricular fibers are damaged, because the fibers recover and begin again to secrete vasopressin. The

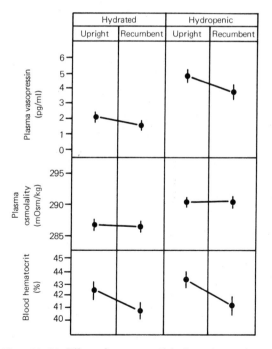

Figure 14–11. Effect of posture and hydropenia on plasma vasopressin in normal humans. Hydrated subjects drank fluids ad libitum. Hydropenic subjects had been deprived of fluids for 17–25 hours. (Modified from Robertson & Athar: The interaction of blood osmolality and blood volume in regulating plasma vasopressin in man. J Clin Endocrinol Metab 42:613, 1976.)

symptoms are passage of large amounts of dilute urine (**polyuria**) and the drinking of large amounts of fluid (**polydipsia**), provided the thirst mechanism is intact. It is the polydipsia that keeps these patients healthy. If their sense of thirst is depressed for any reason and their intake of dilute fluid decreases, they develop dehydration that can be fatal. The amelioration of diabetes insipidus produced by the development of concomitant anterior pituitary insufficiency is due to a decrease in the osmotic load presented to the kidneys for excretion.

Oxytocin

In mammals the principal physiologic effect of oxytocin is on the **myoepithelial cells,** smooth muscle-like cells that line the ducts of the breast. The hormone makes these cells contract, squeezing milk out of the alveoli of the lactating breast into the large ducts (sinuses), and thence out of the nipple **(milk ejection).** Many hormones acting in concert are responsible for breast growth and the secretion of milk into the ducts, but milk ejection in most species requires oxytocin.

The Milk Ejection Reflex

Milk ejection is normally initiated by a neuroendocrine reflex. The receptors involved are the touch receptors, which are plentiful in the breast—especially around the nipple. Impulses generated in these receptors are relayed from the somatic touch pathways via the bundle of Schütz and mammillary peduncle to the supraoptic and paraventricular nuclei. Discharge of the oxytocin-containing neurons causes liberation of oxytocin from the posterior pituitary. The infant suckling at the breast stimulates the touch receptors, the nuclei are stimulated, oxytocin is released, and the milk is expressed into the sinuses, ready to flow into the mouth of the waiting infant. In lactating women, genital stimulation and emotional stimuli also produce oxytocin secretion, sometimes causing milk to spurt from the breast.

Other Actions of Oxytocin

Oxytocin causes contraction of the smooth muscle of the uterus. The sensitivity of the uterine musculature to oxytocin varies. It is enhanced by estrogen and inhibited by progesterone. In late pregnancy, the uterus becomes very sensitive to oxytocin, and oxytocin secretion is increased during labor. After dilatation of the cervix, descent of the fetus down the birth canal probably initiates impulses in the afferent nerves which are relayed to the supraoptic and paraventricular nuclei, causing secretion of sufficient oxytocin to enhance labor. Oxytocin may also play some role in initiating labor. However, the mechanisms controlling the onset of labor are immensely complex, and neuroendocrine reflexes are certainly not the only mechanisms responsible for delivery.

Oxytocin may also act on the nonpregnant uterus to facilitate sperm transport. The passage of sperm up the female genital tract to the fallopian tubes where fertilization normally takes place depends not only on the motile powers of the sperm but, at least in some species, on uterine contractions as well. The genital stimulation involved in coitus releases oxytocin, but it has not been proved that it is oxytocin that initiates the rather specialized uterine contractions that transport the sperm. The secretion of oxytocin, like that of vasopressin, is inhibited by alcohol.

Site of Origin of Posterior Pituitary Hormones

When the hypothalamus and pituitary are treated with the Gomori stain or a number of other special stains, large granules made up of posterior lobe hormones bound to neurophysins (Herring bodies) are seen in nerve endings in the posterior pituitary. There are similar granules along the axons of the supraoptic and paraventricular neurons, and in their cell bodies. The granules in both locations are depleted by stimuli known to increase the secretion of posterior pituitary hormones. After section of the pituitary stalk, they disappear below the section and pile up above it. These observations and considerable additional evidence make it clear that vasopressin and oxytocin and their respective neurophysins are manufactured in the cell bodies of the supraoptic and paraventricular neurons and transported down their axons to the endings in the posterior pituitary. There they are stored until released to the ECF by exocytosis in response to action potentials in the neurons. Although it has not been proved, the posterior pituitary hormone-neurophysin complexes may well be formed in the cell bodies as single molecules and consequently represent examples of prohormones. The peptides are then split from the neurophysins before secretion.

Neurosecretion

Neurons which contain granules that stain with the Gomori stain are generally called neurosecretory neurons, and the secretion of chemical substances at their endings is called "neurosecretion." The supraoptic and paraventricular neurons are the only neurons that normally contain abundant Gomori-positive granules in mammals. However, all neurons appear to liberate chemical agents. Most neurons secrete transmitter substances (see Chapter 4) that cross the synaptic clefts and act on the membranes of the postsynaptic cells. Others secrete substances that pass through the blood stream to affect distant organs. Some of these neurons contain Gomori-positive neurosecretory granules, but others do not. To avoid confusion, it seems wise to abandon the term **neurosecretion** or at least to redefine it as the secretion into the circulating body fluids by the endings of a neuron of chemical substances that act on other cells some distance away, whether or not the neuron contains Gomori-positive granules.

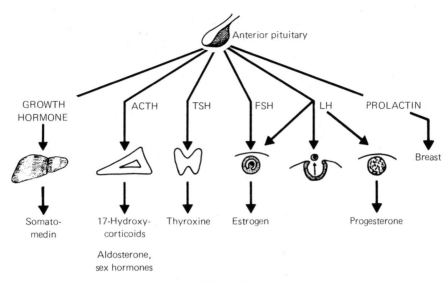

Figure 14–12. Anterior pituitary hormones. In women, FSH and LH act in sequence on the ovary to produce growth of the ovarian follicle, which secretes estrogen, ovulation; and formation and maintenance of the corpus luteum, which secretes estrogen and progesterone. In men, FSH and LH control the functions of the testes. Prolactin stimulates lactation.

CONTROL OF ANTERIOR PITUITARY SECRETION

Anterior Pituitary Hormones

The anterior pituitary secretes 6 hormones: **adrenocorticotropic hormone** (corticotropin, ACTH), **thyroid-stimulating hormone** (thyrotropin, TSH), **growth hormone, follicle-stimulating hormone (FSH), luteinizing hormone (LH),** and **prolactin** (luteotropic hormone, LTH). The actions of these hormones are summarized in Fig 14–12. They are discussed in detail in the chapters on the endocrine system. Other anterior pituitary hormones, including a lipid-mobilizing factor, may exist, but their existence has not been proved. Five of the hormones are **tropic hormones,** ie, they stimulate the secretion of substances from other glands. Prolactin promotes the formation of milk in the breast. The hypothalamus plays an important stimulatory role in regulating the secretion of ACTH, TSH, growth hormone, FSH, and LH. It also regulates prolactin secretion, but its effect is predominantly inhibitory rather than stimulatory.

Nature of Hypothalamic Control

There are probably a few nerve fibers that pass directly from the brain to the anterior pituitary, but they do not control anterior pituitary function. Instead, anterior pituitary secretion is controlled by chemical agents carried in the portal hypophysial vessels from the hypothalamus to the pituitary. These substances have generally been referred to as releasing and inhibiting factors, but they are now commonly called hormones. The latter term seems appropriate, since they are secreted into the blood stream and act at a distance from their site of origin. Furthermore, several of them have been synthesized, and the synthetic factors used clinically are called hormones. Consequently, the term hormone is used in this book. There are 8 relatively well established hypothalamic releasing and inhibiting hormones: **corticotropin releasing hormone (CRH); thyrotropin releasing hormone (TRH); growth hormone releasing hormone (GRH); growth hormone inhibiting hormone (GIH;** also called **somatostatin); follicle-stimulating hormone releasing hormone (FRH); luteinizing hormone releasing hormone (LRH); prolactin releasing hormone (PRH);** and **prolactin inhibiting hormone (PIH).** TRH is a tripeptide (Fig

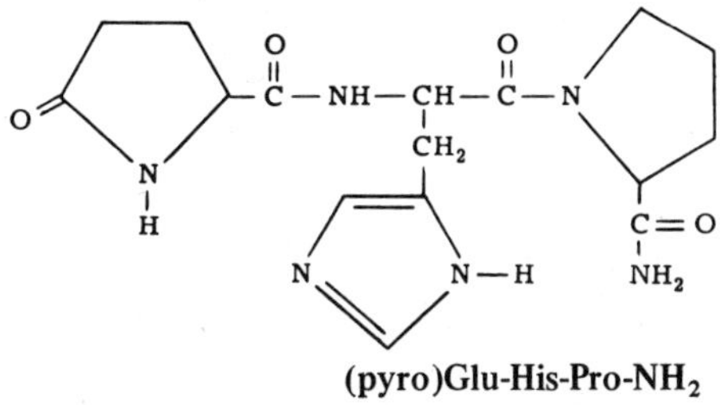

(pyro)Glu-His-Pro-NH₂

Figure 14–13. Structure of human, porcine, and bovine TRH.

(pyro)Glu-His-Trp-Ser-Tyr-Gly-Leu-Arg-Pro-Gly-NH₂
   1   2   3   4   5   6   7   8   9 10

Ala-Gly-Cys-Lys-Asn-Phe-Phe-Trp-Lys-Thr-Phe-Thr-Ser-Cys
 1   2   3   4   5   6   7   8   9 10 11 12 13 14

Figure 14–14. Porcine LRH *(top)* and ovine somatostatin *(bottom).*

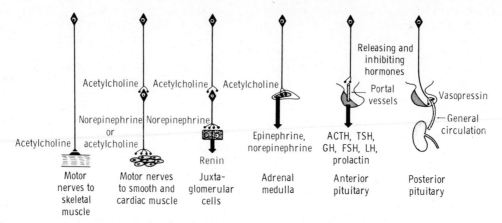

Figure 14—15. Diagrammatic representation of 6 situations in which humoral substances are released by neurons. The last 2 are examples of neurosecretion as this term is defined in the text. (Modified from Harris in: *Handbook of Physiology*. Field J, Magoun HW [editors]. Washington: The American Physiological Society, 1960. Section 1, pp 1007—1038.)

14—13), LRH is a decapeptide, and somatostatin is a tetradecapeptide which contains a disulfide bridge (Fig 14—14). LRH stimulates the secretion of FSH as well as LH, and some have argued that there is no separate FRH. The structures of the other hormones are not yet known, although they are probably small peptides. A possible exception is PIH, which may well be dopamine secreted by the dopaminergic neurons in the hypothalamus (see Chapter 15).

The area from which the hypothalamic releasing and inhibiting hormones are secreted is the median eminence of the hypothalamus (Fig 14—4). This region contains few nerve cell bodies, but there are many nerve endings in close proximity to the capillary loops from which the portal vessels originate. The hormones are secreted from these endings. Their release is therefore an example of neurosecretion as defined above. This type of neuroendocrine regulation is intermediate

between that in the adrenal medulla, where nerve fibers stimulate gland cells, and that in the posterior pituitary, where substances secreted by neurons pass into the general circulation (Fig 14—15).

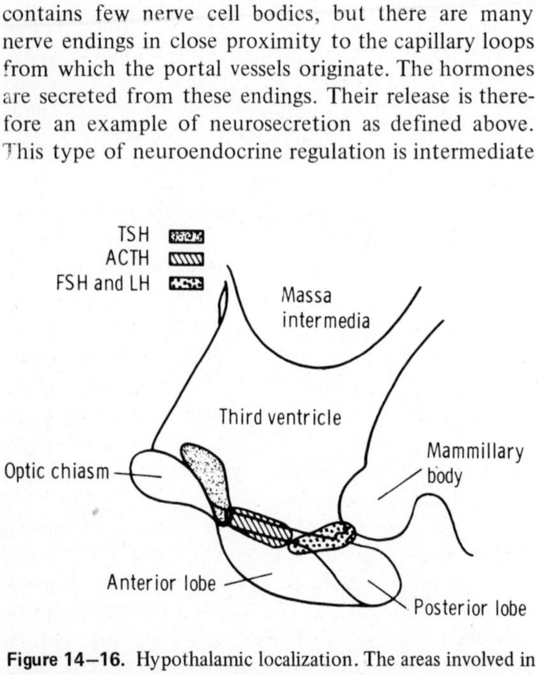

There is considerable evidence in experimental animals that the various hormones of the hypothalamus are secreted from separate zones within the median eminence. In dogs, for example, TRH is secreted anteriorly, CRH in the middle portion, and the gonadotropin-regulating hormones posteriorly (Fig 14—16). A similar hypothalamic localization in humans has not been proved, but there is circumstantial evidence that the arrangement is similar to that in dogs.

The location of the cell bodies of the neurons that secrete hypothalamic hormones is an incompletely resolved problem. The LRH-secreting neurons are located in the preoptic area and neighboring portions of the anterior hypothalamus. The CRH-secreting neurons appear to have their cell bodies throughout the ventral hypothalamus. TRH-secreting neurons are located primarily in the anterior hypothalamus, and GRH-secreting neurons are probably located in the median eminence and preoptic area. There is evidence that anterior pituitary hormones and, in the case of the gonadotropins, gonadal steroids feed back on the hypothalamus to inhibit the secretion of the hypothalamic hormones. The hypothalamic hormone-secreting neurons receive multiple neural inputs, and the transmitters secreted by these converging afferent fibers probably include norepinephrine and serotonin (see Chapter 15).

Figure 14—16. Hypothalamic localization. The areas involved in the control of anterior pituitary secretion in the dog are projected on a midsagittal section of the hypothalamus. (Redrawn and reproduced, with permission, from Ganong in: *Comparative Endocrinology*. Gorbman A [editor]. Wiley, 1959.)

Significance & Clinical Implications

The research delineating the multiple neuroendocrine regulatory functions of the hypothalamus is important because it explains how endocrine secretion is made appropriate to the demands of a changing environment. The nervous system receives information about changes in the internal and external environment from the sense organs. We now know that it brings about adjustments to these changes through effector mechanisms that include not only somatic movement but also changes in the rate at which hormones are secreted. There are many examples of the operation of the neuroendocrine effector pathways. In birds and many mammals, the increasing hours of daylight in the spring stimulate gonadotropin secretion, activating the quiescent gonads and starting the breeding season. In some avian species, the sight of a member of the opposite sex in a mating dance apparently produces the gonadotropin secretion necessary to cause ovulation. It has been claimed that Eskimo women cease to ovulate during the long winter night and that regular menstrual cycles and sexual vigor return in the spring. In more temperate climates, menstruation in women is a year-round phenomenon, but its regularity can be markedly affected by somatic and emotional stimuli. The disappearance of regular periods when young girls move away from home (sometimes called "boarding school amenorrhea") and the inhibition of menstruation that can be produced by fear of pregnancy are examples of the many ways that psychic phenomena affect endocrine secretion.

Hypothalamic disease is not common, but it does occur. Its manifestations are neurologic defects, endocrine changes, and metabolic abnormalities such as hyperphagia and hyperthermia. The relative frequencies of the signs and symptoms of hypothalamic disease in one large series of cases are shown in Table 14–4. The possibility of hypothalamic pathology should be kept in mind in evaluating all patients with pituitary dysfunction, especially those with isolated deficiencies of single pituitary tropic hormones. Many of these deficiencies are proving to be due to hypothalamic rather than primary pituitary disease.

Other Actions of Hypothalamic Hormones

It is worth noting that the hypothalamic hormones that have been synthesized affect the secretion of more than one anterior pituitary hormone. The FSH-stimulating activity of LRH has been mentioned above. TRH stimulates the secretion of prolactin as well as TSH. Somatostatin inhibits the secretion of TSH as well as growth hormone. It does not normally inhibit the secretion of the other anterior pituitary hormones, but it does inhibit the abnormally elevated secretion of ACTH in patients with Nelson's syndrome, a condition characterized by hypersecretion of ACTH following bilateral adrenalectomy for Cushing's syndrome.

Appreciable quantities of LRH and somatostatin are found not only in the median eminence but also in other circumventricular organs (see Chapter 17). Their function in these locations is unknown. Somatostatin and TRH are also found in neural tissue in other parts of the brain, and somatostatin has recently been demonstrated by immunocytochemical technics to be present in the dorsal horn region of the spinal cord, possibly in small diameter primary afferent fibers. These observations suggest that hypothalamic hormones may function as synaptic transmitters as well as regulators of anterior pituitary secretion.

Somatostatin has been found to be present in the pancreas and the gastric and intestinal mucosa as well as the brain. In addition to its action on anterior pituitary secretion, it inhibits the secretion of insulin and glucagon and the gastrointestinal hormones gastrin, secretin, VIP, GIP, and motilin. It also inhibits gastric acid secretion and motility and the exocrine secretion of the pancreas. Thus, it is clear that this hypothalamic hormone has very widespread effects in the body.

Table 14–4. Symptoms and signs in 60 autopsied cases of hypothalamic disease.*

	Percentage of Cases
Endocrine and metabolic findings	
Precocious puberty	40
Hypogonadism	32
Diabetes insipidus	35
Obesity	25
Abnormalities of temperature regulation	22
Emaciation	18
Bulimia	8
Anorexia	7
Neurologic findings	
Eye signs	78
Pyramidal and sensory deficits	75
Headache	65
Extrapyramidal signs	62
Vomiting	40
Psychic disturbances, rage attacks, etc	35
Somnolence	30
Convulsions	15

*Data from Bauer: Endocrine and other manifestations of hypothalamic disease. J Clin Endocrinol 14:13, 1954. See also Kahana & others: Endocrine manifestations of intracranial extrasellar lesions. J Clin Endocrinol 22:304, 1962.

TEMPERATURE REGULATION

In the body, heat is produced by muscular exercise, assimilation of food, and all the vital processes that contribute to the basal metabolic rate (see Chapter 17). It is lost from the body by radiation, conduction, and vaporization of water in the respiratory passages and on the skin. Small amounts of heat are also removed in the urine and feces. The balance between heat production and heat loss determines the body temperature. Because the speed of chemical reactions varies with the temperature and because the enzyme systems of the body have narrow temperature ranges in which their function is optimal, normal body function depends upon a relatively constant body temperature.

Invertebrates generally cannot adjust their body temperatures and so are at the mercy of the environment. In vertebrates, mechanisms for maintaining body temperature by adjusting heat production and heat loss have evolved. In reptiles, amphibia, and fish, the adjusting mechanisms are relatively rudimentary, and these species are called "cold-blooded" or **poikilothermic** because their body temperature fluctuates over a considerable range. In birds and mammals, the "warm-blooded" or **homeothermic** animals, a group of reflex responses that are primarily integrated in the hypothalamus operate to maintain body temperature within a narrow range in spite of wide fluctuations in environmental temperature. The hibernating mammals are a partial exception. While awake, they are homeothermic, but during hibernation their body temperature falls.

Normal Body Temperature

In homeothermic animals the actual temperature at which the body is maintained varies from species to species and, to a lesser degree, from individual to individual. In humans, the traditional normal value for the oral temperature is 37° C (98.6° F), but in one large series of normal young adults the morning oral temperature averaged 36.7° C, with a standard deviation of 0.2°. Therefore, 95% of all young adults would be expected to have a morning oral temperature of 36.3–37.1° C, or 97.3–98.8° F (mean ± 1.96 standard deviations; see Appendix). Various parts of the body are at different temperatures, and the magnitude of the temperature difference between the parts varies with the environmental temperature (Fig 14–17). The extremities are generally cooler than the rest of the body. The rectal temperature is representative of the temperature at the core of the body and varies least with changes in environmental temperature. Oral temperature is normally 0.5° C lower than the rectal

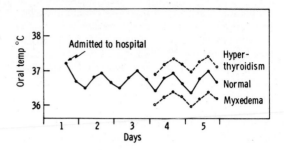

Figure 14–18. Typical temperature chart of a hospitalized patient who does not have a febrile disease. Note the slight rise in temperature, due to excitement and apprehension, at the time of admission to the hospital, and the regular diurnal temperature cycle.

temperature, but it is affected by many factors, including ingestion of hot or cold fluids, gum-chewing, smoking, and mouth breathing.

The normal human core temperature undergoes a regular diurnal fluctuation of 0.5–0.7° C. In individuals who sleep at night and are awake during the day (even when hospitalized at bed rest), it is lowest at about 6:00 a.m. and highest in the evenings (Fig 14–18). It is lowest during sleep, slightly higher in the awake but relaxed state, and rises with activity. In women there is an additional monthly cycle of temperature variation characterized by a rise in basal temperature at the time of ovulation. Temperature regulation is less precise in young children, and they may normally have a temperature that is 0.5° C or so above the established norm for adults.

During exercise the heat produced by muscular contraction accumulates in the body, and rectal temperature normally rises as high as 40° C (104° F). This rise is due in part to the inability of the heat-dissipating mechanisms to handle the greatly increased amount of heat that is produced, but there is evidence that in addition there is an elevation of the body temperature

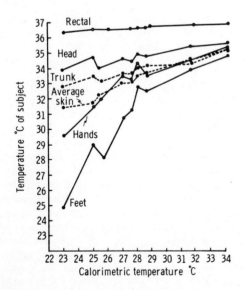

Figure 14–17. Temperature of various parts of the body of a naked subject at various ambient temperatures in a calorimeter. (Redrawn and reproduced, with permission, from Hardy & DuBois: Basal metabolism, radiation, convection and vaporization at temperatures of 22–35° C. J Nutr 15:477, 1938.)

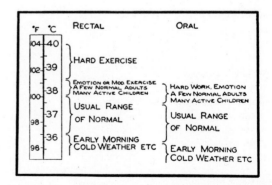

Figure 14–19. Ranges in rectal and oral temperatures seen in normal humans. (Reproduced, with permission, from DuBois: *Fever and the Regulation of Body Temperature.* Thomas, 1948.)

at which the heat-dissipating mechanisms are activated during exercise. Body temperature also rises slightly during emotional excitement, probably due to unconscious tensing of the muscles (Figs 14–18 and 14–19). It is chronically elevated by as much as 0.5° C when the metabolic rate is high, as in hyperthyroidism, and lowered when the metabolic rate is low, as in myxedema. Some apparently normal adults chronically have a temperature above the normal range (constitutional hyperthermia).

Heat Production

A variety of basic chemical reactions contribute to body heat production. Ingestion of food increases heat production because of the specific dynamic action of the food, but the major source of heat is the contraction of skeletal muscle (Table 14–5). Heat production can be varied in the absence of food intake or muscular exertion by endocrine mechanisms. Epinephrine and norepinephrine produce a rapid but short-lived increase in heat production; thyroxine causes a slowly developing but prolonged increase.

A source of considerable heat in human infants is a special type of fat, **brown fat**, which is located between and around the scapulas. This fat has a high rate of metabolism, and its function has been likened to that of an electric blanket. Brown fat is also found in a variety of animals, but, unlike ordinary white fat, it is not found in adult humans.

Heat Loss

The processes by which heat is lost from the body when the environmental temperature is below body temperature are listed in Table 14–5. **Radiation** is the transfer of heat from one object to another with which it is not in contact. **Conduction** is heat exchange between objects at different temperatures that are in contact with one another. The amount of heat transferred by conduction is proportionate to the temperature difference between the 2 objects (**thermal gradient**). **Convection,** the movement of the molecules of a gas or a liquid at one temperature to another location which is at a different temperature, aids conduction. When an individual is in a cold environment, he loses

Table 14–5. Body heat production and heat loss.

Body heat is produced by:
  Basic metabolic processes
  Food intake (specific dynamic action)
  Muscular activity

Body heat is lost by:	Percentage of Heat Lost at 21° C
Radiation and conduction	70
Vaporization of sweat	27
Respiration	2
Urination and defecation	1

heat by conduction to the air around him and by radiation to cool objects in the vicinity. When he is in a hot environment, heat is transferred to him by these processes and adds to his heat load. Thus, in a sense, radiation and conduction work against the maintenance of body temperature. On a cold but sunny day, the heat of the sun reflected off bright objects exerts an appreciable warming effect. It is the heat reflected from the snow, for example, that makes it possible to ski in fairly light clothes even though the air temperature is below freezing.

Since conduction occurs from the surface of one object to the surface of another, the temperature of the skin determines to a large extent the degree to which body heat is lost or gained. The amount of heat reaching the skin from the deep tissues can be varied by changing the blood flow to the skin. When the cutaneous vessels are dilated, warm blood wells up into the skin, whereas in the maximally vasoconstricted state heat is held centrally in the body. The rate at which heat is transferred from the deep tissues to the skin is called the **tissue conductance.** Birds have a layer of feathers next to the skin, and most mammals have a significant layer of hair or fur. Heat is conducted from the skin to the air trapped in this layer, and from the trapped air to the exterior. When the thickness of the trapped layer is increased by fluffing the feathers or erection of the hairs (**horripilation**), heat transfer across the layer is reduced and heat losses (or, in a hot environment, heat gains) are decreased. "Goose pimples" are the result of horripilation in humans; they are the visible manifestation of cold-induced contraction of the piloerector muscles attached to the rather meager hair supply. Humans usually supplement this layer of hair with a layer of clothes. Heat is conducted from the skin to the layer of air trapped by the clothes, from the inside of the clothes to the outside, and from the outside of the clothes to the exterior. The magnitude of the heat transfer across the clothing, a function of its texture and thickness, is the most important determinant of how warm or cool the clothes feel, but other factors, especially the size of the trapped layer of warm air, are important also. Dark clothes absorb radiated heat, and light-colored clothes reflect it back to the exterior.

The other major process transferring heat from the body in humans and those animals that sweat is vaporization of water on the skin and mucous membranes of the mouth and respiratory passages. Vaporization of 1 g of water removes about 0.6 kcal of heat. A certain amount of water is vaporized at all times. This **insensible water loss** amounts to 50 ml/hour in humans. When sweat secretion is increased, the degree to which the sweat vaporizes depends upon the humidity of the environment. It is common knowledge that one feels hotter on a humid day. This is due in part to the decreased vaporization of sweat, but even under conditions in which vaporization of sweat is complete an individual in a humid environment feels warmer than an individual in a dry environment. The reason for this difference is not known, but it seems related to the fact that in the humid environment sweat spreads over a greater area of skin before it evaporates. During muscular exertion in a hot environment, sweat secretion reaches values as high as 1600 ml/hour, and in a dry atmosphere most of this sweat is vaporized. Heat loss by vaporization of water therefore varies from 30 to over 900 kcal/hour.

Some mammals lose heat by **panting**. This rapid, shallow breathing greatly increases the amount of water vaporized in the mouth and respiratory passages, and therefore the amount of heat lost. Because the breathing is shallow, it produces relatively little change in the composition of alveolar air.

The relative contribution of each of the processes that transfer heat away from the body (Table 14–5) varies with the environmental temperature. At 21° C, vaporization is a minor component in a man at rest. As the environmental temperature approaches body temperature, radiation losses decline and vaporization losses increase.

Temperature-Regulating Mechanisms

The reflex and semireflex thermoregulatory responses are listed in Table 14–6. They include autonomic, somatic, endocrine, and behavioral changes. One group of responses increases heat loss and decreases heat production; the other decreases heat loss and increases heat production.

Curling up "in a ball" is a common reaction to cold in animals and has a counterpart in the position some people assume on climbing into a cold bed. Curling up decreases the body surface exposed to the environment. Shivering is an involuntary response of the skeletal muscles, but cold also causes a semiconscious general increase in motor activity. Examples include foot stamping and dancing up and down on a cold day. Increased catecholamine secretion is an important

Table 14—6. Temperature regulating mechanisms.

Mechanisms activated by cold:	
Shivering	
Hunger	Increase
Increased voluntary activity	heat
Increased secretion of norepi- nephrine and epinephrine	production
Cutaneous vasoconstriction	Decrease
Curling up	heat
Horripilation	loss

Mechanisms activated by heat:	
Cutaneous vasodilatation	Increase
Sweating	heat
Increased respiration	loss
Anorexia	Decrease
Apathy and inertia	heat
	production

endocrine response to cold; adrenal medullectomized rats die faster than normal controls when exposed to cold. TSH secretion is increased by cold and decreased by heat in laboratory animals, but the change in TSH secretion produced by cold in adult humans is small and of questionable significance. It is common knowledge that activity is decreased in hot weather—the "it's too hot to move" reaction.

The reflex responses activated by cold are controlled from the posterior hypothalamus. Those activated by warmth are primarily controlled from the anterior hypothalamus, although some thermoregulation against heat still occurs after decerebration at the level of the rostral midbrain. Stimulation of the anterior hypothalamus causes cutaneous vasodilatation and sweating, and lesions in this region cause hyperthermia, with rectal temperatures sometimes reaching 43° C (109.4° F). Posterior hypothalamic stimulation causes shivering, and the body temperature of animals with posterior hypothalamic lesions falls toward that of the environment. There is some evidence that serotonin is a synaptic mediator in the centers controlling the mechanisms activated by cold, and norepinephrine may play a similar role in those activated by heat.

Afferents

The signals which activate the hypothalamic temperature-regulating centers come from 2 sources:

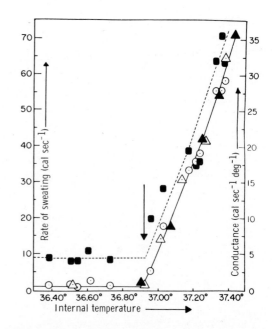

Figure 14—20. Quantitative relations in humans between the temperature of the interior of the head (internal temperature) and cutaneous blood flow (squares, scale at the right), and sweating (circles and triangles, scale at the left). The arrow points to the sharp threshold at which these parameters start to rise. In this subject, the threshold was at 36.9° C. (Reproduced, with permission, from Benzinger: Receptor organs and quantitative mechanisms of human temperature control in a warm environment. Fed Proc 19:32, 1960.)

temperature-sensitive cells in the anterior hypothalamus, and cutaneous temperature receptors, especially cold receptors. Present evidence indicates that the stimuli which activate the defenses against high temperatures in humans come mainly from the temperature-sensitive cells in the hypothalamus. This conclusion grew out of research in which the temperature of the back of the nasal cavity and the interior of the ear, near the hypothalamus, was correlated with thermoregulatory responses to changing environmental temperatures (Fig 14–20). This "head temperature" does not always correlate with rectal "body core" temperature, a fact which was often overlooked in previous research. The response of body heat production to cooling is modified by interactions between cutaneous and central stimuli. Heat production is increased when head temperature falls below a given threshold value, but the threshold for the response is lower and its magnitude decreased when the skin temperature is increased.

Fever

Fever is perhaps the oldest and most universally known hallmark of disease. When an individual develops a fever, his thermoregulatory mechanisms behave as if they were adjusted to maintain his body temperature at a higher than normal level, ie, "as if his thermostat had been reset" to a new set point above 37° C. His temperature receptors then signal that his actual temperature is below the new set point, and temperature-raising mechanisms are activated, producing chilly sensations due to cutaneous vasoconstriction and occasionally enough shivering to produce a shaking chill. Salicylates such as aspirin appear to relieve fever by reducing the set point of the thermoregulatory mechanisms back toward normal.

Fever is produced in various ways. Many infections cause fever by causing the production of **endogenous pyrogen** from polymorphonuclear leukocytes in the blood. This fever-producing substance acts directly on the thermoregulatory centers in the hypothalamus to reset them. Other cells in the body can also release endogenous pyrogens, including monocytes, lymphocytes, and the Kupffer cells of the reticuloendothelial system. The endogenous pyrogens are proteins with molecular weights of 10,000–20,000. They are released from cells in response to viruses, antigens,

antigen-antibody complexes, and even steroid hormones. They are also released in response to the endotoxin produced by some bacteria and as a result of phagocytosis of bacteria by endogenous pyrogen-producing cells.

The benefit of fever to the organism is unknown, although it is presumably beneficial in some way because it has evolved and persisted as a response to infections and other diseases in all homeothermic animals. Before the advent of antibiotics, fevers were artificially induced for the treatment of neurosyphilis. However, it is uncertain whether fever helps to kill the microorganisms that cause other infectious diseases. Very high temperatures are harmful. When the rectal temperature is over 41° C (106° F) for prolonged periods, some permanent brain damage results. When it is over 43° C, heat stroke develops and death is common.

Hypothermia

In hibernating mammals, body temperature drops to low levels without causing any ill effects which are demonstrable upon subsequent arousal. This observation led to experiments on induced hypothermia. When the skin or the blood is cooled enough to lower the body temperature in nonhibernating animals and in humans, metabolic and physiologic processes slow down. Respiration and heart rate are very slow, blood pressure is low, and consciousness is lost. At rectal temperatures of about 28° C, ability to spontaneously return the temperature to normal is lost, but the individual continues to survive and, if rewarmed with external heat, returns to a normal state. If care is taken to prevent the formation of ice crystals in the tissues, the body temperature of experimental animals can be lowered to subfreezing levels without producing any damage that is detectable after subsequent rewarming.

Humans tolerate body temperatures of 21–24° C (70–75° F) without permanent ill effects, and induced hypothermia has been used extensively in surgery. In hypothermic patients the circulation can be stopped for relatively long periods because the O_2 needs of the tissues are greatly reduced. Blood pressure is low, and bleeding is minimal. It is possible under hypothermia to stop and open the heart and to perform other procedures, especially brain operations, that would have been impossible without cooling.

15...
Neurophysiologic Basis of Instinctual Behavior & Emotions

Emotions have both mental and physical components. They involve **cognition**, an awareness of the sensation and usually its cause; **affect**, the feeling itself; **conation**, the urge to take action; and **physical changes** such as hypertension, tachycardia, and sweating. Physiologists have been concerned for some time with the physical manifestations of emotional states, while psychologists have been concerned with emotions themselves. However, their interests merge in the hypothalamus and limbic systems since these parts of the brain are now known to be intimately concerned not only with emotional expression but with the genesis of emotions as well.

ANATOMIC CONSIDERATIONS

The term **limbic lobe** or **limbic system** is now generally applied to the part of the brain formerly called the rhinencephalon because it has become clear that only a small portion of this part of the brain is directly concerned with smell. Each limbic lobe consists of a rim of cortical tissue around the hilus of the cerebral hemisphere and a group of associated deep structures—the amygdala, the hippocampus, and the septal nuclei (Figs 15–1 and 15–2).

Histology

The limbic cortex is phylogenetically the oldest part of the cerebral cortex. Histologically, it is made up of a primitive type of cortical tissue called **allocortex,** surrounding the hilus of the hemisphere, and a second ring of a transitional type of cortex called **juxtallocortex** between the allocortex and the rest of the cerebral hemisphere. The cortical tissue of the remaining nonlimbic portions of the hemisphere is called **neocortex.** The neocortex is the most highly developed type, and is characteristically 6-layered. The actual extent of the allocortical and juxtallocortical

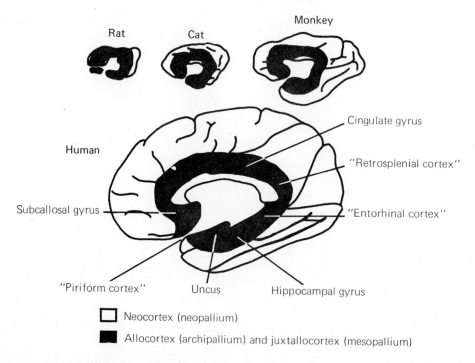

Figure 15–1. Relation of the limbic cortex in rats, cats, monkeys, and humans. (Redrawn and reproduced, with permission, from MacLean: The limbic system and its hippocampal formation. J Neurosurg 11:29, 1954.)

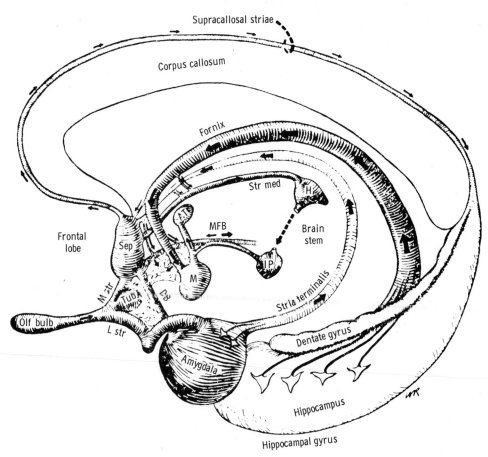

Figure 15–2. Diagram of the principal connections of the limbic system. M str, L str, medial and lateral olfactory striae; Str med, stria medullaris; Tub, olfactory tubercle; DB, diagonal band of Broca; Sep, septum; AT, anterior nucleus of the thalamus; M, mammillary body; H, habenula; IP, interpeduncular nucleus; MFB, medial forebrain bundle. (After Krieg. Reproduced, with permission, from MacLean: Psychosomatic disease and the visceral brain. Psychosom Med 11:338, 1949.)

areas has changed little as mammals have evolved, but these regions have been overshadowed by the immense growth of the neocortex, which reaches its greatest development in humans (Fig 15–1).

Afferent & Efferent Connections

The major connections of the limbic system are shown in Fig 15–2. The fornix connects the hippocampus to the mammillary bodies, which are in turn connected to the anterior nuclei of the thalamus by the mammillothalamic tract of Vicq d'Azyr. The anterior nuclei of the thalamus project to the cingulate cortex, and from the cingulate cortex there are connections to the hippocampus, completing a complex closed circuit. This circuit was originally described by Papez, and has been called the Papez circuit.

Correlations Between Structure & Function

One characteristic of the limbic system is the paucity of the connections between it and the neocortex. Nauta has aptly stated that, "The neocortex sits astride the limbic system like a rider on a horse without reins." Actually, there are a few reins; there are

fibers from the frontal lobe to adjacent limbic structures, and probably some indirect connections via the thalamus. From a functional point of view, neocortical activity does modify emotional behavior and vice versa. However, one of the characteristics of emotion is that it cannot be turned on and off at will.

Another characteristic of limbic circuits is their prolonged afterdischarge following stimulation. This may explain in part the fact that emotional responses are generally prolonged rather than evanescent, and outlast the stimuli that initiate them.

LIMBIC FUNCTIONS

Stimulation and ablation experiments indicate that in addition to its role in olfaction (Chapter 10), the limbic system is concerned with feeding behavior. Along with the hypothalamus, it is also concerned with sexual behavior, the emotions of rage and fear, and motivation.

Autonomic Responses & Feeding Behavior

Limbic stimulation produces autonomic effects, particularly changes in blood pressure and respiration. These responses are elicited from many limbic structures, and there is little evidence of localization of autonomic responses. This suggests that the autonomic effects are part of more complex phenomena, particularly emotional and behavioral responses. Stimulation of the amygdaloid nuclei causes movements such as chewing and licking and other activities related to feeding. Lesions in the amygdala cause moderate hyperphagia, with indiscriminate ingestion of all kinds of food. The relation of this type of omniphagia to the hypothalamic mechanisms regulating appetite is discussed in Chapter 14.

SEXUAL BEHAVIOR

Mating is a basic but complex phenomenon in which many parts of the nervous system are involved. Copulation itself is made up of a series of reflexes integrated in spinal and lower brain stem centers, but the behavioral components that accompany it, the urge to copulate, and the coordinated sequence of events in the male and female that lead to pregnancy are regulated to a large degree in the limbic system and hypothalamus. Learning plays a part in the development of mating behavior, particularly in primates and humans, but in lower animals courtship and successful mating can occur with no previous sexual experience. The basic responses are therefore innate and are undoubtedly present in all mammals. However, in humans the sexual functions have become extensively encephalized and conditioned by social and psychic factors. The basic physiologic mechanisms of sexual behavior in animals will therefore be considered first and then compared to the responses in humans.

Relation to Endocrine Function

In animals other than humans, removal of the gonads leads eventually to decreased or absent sexual activity in both the male and the female—although the loss is slow to develop in the males of some species. Injections of gonadal hormones in castrate animals revive sexual activity. Testosterone in the male and estrogen in the female have the most marked effect. Large doses of progesterone are also effective in the female, while in the presence of smaller doses of progesterone the dose of estrogen necessary to produce sexual activity is lowered. Large doses of testosterone and other androgens in castrate females initiate female behavior, and large doses of estrogens in castrate males trigger male mating responses. It is unsettled why responses appropriate to the sex of the animal occur when the hormones of the opposite sex are injected.

Clinical Correlates

In adult women, ovariectomy does not necessarily reduce libido (defined in this context as sexual interest and drive) or sexual ability. Postmenopausal women continue to have sexual relations, often without much change in frequency from their premenopausal pattern. Some investigators claim that this persistence is due to continued secretion of estrogens and androgens from the adrenal cortex, but it is more likely due to the greater degree of encephalization of sexual functions in humans and their relative emancipation from instinctual and hormonal control. However, treatment with sex hormones increases sexual interest and drive in humans. Testosterone, for example, increases libido in males, and so does estrogen used to treat diseases such as carcinoma of the prostate. The behavioral pattern present before treatment is stimulated but not redirected. Thus, administration of testosterone to homosexuals intensifies their homosexual drive but does not convert it to a heterosexual drive.

Neural Control in the Male

In male animals, removal of the neocortex generally inhibits sexual behavior. Partial cortical ablations also produce some inhibition, the degree of the inhibition being independent of the coexisting motor deficit and most marked when the lesions are in the frontal lobes. On the other hand, cats and monkeys with bilateral limbic lesions localized to the piriform cortex

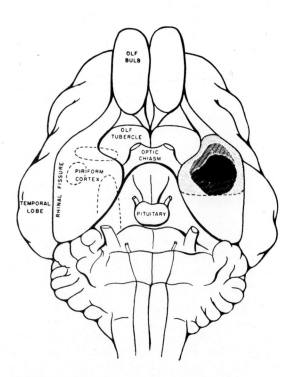

Figure 15–3. Site of lesions producing hypersexuality in male cats. When the black area was destroyed, hypersexuality was always present. The incidence of hypersexuality in animals with lesions in the surrounding lighter zones was not so high. Olf, olfactory. (Reproduced, with permission, from Green & others: Rhinencephalic lesions and behavior in cats. J Comp Neurol 108:505, 1957.)

overlying the amygdala (Fig 15—3) develop a marked intensification of sexual activity. These animals not only mount adult females; they also mount immature females and other males, and attempt to copulate with animals of other species and with inanimate objects. Despite some claims to the contrary, such behavior is clearly abnormal in the species studied. The behavior is dependent upon the presence of testosterone but is not due to any increase in its secretion.

The hypothalamus is also involved in the control of sexual activity in males. Stimulation along the medial forebrain bundle and in neighboring hypothalamic areas causes penile erection with considerable emotional display in monkeys. In castrated rats, intrahypothalamic implants of testosterone restore the complete pattern of sex behavior; and in intact rats, appropriately placed anterior hypothalamic lesions abolish interest in sex. It has been reported that lesions in the mammillary region in male rats lead to increased sexual activity.

Sexual Behavior in the Female

In mammals, the sexual activity of the male is more or less continuous, but in most species the sexual activity of the female is cyclic. Most of the time, the female avoids the male and repulses his sexual advances. Periodically, however, there is an abrupt change in behavior and the female seeks out the male, attempting to mate. These short episodes of **heat** or **estrus** are so characteristic that the sexual cycle in mammalian species that do not menstruate is named the **estrous cycle.**

This change in female sexual behavior is brought on by a rise in the circulating blood estrogen level. Some animals, notably the rabbit and the ferret, come into heat and remain estrous until pregnancy or pseudopregnancy results. In these species, ovulation is due to a neuroendocrine reflex. Stimulation of the genitalia and other sensory stimuli at the time of copulation provokes release from the pituitary of the gonadotropin that makes the ovarian follicles rupture. In many other species, spontaneous ovulation occurs at regular intervals, and the periods of heat coincide with its occurrence. This is true in monkeys and apes. In captivity, these species mate at any time; but in the wild state the females accept the male more frequently at the time of ovulation.

In monkeys, the sex drive of the male is greater when he is exposed to a female at the time of ovulation than when he is exposed to a female at another time of her cycle. The "message" sent by the female to the male in this situation is olfactory, and the substances responsible are certain fatty acids in the vaginal secretions. These fatty acids are also found in increased amounts in human vaginal secretions at about midcycle. Substances produced by an animal that act at a distance to produce behavioral or other physiologic changes in another animal of the same species have been called **pheromones.** The sex attractants of certain insects are particularly well known examples, but it appears from the evidence cited above that phero-

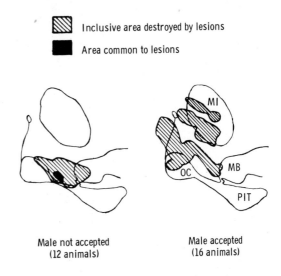

Inclusive area destroyed by lesions

Area common to lesions

Male not accepted (12 animals)

Male accepted (16 animals)

Figure 15—4. Sites of hypothalamic lesions which blocked behavioral heat without affecting ovarian cycles in ewes. MI, massa intermedia; MB, mammillary body; OC, optic chiasm; PIT, pituitary. (From data of Clegg & Ganong.)

mones also operate in the regulation of sexual behavior in primates.

Neural Control in the Female

In female animals, removal of the neocortex and the limbic cortex abolishes active seeking out of the male ("enticement reactions") during estrus, but other aspects of heat are unaffected. Amygdaloid and periamygdaloid lesions do not produce hypersexuality in females as they do in the male. However, discrete anterior hypothalamic lesions abolish behavioral heat (Fig 15—4) without affecting the regular pituitary-ovarian cycle.

Implantation of minute amounts of estrogen in the anterior hypothalamus causes heat in ovariectomized rats. Implantation of estrogen into other parts of the brain and outside the brain does not have this effect. Apparently, therefore, some element in the hypothalamus is sensitive to the circulating estrogen titer and is stimulated by a high titer to initiate estrous behavior.

Effects of Sex Hormones in Infancy on Adult Behavior

In female experimental animals, exposure to sex steroids in utero or during early postnatal development causes marked abnormalities of sexual behavior when the animals reach adulthood. Female rats treated with a single relatively small dose of androgen before the fifth day of life do not have normal heat periods when they mature; they generally will not mate, even though they have cystic ovaries that secrete enough estrogen to cause the animals to have a persistently estrous type of vaginal smear. These rats do not show the cyclic release of pituitary gonadotropins characteristic of the adult female, but rather the tonic, steady secretion characteristic of the adult male; their brains have been "masculinized" by the single brief exposure to androgens. Conversely, male rats castrated at birth develop the female pattern of cyclic gonadotropin secretion and show considerable female sexual behavior when given doses of ovarian hormones that do not have this effect in intact males. Thus, the development of a "female hypothalamus" depends simply on the absence of androgens in early life rather than on exposure to female hormones.

Rats are particularly immature at birth, and animals of other species in which the young are more fully developed at birth do not show these changes when exposed to androgens during the postnatal period. However, these animals develop genital abnormalities when exposed to androgens in utero. Monkeys exposed to androgens in utero do not lose the female pattern of gonadotropin secretion, but such monkeys do develop abnormalities of sexual behavior in adulthood.

Clinical Correlates

The extent to which the findings in male animals with periamygdaloid lesions are applicable to men is, of course, difficult to determine, but there are reports of hypersexuality in men with bilateral lesions in the region of the amygdaloid nuclei.

In women, sexual activity is generally not confined to any period of heat, although some studies indicate an increase at about the time of ovulation. Others show some increase near the menses. There are reports of transient hypersexuality in women after surgical procedures involving manipulation of the anterior hypothalamus and neighboring structures. Because these reported effects were short-lived, they were probably due to inadvertent stimulation of diencephalic structures.

Early exposure to androgens in human females does not change the cyclic pattern of gonadotropin secretion in adulthood. However, there is evidence that masculinizing effects on behavior do occur.

Maternal Behavior

Maternal behavior is depressed by lesions of the cingulate and retrosplenial portions of the limbic cortex in animals. Hormones do not appear to be necessary for its occurrence, but certain hormones may facilitate its appearance. Prolactin from the anterior pituitary, which is secreted in large amounts during lactation, may exert a facilitatory effect by acting directly on the brain.

FEAR & RAGE

Fear and rage are in some ways closely related emotions. The external manifestations of the **fear, fleeing,** or **avoidance reaction** in animals are autonomic responses such as sweating and pupillary dilatation,

cowering, and turning the head from side to side to seek escape. The **rage, fighting,** or **attack reaction** is associated in the cat with hissing, spitting, growling, piloerection, pupillary dilatation, and well-directed biting and clawing. Both reactions—and sometimes mixtures of the two—can be produced by hypothalamic stimulation. When an animal is threatened, it usually attempts to flee. If cornered, an animal fights. Thus, fear and rage reactions are probably related instinctual protective responses to threats in the environment.

Fear

The fear reaction can be produced in conscious animals by stimulation of the hypothalamus and the amygdaloid nuclei. Conversely, the fear reaction and its autonomic and endocrine manifestations are absent in situations in which they would normally be evoked when the amygdalae are destroyed. A dramatic example is the reaction of monkeys to snakes. Monkeys are normally terrified by snakes. After bilateral temporal lobectomy, monkeys approach snakes without fear, pick them up, and even eat them.

Rage & Placidity

Most animals and humans maintain a balance between rage and its opposite, the emotional state which for lack of a better name is called here placidity. Major irritations make the normal individual "lose his temper," but minor stimuli are ignored. In animals with certain brain lesions, this balance is altered. Some lesions produce a state in which the most minor stimuli evoke violent episodes of rage; others produce a state in which the most traumatic and anger-provoking stimuli fail to ruffle the animal's abnormal calm.

Rage responses to minor stimuli are observed after removal of the neocortex and after lesions of the ventromedial hypothalamic nuclei and septal nuclei in animals with intact cerebral cortices. On the other hand, bilateral destruction of the amygdaloid nuclei causes in monkeys a state of abnormal placidity. Similar responses are usually seen in cats and dogs. Wild rats which are vicious in captivity are transformed by this operation into animals that are as tractable and calm as ordinary laboratory white rats. Stimulation of some parts of the amygdala in cats produces rage. The placidity produced by amygdaloid lesions in animals is converted into rage by subsequent destruction of the ventromedial nuclei of the hypothalamus.

Rage can also be produced by stimulation of an area extending back through the lateral hypothalamus to the central gray area of the midbrain, and the rage response usually produced by amygdaloid stimulation is abolished by ipsilateral lesions in the lateral hypothalamus or rostral midbrain.

Gonadal hormones appear to affect aggressive behavior. In animals, aggression is decreased by castration and increased by androgens. It is also conditioned by social factors; it is more prominent in males that live with females, and increases when a stranger is introduced into an animal's territory.

"Sham Rage"

It was originally thought that rage attacks in animals with diencephalic and forebrain lesions represented only the physical, motor manifestations of anger, and the reaction was therefore called "sham rage." This now appears to be incorrect. Although rage attacks in animals with diencephalic lesions are induced by minor stimuli, they are usually directed with great accuracy at the source of the irritation. Furthermore, hypothalamic stimulation which produces the fear-rage reaction is apparently unpleasant to animals because they become conditioned against the place where the experiments are conducted and try to avoid the experimental sessions. They can easily be taught to press a lever or perform some other act to avoid a hypothalamic stimulus that produces the manifestations of fear or rage. It is difficult if not impossible to form conditioned reflex responses (see Chapter 16) by stimulation of purely motor systems, and it is also difficult if the unconditioned stimulus does not evoke either a pleasant or unpleasant feeling. The fact that hypothalamic stimulation is a potent unconditioned stimulus for the formation of conditioned avoidance responses and the fact that the avoidance responses are extremely persistent indicates that the stimulus is unpleasant. There is therefore little doubt that rage attacks include the mental as well as the physical manifestations of rage, and the term "sham rage" should be dropped.

Significance & Clinical Correlates

It is tempting on the basis of the evidence cited above to speculate that there are 2 intimately related mechanisms in the hypothalamus and limbic system, one promoting placidity and the other rage. If this is true, the emotional state is probably determined by afferent impulses which adjust the balance between them. An arrangement of this sort would be analogous to the systems controlling feeding and body temperature.

Although emotional responses are much more complex and subtle in humans than in animals, the neural substrates are probably the same. It is doubtful if placidity would be recognized as a clinical syndrome in our culture, but rage attacks in response to trivial stimuli have been observed many times in patients with brain damage. They are a complication of pituitary surgery when there is inadvertent damage to the base of the brain. They also follow a number of diseases of the nervous system, especially epidemic influenza and encephalitis, which destroy neurons in the limbic system and hypothalamus. Stimulation of the amygdaloid nuclei and parts of the hypothalamus in conscious humans produces sensations of anger and fear. In Japan, bilateral amygdaloid lesions have been produced in agitated, aggressive mental patients. The patients are said to have become placid and manageable, and it is of some interest that they were reported not to have developed hypersexuality or memory loss.

MOTIVATION

If an animal is placed in a box with a pedal or bar that can be pressed, the animal sooner or later accidentally presses it. Olds and his associates have shown that if the bar is connected in such a way that each press delivers a stimulus to an electrode implanted in certain parts of the brain (Fig 15–5), the animal returns to the bar and presses it again and again. Pressing the bar soon comes to occupy most of the animal's time. Some animals go without food and water to press the bar for brain stimulation, and some will continue until they fall over exhausted. Rats press the bar 5000–12,000 times per hour, and monkeys have been clocked at 17,000 bar presses per hour. On the other hand, when the electrode is in certain other areas the animals avoid pressing the bar, and stimulation of these areas is a potent unconditioned stimulus for the development of conditioned avoidance responses.

The points where stimulation leads to repeated bar pressing are located in a medial band of tissue passing from the amygdaloid nuclei through the hypothalamus to the midbrain tegmentum (Fig 15–6). The highest rates are generally obtained from points in the tegmentum, posterior hypothalamus, and septal nuclei. The points where stimulation is avoided are in the lateral portion of the posterior hypothalamus and dorsal midbrain and in the entorhinal cortex. The latter points are sometimes close to points where bar pressing is repeated, but they are part of a separate system. The areas where bar pressing is repeated are much more extensive than those where it is avoided. It

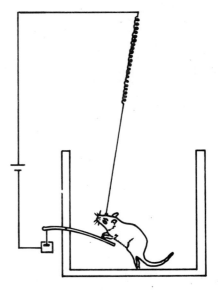

Figure 15–5. Diagram of the apparatus in self-stimulation experiments. Each time the animal steps on the pedal, the electrical circuit is closed and a single current pulse is delivered to its brain through implanted electrodes. (Modified from Olds, in: *Electrical Stimulation of the Unanesthetized Brain.* Ramey E, O'Doherty J [editors]. Hoeber, 1960.)

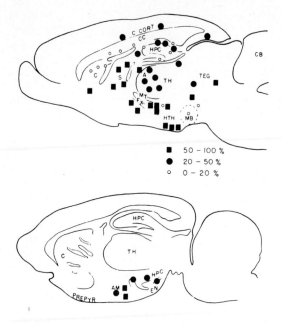

■ 50 – 100 %
● 20 – 50 %
○ 0 – 20 %

Figure 15–6. Location of electrodes in self-stimulation studies, projected on parasagittal sections of the rat brain. The figures in the legend are percentages of time spent pressing the bar in a 6-hour test period. C, caudate; HPC, hippocampus; AM, amygdala; TH, thalamus; HTH, hypothalamus; MB, mammillary bodies; FX, fornix; TEG, tegmentum; S, septum; CB, cerebellum; EN, entorhinal cortex; CC, corpus callosum; C CORT, cerebral cortex; A, anterior commissure; MT, mammillothalamic tract; PREPYR, prepiriform cortex. (Reproduced, with permission, from Olds: A preliminary mapping of electrical reinforcing effects in the rat brain. J Comp Physiol Psychol 49:281, 1956.)

has been calculated that in rats repeated pressing is obtained from 35% of the brain, avoidance from 5%, and indifferent responses (neither repetition nor avoidance) from 60%.

It is obvious that some effect of the stimulation causes the animals to stimulate themselves again and again, but what the animals feel is, of course, unknown. There are a number of reports of bar-pressing experiments in humans with chronically implanted electrodes. Most of the subjects were schizophrenics or epileptics, but a few were patients with visceral malignancies and intractable pain. Like animals, humans press the bar repeatedly. They generally report that the sensations evoked are pleasurable, using phrases like "relief of tension" and "a quiet, relaxed feeling" to describe the experience. However, they rarely report "joy" or "ecstasy," and some persons with the highest self-stimulation rates cannot tell why they keep pushing the bar. When the electrodes are in the areas where stimulation is avoided, patients report sensations ranging from vague fear to terror. It is probably wise, therefore, to avoid vivid terms and call the brain systems involved the **reward** or **approach system** and the **punishment** or **avoidance system**.

Stimulation of the approach system provides a potent motivation for learning mazes or performing

other tasks. Hungry rats will cross an electrified grid to obtain food only when the current in the grid is less than 70 microamperes, but when self-stimulation is the reward they will brave currents of 300 microamperes or more. A rat may even take a shock so strong that it will be stunned, but when it recovers consciousness will roll over and again struggle toward the bar.

To a certain extent, the reward system can be broken down into subsystems. In rats with certain lateral hypothalamic electrode placements, for example, self-stimulation rates are higher when the animals are hungry than when they are sated. In other hypothalamic locations, especially in the medial forebrain bundle, castration decreases and androgen treatment increases the self-stimulation rate. However, feeding and androgen treatment do not modify the responses in other locations.

Studies of the kind described above provide physiologic evidence that behavior is motivated not only by reduction or prevention of an unpleasant affect but also by primary rewards such as those produced by stimulation of the approach system of the brain. The implications of this fact are great in terms of the classical drive-reduction theory of motivation, in terms of the disruption and facilitation of ongoing behavior, and in terms of normal and abnormal emotional responses.

BRAIN CHEMISTRY, BEHAVIOR, & SYNAPTIC TRANSMISSION IN THE CNS

Drugs that modify human behavior include **psychotomimetic agents,** drugs that produce hallucinations and other manifestations of the psychoses; **tranquilizers,** drugs that allay anxiety and various psychiatric symptoms; and **psychic energizers,** antidepressant drugs that elevate mood and increase interest and drive. Many of these drugs appear to act by modifying transmission at synaptic junctions in the brain, and their discovery has stimulated great interest in the nature and properties of the transmitter agents involved.

Various agents have been suspected of being transmitters. Uneven distribution of a given substance in the various parts of the CNS and a parallel distribution of the enzymes responsible for the substance's synthesis and catabolism suggest that it may play a transmitter role. A change in behavior or some other CNS function coincident with a drug-induced change in the concentration of a substance is also indirect evidence that the substance is a transmitter. More direct evidence is provided by differential centrifugation of brain tissue, which has demonstrated the presence of a number of suspected mediators in fractions known to contain nerve endings. Agents found in nerve ending fractions in the CNS include acetylcholine, norepinephrine, dopamine, and serotonin. Additional evidence is provided by histochemical localization, which is now available for norepinephrine, epinephrine, serotonin, and dopamine. It has also been shown that certain of the suspected mediators are liberated from the brain in vitro, and that acetylcholine, glutamic acid, and some other suspected CNS mediators excite single neurons when applied to their membranes by means of a micropipet (**microelectrophoresis**). The substances currently known or suspected of being released from nerve endings are summarized in Table 15—1.

Serotonin

Serotonin (5-hydroxytryptamine, 5-HT) is present in highest concentration in blood platelets and in the gastrointestinal tract, where it is found in the enterochromaffin cells and the myenteric plexus. Lesser amounts are found in the brain, particularly in the hypothalamus (Table 15—2), and in the retina (see Chapter 8).

The monoamines in tissues can be demonstrated histochemically. The method makes serotonin, norepinephrine, epinephrine, and dopamine all fluoresce, but comparing the histologic pictures in animals treated with drugs that selectively deplete the various amines makes it possible to identify each amine. With this technic, it has been demonstrated that serotonin, norepinephrine, and dopamine are all localized in nerve endings. Serotonin is found in relatively high concentrations in the lateral gray horns of the spinal cord and

in a number of areas in the brain. Histochemically, it can be shown that there is a system of serotonin-containing neurons that have their cell bodies in the raphe nuclei of the brain stem and project to portions of the hypothalamus, the limbic system, and the neocortex (Fig 15—7).

Serotonin is formed in the body by hydroxylation and decarboxylation of the essential amino acid tryptophan (Fig 15—8). It is inactivated principally by monoamine oxidase (Fig 15—9) to form 5-hydroxyindoleacetic acid (5-HIAA). This substance is the principal urinary metabolite of serotonin, and the urinary output of 5-HIAA is used as an index of the rate of serotonin metabolism in the body. In the pineal gland, serotonin is converted to the hormone melatonin.

The psychotomimetic agent lysergic acid diethylamide (LSD) is a serotonin antagonist. The transient hallucinations and other mental aberrations produced by this drug were discovered when the chemist who synthesized it inhaled some by accident. Although the relation of LSD to brain serotonin remains unsettled, its discovery called attention to the correlation between behavior and variations in brain serotonin content. Several substances which, like serotonin, are derivatives of tryptamine have psychotomimetic actions; psilocybin, a hallucinogenic agent found in certain mushrooms, is the best known of these compounds. The tranquilizing drug reserpine causes a

Table 15—1. Known and suspected synaptic transmitter agents and "neural hormones" in mammals.

| Substance | Locations Where Substance Is Secreted | |
	Known	Suspected
Acetylcholine	Myoneural junction Preganglionic autonomic endings Postganglionic parasympathetic endings Postganglionic sweat gland and muscle vasodilator endings Many parts of brain	Retina
Norepinephrine	Postganglionic sympathetic endings Cerebral cortex, hypothalamus, brain stem, cerebellum, spinal cord	
Dopamine	Caudate nucleus, putamen, hypothalamus, limbic system, cerebral cortex	Retina
Epinephrine	Hypothalamus	
Serotonin	Hypothalamus, limbic system, cerebellum, spinal cord	Retina
Substance P	Substantia gelatinosa, many other parts of brain	Retina, intestine
Histamine		Hypothalamus
Vasopressin	Posterior pituitary	
Oxytocin	Posterior pituitary	
Hypothalamic releasing and inhibiting hormones (CRH, TRH, GRH, GIH, LRH, FRH, PRH, PIH; see Chapter 14)	Median eminence of hypothalamus	Other parts of brain, spinal cord
Glycine		Neurons mediating direct inhibition in spinal cord
Gamma-aminobutyric acid (GABA)	Cerebellum, cerebral cortex; neurons mediating presynaptic inhibition in spinal cord; retina	
Glutamic acid (glutamate)		Excites many mammalian neurons
Enkephalins, endorphins		Many parts of CNS, gastrointestinal tract

Table 15—2. Brain content of GABA and a number of probable transmitter agents at synapses in the CNS.

	DOG					RAT
	Acetyl-choline ($\mu g/g*$)	Substance P (units/g*)	Sero-tonin ($\mu g/g*$)	Norepi-nephrine ($\mu g/g*$)	Hista-mine ($\mu g/g*$)	GABA ($\mu g/g\dagger$)
Cerebral cortex—somesthetic	2.8	‡	‡	0	0	} 210
Cerebral cortex—motor	4.5	19	0.02	0.18	0	
Caudate nucleus	2.7	46	0.10	0.06	0	‡
Thalamus	3.0	13	0.02	0.16	0	‡
Hypothalamus	1.8	70	0.25	1.03	30	380
Hippocampus	‡	15	0.05	‡	‡	‡
Medulla	1.6	25	0.03	‡	‡	200
Cerebellum	0.2	2	0.01	0.07	0	160
Spinal cord	1.6	29	0	‡	0	‡
Sympathetic ganglia	30.0	7	0	6.00	5	‡
Area postrema	‡	460	0.24	1.04	‡	‡

*Data on dog from various authors, compiled by Paton: Annu Rev Physiol 20:431, 1958.
†Data on rat GABA (gamma-aminobutyric acid) from Berl & Waelsch: J Neurochem 3:161, 1958.
‡No data.

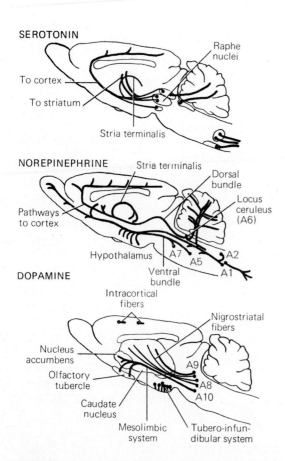

Figure 15—7. Aminergic pathways in a rat's brain. The numbers and letters (A1, A2, etc) refer to specific groups of catecholamine-containing cell bodies. The pathways in humans are similar. (Modified and reproduced, with permission, from Ungerstedt: Stereotaxic mapping of the monoamine pathways in the rat brain. Acta Physiol Scand [Suppl] 367:1, 1971.)

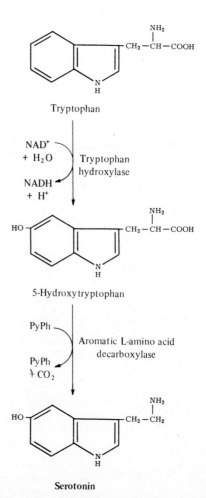

Figure 15—8. Biosynthesis of serotonin. PyPh = pyridoxal phosphate. Note that the same enzyme catalyzes the decarboxylation of 5-hydroxytryptophan and dopa (see Fig 13—3).

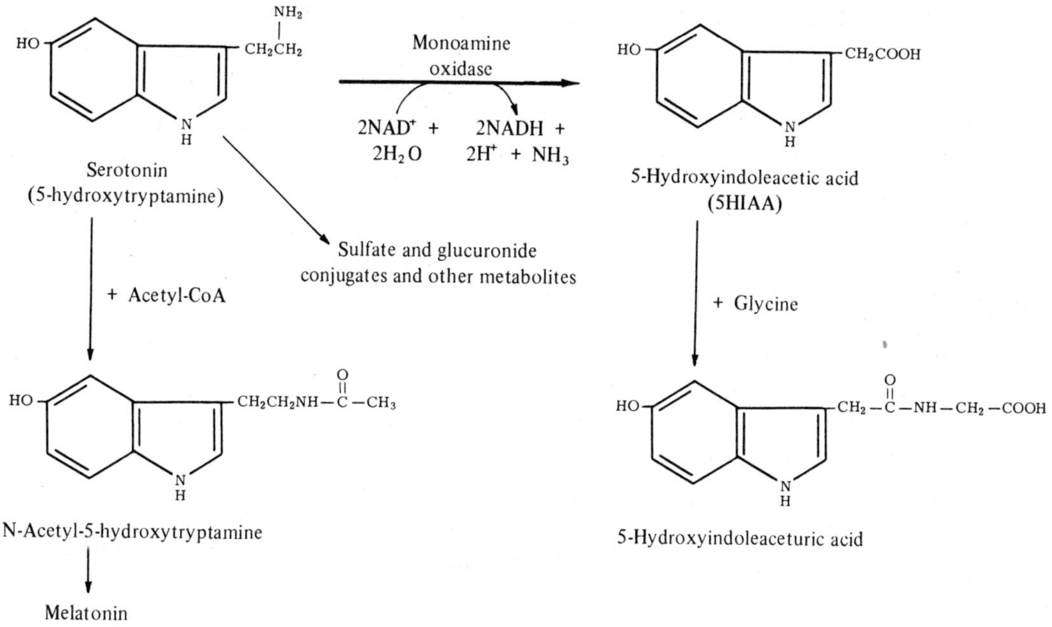

Figure 15–9. Catabolism of serotonin. In oxidative deaminations catalyzed by monoamine oxidase, an aldehyde is formed first and then oxidized to the corresponding acid. Some of the aldehyde is also reduced to the corresponding alcohol. The heavy arrow indicates the major metabolic pathway.

pronounced depletion of serotonin from body stores, including the brain; and if serotonin depletion is prevented the drug's tranquilizing action is blocked. However, reserpine also depletes brain norepinephrine and dopamine, and it is difficult to decide which of its effects are due to serotonin depletion and which to catecholamine depletion. Monoamine oxidase inhibitors, which are psychic energizers, increase brain serotonin, but they also increase brain norepinephrine and dopamine. Selective depletion of brain serotonin can be produced by administering *p*-chlorophenylalanine, a compound that blocks conversion of tryptophan to 5-hydroxytryptophan (Fig 15–8). This is the rate-limiting step in serotonin biosynthesis. In animals, *p*-chlorophenylalanine produces prolonged wakefulness, suggesting (along with other evidence) that serotonin plays a role in sleep. However, wakefulness is

not produced in humans, and no clear-cut psychic changes are produced even by large doses. Thus, the relation of serotonin to mental function remains uncertain. Serotonin may play a role in the regulation of the secretion of growth hormone and other anterior pituitary hormones. There is some evidence that serotonin is a mediator in descending fiber systems that inhibit the initiation of autonomic impulses in the lateral gray columns of the spinal cord. In addition, there is a prominent serotoninergic innervation of the suprachiasmatic nuclei of the hypothalamus, and serotonin may play some role in the regulation of circadian rhythms (see Chapter 14).

Norepinephrine

The distribution of norepinephrine in the brain parallels that of serotonin (Tables 15–2 and 15–3).

Table 15–3. Amine and substance P content of selected portions of the human brain.
Data compiled from various authors.

	Norepinephrine	Dopamine	Serotonin	Histamine	Substance P (units/g)
	(μg/g fresh tissue)				
Amygdala	0.21	0.6	0.26	*	*
Caudate nucleus	0.09	3.5	0.33	0.5	85
Putamen	0.12	3.7	0.32	0.7	*
Globus pallidus	0.15	0.5	0.23	0.6	*
Thalamus	0.13	0.3	0.26	0.4	12
Hypothalamus	1.25	0.8	0.29	2.5	102
Substantia nigra	0.21	0.9	0.55	*	699

*No data.

The cell bodies of most if not all of the norepinephrine-containing neurons are located in the locus ceruleus and other nuclei in the pons and medulla. Some of the axons descend in the spinal cord, innervating the dorsal and ventral horns and lateral gray columns. Some enter the cerebellum. Some ascend in the ventral bundle (Fig 15–7) to innervate the hypothalamus, and some ascend in the dorsal bundle to innervate the dorsal hypothalamus, limbic system, and neocortex.

Evidence has now accumulated that the norepinephrine in the brain is related to mental function. It has been known for some time that reserpine can produce depression and that monoamine oxidase inhibitors are psychic energizers. These drugs affect brain serotonin as well as brain catecholamines, but recent research with compounds that affect norepinephrine selectively indicates that mood is related to the amount of free norepinephrine available at synapses in the brain. When too little norepinephrine is available, depression results; and drugs such as monoamine oxidase inhibitors and amphetamine, which increase free norepinephrine, elevate mood. The tricyclic antidepressants such as desipramine appear to act in the same way; they decrease the reuptake of liberated norepinephrine (see Chapter 13), thus leaving more available to act on the postsynaptic structures.

In the cerebellum, adrenergic neurons inhibit Purkinje cells, and there is evidence that these inhibitory effects are mediated via β receptors and cyclic AMP.

The norepinephrine-containing neurons in the hypothalamus are involved in regulation of the secretion of anterior pituitary hormones (see Chapter 14), and they appear to inhibit the secretion of vasopressin and oxytocin. There is some evidence that norepinephrine is involved in the control of food intake and self-stimulation. Along with serotonin, it appears to be involved in the regulation of body temperature. An inhibitory effect on autonomic discharge from the spinal cord has also been suggested.

There is a system of PNMT-containing neurons with cell bodies in the medulla that project to the hypothalamus. Those neurons secrete epinephrine, but their function is uncertain. The biosynthesis and metabolism of norepinephrine and epinephrine are discussed in Chapter 13. There are appreciable quantities of tyramine in the CNS, but no function has been assigned to this agent.

Dopamine

Dopamine is the immediate precursor of norepinephrine (Fig 13–3). In certain parts of the brain, the concentration of norepinephrine is low and that of dopamine is very high (Table 15–3). These regions contain most of the enzymes found in parts of the brain that are rich in norepinephrine, but their dopamine β-hydroxylase activity is low. This is the enzyme that catalyzes the conversion of dopamine to norepinephrine; consequently, catecholamine synthesis stops at dopamine.

Dopamine is inactivated by monoamine oxidase

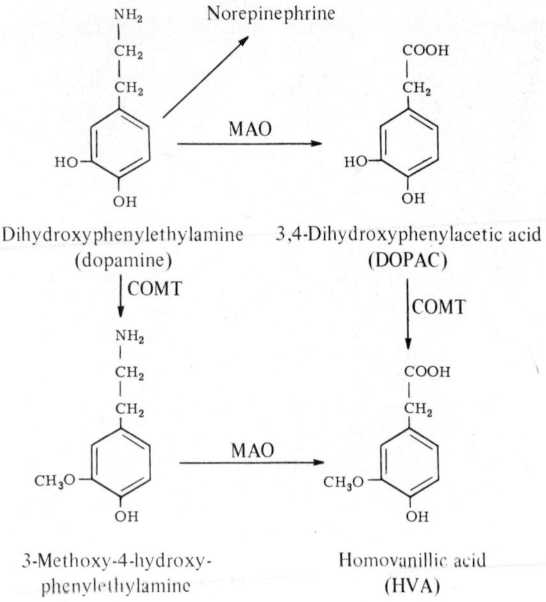

Figure 15–10. Catabolism of dopamine. MAO, monoamine oxidase; COMT, catechol-O-methyltransferase. See legend of Fig 15–9.

and by catechol-O-methyltransferase (Fig 15–10) in a manner analogous to the inactivation of norepinephrine (Fig 13–5).

Many dopaminergic neurons have their cell bodies in the midbrain (Fig 15–7). They project from the substantia nigra to the striatum (**nigrostriatal system**) and from other portions of the midbrain to the olfactory tubercle, nucleus accumbens, and related limbic areas (**mesolimbic system**). A separate intrahypothalamic system of dopaminergic neurons (**tuberoinfundibular system**) projects from cell bodies in the arcuate nucleus to the external layer of the median eminence of the hypothalamus (Fig 15–11). Dopaminergic neurons are also found in the cerebral cortex.

Evidence is accumulating that dopamine is related in some way to motor function. In Parkinson's disease (see Chapter 12), the dopamine content of the caudate nucleus and putamen is about 50% of normal. Hypothalamic norepinephrine is also reduced, but not to so great a degree. Several drugs that produce parkinsonism-like states as undesirable side-effects have been shown to alter the metabolism of dopamine or block dopamine receptors in the brain. On the other hand, L-dopa (levodopa) has been found to be very effective in the treatment of Parkinson's disease when administered in large doses. This compound, unlike dopamine, crosses the blood-brain barrier (see Chapter 17) and produces an increase in brain dopamine content.

Dopamine is also involved in the control of prolactin secretion. L-Dopa inhibits prolactin secretion in experimental animals and humans and has been used in the treatment of conditions in which there is abnormal milk secretion (galactorrhea). On the other hand, drugs

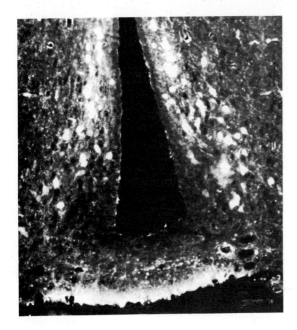

Figure 15—11. Dopaminergic neurons in the hypothalamus of the rat. *a*-Methylnorepinephrine injected before sacrifice to intensify fluorescence. Transverse section. Cell bodies can be seen above, in the arcuate nucleus on either side of the third ventricle, and the dense nerve terminals can be seen below in the external layer of the median eminence. (Reproduced, with permission, from Hökfelt & Fuxe: On the morphology and the neuroendocrine role of the hypothalamic catecholamine neurons. In: *Brain-Endocrine Interaction.* Knigge K, Scott D, Weindl A [editors] . Karger, 1972.)

such as reserpine which deplete brain catecholamines can cause galactorrhea. Dopamine can act directly on the anterior pituitary to inhibit prolactin secretion and has been found in portal hypophysial blood. Thus, it may well be the hypothalamic prolactin inhibiting hormone. However, there is some evidence for an additional polypeptide PIH.

There is increasing evidence that dopamine is involved in the pathogenesis of schizophrenia. Amphetamine, which stimulates dopamine secretion, produces a psychosis which resembles schizophrenia when administered in large doses, and several dopamine derivatives are hallucinogens. On the other hand, the phenothiazine tranquilizers are effective in the relief of many of the symptoms of schizophrenia, and their antipsychotic activity parallels their ability to block dopamine receptors.

Acetylcholine

Acetylcholine is distributed throughout the CNS with the highest concentrations in the motor cortex and the thalamus (Tables 15—1 and 15—2). The distribution of choline acetyltransferase and acetylcholinesterase parallels that of acetylcholine. Most of the acetylcholinesterase is in neurons, but some is found in glia. Pseudocholinesterase is found in many parts of the CNS.

Acetylcholine has been linked directly or indirectly to a variety of brain functions. Many cholinergic neurons in the CNS form a large ascending system. The cell bodies of these neurons are in the reticular formation and their axons radiate to all parts of the forebrain, including the hypothalamus, thalamus, visual pathways, basal ganglia, hippocampus, and neocortex. This system appears to be the ascending reticular activating system, which produces EEG arousal and maintains consciousness (see Chapter 11).

A number of hallucinogenic agents are derivatives of atropine, a drug which blocks muscarinic cholinergic receptors. Injections of acetylcholine into the hypothalamus and parts of the limbic system cause drinking. Application of acetylcholine to the supraoptic nucleus in dogs causes increased secretion of vasopressin. In blinded rats, acetylcholinesterase activity is decreased in the superior colliculi and elevated in the occipital cortex. Cortical levels of acetylcholinesterase are greater in rats raised in a complex environment than in rats raised in isolation, but the significance of this type of correlation is uncertain. Acetylcholine is an excitatory transmitter in the basal ganglia, whereas dopamine is an inhibitory transmitter in these structures. In parkinsonism, the loss of dopamine alters the cholinergic-dopaminergic balance, and anticholinergic drugs are of benefit along with L-dopa in the treatment of the disease.

Gamma-Aminobutyric Acid & Other Amino Acids

Gamma-aminobutyric acid (GABA) has been proved to be the synaptic transmitter at the inhibitory neuromuscular junctions in crustaceans. In mammals, it appears to be the mediator for presynaptic inhibition in the spinal cord (see Chapter 4) and an inhibitory mediator in the brain and in the retina. Its action is antagonized by picrotoxin. There is an increase in the amount of GABA released from the brain when the EEG pattern is that of slow wave sleep.

GABA is formed by decarboxylation of glutamic acid, and it can reenter the citric acid cycle by conversion to succinic acid (Fig 15—12). Glutamic decarboxylase has been demonstrated by immunocytochemical technics to be localized in nerve endings. The citric acid cycle is the major pathway by which intermediates formed in the catabolism of carbohydrates, proteins, and fats are metabolized to CO_2 and H_2O. Pyridoxal phosphate, a derivative of the B complex vitamin pyridoxine, is a cofactor for the decarboxylase that catalyzes the formation of GABA from glutamic acid. The transaminases responsible for the formation of glutamic acid and for the formation of succinic semialdehyde are also pyridoxine-dependent. However, the decarboxylation, unlike the transaminations, is essentially irreversible. Consequently, the GABA content of the brain is reduced in pyridoxine deficiency. Pyridoxine deficiency is associated with signs of neural hyperexcitability and convulsions, although pyridoxine treatment is unfortunately of no value in most clinical cases of idiopathic epilepsy.

Glutamic acid (glutamate) has been shown to be

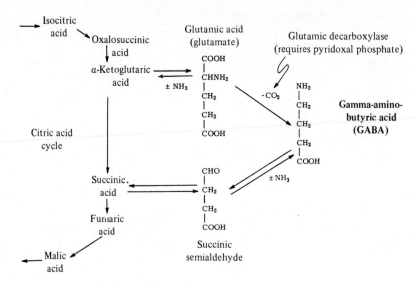

Figure 15–12. Formation and metabolism of gamma-aminobutyric acid.

the excitatory mediator at myoneural junctions in certain insects. Glutamic acid and aspartic acid (aspartate) depolarize mammalian neurons when placed directly on their membranes by microelectrophoresis, but they have not been proved to be transmitters at any specific location in mammals.

Evidence is now accumulating that the ubiquitous amino acid **glycine** is the mediator responsible for direct inhibition in the spinal cord. When applied directly to the membranes of neurons, it produces hyperpolarization, and its action is antagonized by strychnine.

One conceptual objection to glycine and other amino acids as transmitters is the fact that these amino acids probably occur not only in neurons but in most if not all living cells. However, the necessary specificity for chemical transmission is provided not by unique chemicals but by specialized neuronal mechanisms for the storage, release, and postsynaptic action of a particular substance. Thus, almost any small diffusible substance could be a transmitter.

Histamine

There are large amounts of histamine in the anterior and posterior lobes of the pituitary and in the adjacent median eminence of the hypothalamus. The heparin-containing tissue cells called **mast cells** have a high histamine content, and most of the histamine in the posterior pituitary is in mast cells although the histamine in the anterior pituitary and the hypothalamus is not. In other parts of the brain, the histamine content is low, but various parts of the brain have been shown to contain histamine-activated adenylate cyclase. Histamine is formed by decarboxylation of the amino acid histidine (Fig 15–13). The enzyme that catalyzes this step differs from L-aromatic amino acid decarboxylase, which decarboxylates 5-hydroxytryptophan and dopa. Histamine is converted to methylhista-

mine, or alternately, to imidazoleacetic acid. The latter reaction is quantitatively less important in humans. It requires the enzyme **diamine oxidase (histaminase)** rather than monoamine oxidase, even though monoamine oxidase catalyzes the oxidation of methylhistamine to methylimidazoleacetic acid.

So far, there is relatively little evidence other than uneven distribution to suggest that histamine is a synaptic mediator in the brain. However, there are 2 known types of histamine receptors, H_1 and H_2 receptors, and both are found in the brain. The histamine

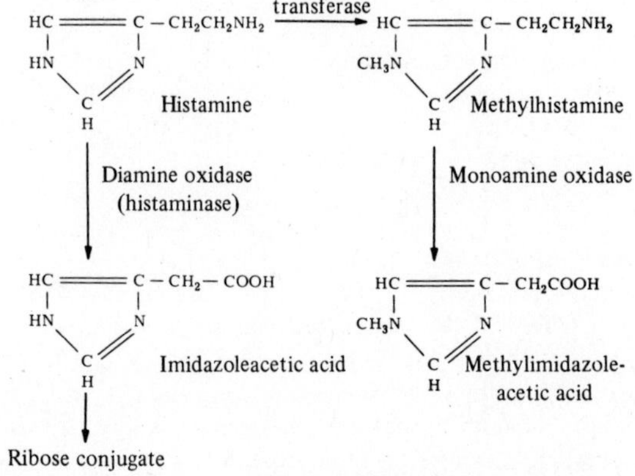

Figure 15–13. Synthesis and catabolism of histamine.

Arg-Pro-Lys-Pro-Gln-Gln-Phe-Phe-Gly-Leu-Met-NH$_2$
 1   2   3   4   5   6   7   8   9   10   11

Figure 15—14. Bovine substance P.

Tyr-Gly-Gly-Phe-Met
Met-enkephalin

Tyr-Gly-Gly-Phe-Leu
Leu-enkephalin

Figure 15—15. The 2 enkephalins found in brain tissue.

content of the brain is increased by the tremor-producing drug tremorine; by the psychotomimetic agent mescaline; and by the tranquilizer chlorpromazine. The content is decreased by reserpine.

Substance P

Substance P (Fig 15—14) is a polypeptide. It is found in appreciable quantities in the intestine, where it may be a chemical mediator in the myenteric reflex. In the nervous system, high concentrations are found in the hypothalamus and the dorsal roots of the spinal nerves, and there are particularly large amounts in the substantia nigra (Tables 15—2 and 15—3). Little is known about the synthesis and catabolism of this polypeptide, although brain tissue apparently contains enzymes that are concerned with both processes. There is considerable evidence that substance P is a transmitter in primary sensory afferents that end in the region of the dorsal horn of the spinal cord.

Other Peptides

The hypothalamic hormones somatostatin and TRH (see Chapter 14) are found in other parts of the brain in addition to the hypothalamus, and somatostatin-containing granules have been reported to be present in primary sensory afferents that are different from those containing substance P. It has recently been reported that the gastrointestinal hormone VIP and a substance resembling CCK are also present in the brain, but their function in this location is not known.

The brain contains receptors that bind morphine,

and 2 closely related pentapeptides called **enkephalins** (Fig 15—15), which bind to these opiate receptors, have been isolated from brain tissue. Their function is as yet unknown, but they do have analgesic activity when injected into the brain stem. Two larger peptides called **endorphins**, which bind to opiate receptors and have analgesic activity, are also found in the body. One contains 17 amino acid residues (a-endorphin) and the other contains these 17 plus 16 additional amino acid residues (β-endorphin). Both contain the amino acid sequence of Met-enkephalin. The amino acid sequence found in β-endorphin is in turn found in a polypeptide called β-lipotropin that has been isolated from the anterior pituitary gland. The significance of this fact is as yet unknown.

Prostaglandins

Prostaglandins—fatty acid derivatives found in high concentration in semen—are also found in the brain. They have been shown to be present in nerve ending fractions of brain homogenates and to be released from the cortex, the cerebellum, and the spinal cord. When administered by microelectrophoresis onto nerve cell membranes, they alter the firing rates of the neurons. This suggests that they may be synaptic mediators. However, it seems more likely that they exert their effects by modulating reactions mediated by cyclic AMP.

16...
"Higher Functions of the Nervous System": Conditioned Reflexes, Learning, & Related Phenomena

In previous chapters, somatic and visceral input to the brain and output from it have been discussed. The functions of the reticular core in maintaining an alert, awake state have been described, and the functions of the limbic-midbrain circuit in the maintenance of homeostatic equilibriums and the regulation of instinctual and emotional behavior have been catalogued (Fig 16—1). There remain the phenomena called, for lack of a better or more precise term, the "higher functions of the nervous system": learning, memory, judgment, language, and the other functions of the mind. As Penfield has said, those who study the neurophysiology of the mind are, ". . . like men at the foot of a mountain. They stand in the clearings they have made

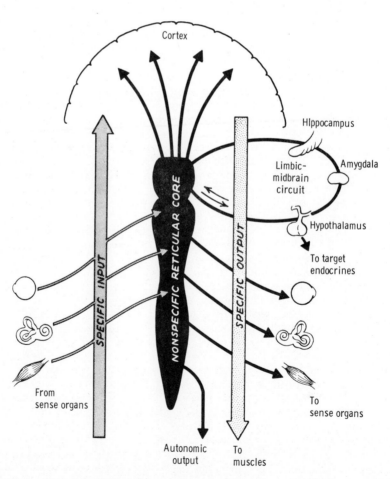

Figure 16—1. Organization of the nervous system. (Modified from Galambos & Morgan, in: *Handbook of Physiology*. Field J, Magoun HW [editors]. Washington: The American Physiological Society, 1960. Section 1, pp 1471—1500.)

on the foothills, looking up at the mountain they hope to scale. But the pinnacle is hidden in eternal clouds."* These "clearings on the foothills" are the subject of this chapter.

Methods

Some of the phenomena of the mind, such as learning and possibly memory, occur in many animal species, whereas others probably only occur to a significant degree in humans. All are hard to study because it is difficult to communicate with animals and because moral and legal considerations rightly limit experimental studies in humans. In general, the available data have been obtained by 5 methods. The oldest method consists of correlating clinical observations in humans with the site and extent of brain pathology discovered at autopsy. Information obtained in this way has been supplemented by studying the effects of stimulation of the exposed cerebral cortex during neurosurgical procedures under local anesthesia. Another method is study of the effects of stimulating subcortical structures with chronically implanted electrodes in patients with parkinsonism, schizophrenia, epilepsy, and incurable malignancies. There has been a good deal of work on changes in brain morphology and chemistry coincident with learning in animals. The fifth approach has been the study of conditioned reflexes.

LEARNING

Learning is sometimes assumed to be a function of the cerebral hemispheres, but it also occurs in many animal species that have no cerebral cortex. It occurs readily in animals such as the octopus; it has been demonstrated in worms; and it may even occur in unicellular organisms. In addition, phenomena resembling learning occur at subcortical and spinal levels in mammals. Post-tetanic potentiation, the facilitation in a synaptic pathway that follows repeated stimulation (see Chapter 4), is such a phenomenon. Another is the long-term response to the injection of formalin into one paw in kittens. The inflammation and other visible effects of such an injection subside within a few weeks. However, it has been reported that if the kitten is decerebrated months or even years later, it develops flexor rather than extensor rigidity in the injected limb, even though the expected extensor response occurs in the other 3 extremities.

The rapidity with which persistent alterations in neural pathways can be produced in the spinal cord is illustrated by experiments on the effect of cord section in rats with unilateral cerebellar lesions. These lesions cause the rats to assume abnormal postures. The postural abnormalities in the limbs and trunk disappear if

*From *Handbook of Physiology*. Field J, Magoun HW (editors). Washington: The American Physiological Society, 1960. Section 1, p 1441.

the spinal cord is transected in the cervical region up to 45 minutes after the production of the lesion. However, if the spinal cord is transected more than 45 minutes after the lesion has been produced, the abnormalities persist.

More advanced types of learning are largely cortical phenomena, but the brain stem is also involved in these processes. Some types of learning have been shown to produce structural changes in the cerebral cortex. For example, rats exposed to visually complex environments and trained to perform various tasks have thicker, heavier cerebral cortices than control rats exposed to monotonously uniform environments. Mice raised in darkness and then exposed to light develop additional spines on the dendrites of their pyramidal cortical cells.

Conditioned Reflexes

Conditioned reflexes are an important type of learning. A conditioned reflex is a reflex response to a stimulus which did not previously elicit the response, acquired by repeatedly pairing the stimulus with another stimulus that normally does produce the response. In Pavlov's classical experiments, the salivation normally induced by placing meat in the mouth of a dog was studied. A bell was rung just before the meat was placed in the dog's mouth, and this was repeated a number of times until the animal would salivate when the bell was rung even though no meat was placed in its mouth. In this experiment the meat placed in the mouth was the **unconditioned stimulus** (US), the stimulus that normally produces a particular innate response. The **conditioned stimulus** (CS) was the bell-ringing. After the CS and US had been paired a sufficient number of times, the CS produced the response originally evoked only by the US. An immense number of somatic, visceral, and other neural phenomena can be made to occur as conditioned reflex responses.

If the CS is presented repeatedly without the US, the conditioned reflex eventually dies out. This process is called **extinction** or **internal inhibition**. If the animal is disturbed by an external stimulus immediately after the CS is applied, the conditioned response may not occur (**external inhibition**). However, if the conditioned reflex is **reinforced** from time to time by again pairing the CS and US, the conditioned reflex persists indefinitely.

When a conditioned reflex is first established, it can be evoked not only by the CS but also by similar stimuli. However, if only the CS is reinforced and the similar stimuli are not, the animal can be taught to discriminate between different signals with great accuracy. The elimination of the response to other stimuli is an example of internal inhibition. By means of such **discriminative conditioning** dogs can be taught, for example, to distinguish between a tone of 800 Hz and one of 812 Hz. Most of the data on pitch discrimination, color vision, and other sensory discriminations in animals have been obtained in this way.

For conditioning to occur, the CS must precede the US. If the CS follows the US, no conditioned response develops. The conditioned response follows the CS by the time interval that separated the CS and US during training. The delay between stimulus and response may be as long as 90 sec. When the time interval is appreciable, the response is called a **delayed conditioned reflex.**

As noted in Chapter 15, conditioned reflexes are difficult to form if the US provokes a purely motor response. They are relatively easily formed if the US is associated with a pleasant or unpleasant affect. Stimulation of the brain reward system is a powerful US (pleasant, or **positive reinforcement**), and so is stimulation of the avoidance system or a painful shock to the skin (unpleasant, or **negative reinforcement**).

Operant conditioning has been the subject of considerable research, especially in the United States. This is a form of conditioning in which the animal is taught to perform some task ("operate on the environment") in order to obtain a reward or avoid punishment. The US is the pleasant or unpleasant event, and the CS is a light or some other signal that alerts the animal to perform the task. Conditioned motor responses that permit an animal to avoid an unpleasant event are called **conditioned avoidance reflexes.** For example, an animal is taught that by pressing a bar it can prevent an electric shock to the feet. Reflexes of this type are extensively used in testing tranquilizers and other drugs that affect behavior.

Physiologic Basis of Conditioned Reflexes

The essential feature of the conditioned reflex is the formation of a new functional connection in the nervous system. In Pavlov's experiment, for example, salivation in response to bell-ringing indicates that a functional connection has developed between the auditory pathways and the autonomic centers controlling salivation. Because decortication depresses or interferes with the formation of many conditioned reflexes, it was originally thought that these new connections were intracortical. However, the effects of cortical ablation on conditioned reflexes are complex. When the CS is a complex sensory stimulus, the cortical sensory area for the sensory modality involved must be present. The rest of the cortex is not necessary, however, and nondiscriminative conditioned responses to simple sensory stimuli can be formed in the absence of the whole cortex. These and other experiments indicate that the new connections are formed in subcortical structures.

Electroencephalographic & Evoked Potential Changes During Conditioning

When a new sensory stimulus is first presented to an animal, it produces diffuse EEG arousal and prominent evoked secondary responses in many parts of the brain. Behaviorally, the human or animal becomes alert and attentive, a response that Pavlov called the **orienting reflex** (the "What is it?" response). If the stimulus is neither pleasurable nor noxious, it evokes less electrical response when repeated, and the EEG and other changes eventually cease to occur; the animal "becomes accustomed to" the stimulus and ignores it. These electrical and behavioral phenomena are thus examples of habituation. Changes in sensory stimuli also provoke arousal. For example, when an animal becomes habituated to a stimulus such as a regularly repeated tone, stopping the tone produces arousal.

If a signal to which an animal has become habituated is paired with another stimulus that evokes EEG arousal, conditioning occurs; after relatively few pairings, the previously neutral stimulus alone evokes desynchronization. This conditioned response to the neutral stimulus is an example of **electrocortical conditioning,** and is sometimes called the **alpha block conditioned reflex.** An example in the human of the alpha block conditioned reflex is shown in Fig 16–2. Electrocortical conditioning is unaffected by cutting the lateral connections of the cortical sensory areas but is prevented by lesions in the nonspecific projection nuclei of the thalamus, which indicates that the new connections involved are formed at or below the thalamic level. If an alpha block conditioned reflex is not reinforced, extinction occurs. Extinction is associated with the development of EEG hypersynchrony (extremely regular, large amplitude waves) in the cortical area concerned with the US that generated the reflex. This observation and various psychologic data suggest that extinction, or "unlearning," is not passive but,

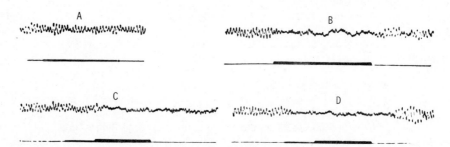

Figure 16–2. Conditioned blocking of the alpha rhythm in the occipital region in a normal human. *A:* Lack of response to a tone to which the subject was habituated (thin black signal). *B:* Unconditioned alpha block (desynchronization) in response to a bright light (heavy black signal). *C:* Failure of the tone to produce desynchronization when first paired with the light. *D:* After ninth pairing of tone and light, the tone produces conditioned alpha block before the light is turned on. (Reproduced, with permission, from Morrell & Ross: Central inhibition in cortical reflexes. Arch Neurol Psychiatry 70:611, 1953.)

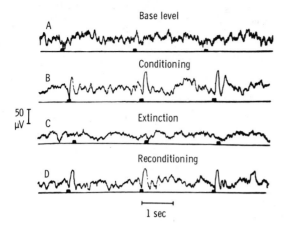

Base level

A

Conditioning

B

50 μV I

C

Extinction

D

Reconditioning

1 sec

Figure 16–3. Records of the electrical activity of the hippo-campus in a monkey exposed repeatedly to a tone stimulus (black signal marks). *A:* Control. *B:* After the tone was paired with a reward of food. *C:* After extinction of this response. *D:* After reconditioning by again pairing the tone with food. (Reproduced, with permission, from Hearst & others: Some electrophysiological correlates of conditioning in the monkey. Electroencephalogr Clin Neurophysiol 12:137, 1960.)

like learning, involves an active process in the nervous system.

A stimulus produces EEG and behavioral arousal and widespread evoked potentials not only if it is new but also if it has been paired with a pleasant or unpleasant experience. For example, if a tone to which the animal has become habituated is paired a few times with an electric shock to the feet, the tone will produce large evoked responses in the brain stem reticular formation and throughout much of the cortex. A similar response is observed if the tone is positively reinforced. An example of these changes in a record of the electrical activity of the hippocampus is shown in Fig 16–3. The hippocampus is not in the direct sensory pathways, but evoked potentials are regularly produced in it by sensory stimuli, presumably via the RAS.

It is common knowledge that, at least at a behavioral level, similar conditioning of the arousal value of stimuli occurs in humans. The mother who sleeps through many kinds of noise but wakes promptly when her baby cries is one example. The intern who is unaware of the calls on the loudspeaker unless his own name is called is another example of a conditioned arousal response to a particular stimulus.

Attention

The generalized arousal response to a stimulus can progress to focused attention. When such focusing occurs, other sensory inputs are inhibited. This inhibition is common knowledge; we have all had the experience of having to say, "I'm sorry, but I didn't hear you. I was reading the newspaper." In animals this inhibition can occur at many levels, from the sense organs themselves to the cortex (see Chapter 11).

Intercortical Transfer of Learning

If a cat or monkey is conditioned to respond to a visual stimulus with one eye covered and then tested with the blindfold transferred to the other eye, it performs the conditioned response. This is true even if the optic chiasm has been cut, making the visual input from each eye go only to the ipsilateral cortex. If, in addition to the optic chiasm, the anterior and posterior commissures and the corpus callosum are sectioned ("split brain animal"), no transfer of learning occurs. This demonstrates that the neural coding necessary for "remembering with one eye what has been learned with the other" has been transferred somehow to the opposite cortex via the commissures. There is evidence for similar transfer of information acquired through other sensory pathways. "Split brain animals" can even be trained to respond to different and conflicting stimuli, one with one eye and another with the other—literally an example of not letting the right side know what the left side is doing. Attempts at such training in normal animals and humans lead to confusion, but they do not faze the animals with split brains. Similar results have been obtained in humans in whom the corpus callosum is congenitally absent or in whom it has been sectioned surgically in an effort to control epileptic seizures.

MEMORY

In discussions of the memory process, it is important to distinguish between remote and recent memories. It now appears that 3 mechanisms interact in the production of memories, one mediating immediate recall of the events of the moment, another mediating memories of events that occurred minutes to hours before, and a third mediating memories of the remote past. Memory for recent events is quite frequently impaired or lost in individuals with neurologic diseases, but remote memories are remarkably resistant and persist in the presence of severe brain damage.

Stimulation of portions of the temporal lobe in patients with temporal lobe epilepsy evokes detailed memories of events that occurred in the remote past, often beyond the power of voluntary recall. This response has not as yet been definitely proved to occur in individuals with normal temporal lobe function, but exposure of the temporal lobe has been carried out in relatively few individuals who were not suffering from temporal lobe disease. The memories produced by temporal lobe stimulation are "flashed back" complete, as if they were replays of a segment of experience. A particular memory is generally evoked by stimulation of a given point; it unfolds as long as the stimulus is applied, and stops when the stimulus is discontinued. For a number of reasons it seems unlikely that the memories themselves are localized in the temporal lobes. Instead, the temporal lobe points are probably "keys" that unlock memory traces stored elsewhere in the brain and the brain stem. Normally, a key is turned by some sort of comparing, associating circuit when there is a similarity between the memory and the current sensory input or stream of thought.

Stimulation of other parts of the temporal lobes sometimes causes a patient to change his interpretation of his surroundings. For example, when the stimulus is applied, he may feel strange in a familiar place or may feel that what is happening now has happened before. The occurrence of a sense of familiarity or a sense of strangeness in appropriate situations probably helps the normal individual adjust to the environment. In strange surroundings one is alert and on guard, whereas in familiar surroundings vigilance is relaxed. An inappropriate feeling of familiarity with new events or in new surroundings is known clinically as the *déjà vu* **phenomenon,** from the French words meaning "already seen." The phenomenon occurs from time to time in normal individuals, but it also may occur as an aura (a sensation immediately preceding a seizure) in patients with temporal lobe epilepsy.

Other data pertinent to the physiology of memory are the clinical and experimental observations showing that there is frequently a loss of memory for the events immediately preceding brain concussion or electroshock therapy **(retrograde amnesia).** In humans this amnesia encompasses longer periods than it does in animals—sometimes days, weeks, and even years—but remote memory is not affected. In animals, acquisition of learned responses—or at least their retrieval—is prevented if, within 5 minutes after each training session, the animals are anesthetized, given electroshock treatment, or subjected to hypothermia. Such treatment 4 hours after the training sessions has no effect on acquisition. It thus appears that there is a period of "encoding" or "consolidation" of memory during which the memory trace is vulnerable. However, following this period a stable and remarkably resistant memory engram exists.

There is considerable evidence that the encoding process involves the hippocampus and its connections. Bilateral destruction of the ventral hippocampus in humans and bilateral lesions of the same area in experimental animals cause striking defects in recent memory. Humans with such destruction have intact remote memory, and they perform adequately as long as they concentrate on what they are doing. However, if they are distracted for even a very short period, all memory of what they were doing and proposed to do is lost. They are thus capable of new learning and retain old memories, but they are deficient in forming new memories.

Additional evidence for the involvement of the hippocampus is the observation that in humans with chronically implanted electrodes, stimuli producing seizures in the hippocampus cause loss of recent memory. The hippocampal neurons are particularly prone to iterative discharge, and hippocampal seizures presumably disrupt the normal function of this structure. Several drugs which impair or alter recent memory produce abnormal electrical discharges in the hippocam-

pus. Some alcoholics with brain damage develop considerable impairment of recent memory, and it has been claimed that the occurrence of this defect correlates well with the presence of pathologic changes in the mammillary bodies.

Ribonucleic Acid (RNA), Protein Synthesis, & Memory

The nature of the stable memory trace is largely unknown, but its resistance to electroshock and concussion suggests that memory might be stored as an actual biochemical change in the neurons. The ability of regenerated planarians to retain learned habits indicates that such changes occur in some animal species. Planarians are flatworms with rudimentary nervous systems and a remarkable ability to regenerate when cut in pieces. They can be taught to avoid certain visual stimuli. If a trained worm is divided in two, not only does the worm regenerated from the head piece retain the response but so does the worm regenerated from the tail.

One possible explanation of this phenomenon is the hypothesis that the acquisition of the learned response is associated with an increase in the synthesis of new ribonucleic acid (RNA) in the cells. RNA provides a template for protein synthesis (see Chapter 1). If learning causes a stable alteration in the RNA, the learning response could conceivably be passed on to the new parts of the regenerated planarians. In support of this idea is the observation that treatment of the cut pieces of conditioned planarians with ribonuclease, the enzyme that destroys RNA, prevents the tail segments from regenerating into fully conditioned worms. Indeed, it has been claimed that if trained planarians are ground up and fed to untrained planarians, the untrained worms acquire with much greater facility than controls the responses the trained worms had learned. It has also been reported that, in goldfish and rats, injection of brain extracts of trained animals improves learning in untrained animals.

There is additional evidence that protein synthesis is involved in some way in the processes responsible for memory. In rats, increased RNA turnover occurs in nerve cells subjected to intense stimulation. In goldfish, the antibiotics puromycin and acetoxycycloheximide prevent the retention of conditioned avoidance responses when given up to 1 hour after the training session, although they have no effect on their acquisition. Puromycin also disrupts recent memory in mice. These antibiotics inhibit protein synthesis. Theoretically, the discharge of neurons during learning sessions could lead to changes in the phosphorylation of nuclear proteins, the methylation of DNA bases, or both. This could in turn enhance synthesis of mRNA and hence the synthesis of particular proteins. These proteins could modify synaptic transmission by affecting transmitter synthesis, membrane permeability, or some other neural process. However, it is a long way from these speculations to an understanding of the relationship of RNA and protein synthesis to the formation of the stable memory trace.

Drugs That Facilitate Learning

A variety of CNS stimulants have been shown to improve learning in animals when administered immediately before or after the learning sessions. These include caffeine, physostigmine, amphetamine, nicotine, and the convulsants picrotoxin, strychnine, and pentylenetetrazol (Metrazol). They seem to act by facilitating consolidation of the memory trace. In senile humans, small doses of pentylenetetrazol appear to improve memory and general awareness. The β-adrenergic blocking drug propranolol has been reported to improve learning in the elderly, and a theory has been advanced that decreased learning in these individuals is related to increased autonomic activity. Another drug that appears to facilitate learning in animals is pemoline (Cylert). This compound is a mild CNS stimulant, but it has attracted attention because it has also been shown to stimulate RNA synthesis.

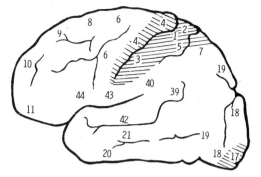

Figure 16–4. Lateral view of the human cerebral cortex, showing various numbered areas of Brodmann. The shaded areas represent the primary sensory and motor areas. The remaining white areas are the association areas. (Reproduced, with permission, from Cobb: *Foundations of Neuropsychiatry,* 6th ed. Williams & Wilkins, 1958.)

FUNCTIONS OF THE NEOCORTEX

Memory and learning are functions of large parts of the brain, but the centers controlling some of the other "higher functions of the nervous system," particularly the mechanisms related to language, are more or less localized to the neocortex. It is interesting that speech and other intellectual functions are especially well developed in humans—the animal species in which the neocortical mantle is most highly evolved.

Anatomic Considerations

There are 3 living species with brains larger than a human's (the porpoise, the elephant, and the whale), but in humans the ratio between brain weight and body weight far exceeds that of any of their animal relatives. From the comparative point of view, the most prominent gross feature of the human brain is the immense growth of the 3 major **association areas**: the **frontal,** in front of the motor cortex; the **temporal,** between the superior temporal gyrus and the limbic cortex; and the **parieto-occipital,** between the somesthetic and visual cortices.

The association areas are part of the 6-layered neocortical mantle of gray matter that spreads over the lateral surfaces of the cerebral hemispheres from the concentric allocortical and juxtallocortical rings around the hilus (see Chapter 15). The minor histologic differences in various portions of the cortex that are the basis for numbering cortical areas (Fig 16–4) are generally but not always correlated with differences in function.

The neuronal connections within the neocortex form a complicated network (Fig 11–2). The descending axons of the larger cells in the pyramidal cell layer give off collaterals that feed back via association neurons to the dendrites of the cells from which they originate, laying the foundation for complex reverbera-

tion. The recurrent collaterals also connect to neighboring cells and some end on inhibitory neurons which in turn end on the original cell, forming loops that mediate negative feedback inhibition (Chapter 4). The large, complex dendrites of the deep cells receive ascending fibers, nonspecific thalamic and reticular afferents and association fibers ending in all layers, and specific thalamic afferents ending in layer 4 of the cortex. The function of the intracortical association fibers is uncertain, but they can be cut with little evident effect. Thus, the term association areas is somewhat misleading; these areas must have a much more complex function than simple interconnection of cortical regions.

Aphasia & Allied Disorders

One group of functions which are more or less localized to the neocortex in humans are those related to language, ie, to understanding the spoken and printed word and to expressing ideas in speech and writing. Abnormalities of these functions which are not due to defects of vision or hearing or to motor paralysis are called **aphasias.** Many different classifications of the aphasias have been published, and the nomenclature in this area is chaotic. In a general way, the aphasias can be divided into **sensory** (or **receptive**) aphasias and **motor** (or **expressive**) aphasias. They can be further subdivided into **word deafness,** inability to understand spoken words; **word blindness,** inability to understand written words; **agraphia,** inability to express ideas in writing; and the defect commonly signified by the term **motor aphasia,** inability to express ideas in speech. Inability to carry out learned motor acts is called **apraxia.** Motor aphasia is divided into **nonfluent aphasia,** in which speech is slow and words hard to come by; and **fluent aphasia,** in which speech is normal or even rapid but key words are missing. Patients with severe degrees of nonfluent aphasia are limited to 2 or 3 words with which they must attempt to express the whole range of meaning and emotion. Sometimes the words retained are those that were being spoken at the

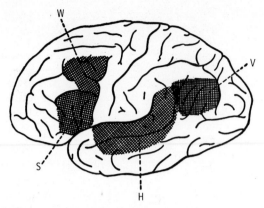

Figure 16–5. One theory of the localization of the language functions. In the hemisphere concerned with language functions, lesions at W are said to cause difficulty in expressing ideas in writing; at S, difficulty in oral expression; at H, difficulty in understanding spoken words; and at V, difficulty in understanding written words. (Reproduced, with permission, from *Physiology and Biophysics,* 19th ed. Ruch TC, Patton HD [editors]. Saunders, 1965.)

time of injury or vascular accident that caused the aphasia. More commonly they are frequently used **automatic words** such as the days of the week, or, for some reason, "dirty" words and swear words.

Only one of the cerebral hemispheres is primarily concerned with the language function (see below). In this hemisphere, the locations said to be associated with the various forms of aphasia are shown in Fig 16–5. In clinical cases, however, more than one form of aphasia is usually present. Frequently, the aphasia is general, or **global,** involving both receptive and expressive functions. Lesions of area 44 in the inferior frontal gyrus (**Broca's area,** area S in Fig 16–5) cause nonfluent aphasia; in patients with fluent aphasia, Broca's area is intact and the lesions are generally in the temporal or parietal lobe.

Complementary Specialization of the Hemispheres vs "Cerebral Dominance"

It is a well-established fact that human language functions depend more on one cerebral hemisphere than on the other. This hemisphere is concerned with categorization and symbolization and has often been called the **dominant hemisphere.** However, it is now clear that the other hemisphere is not simply less developed or "nondominant"; instead, it is specialized in the area of spatiotemporal relations. It is this hemisphere which is concerned, for example, with the recognition of faces, the identification of objects by their form, and the recognition of musical themes. Consequently, the concept of "cerebral dominance" and a dominant and nondominant hemisphere is being replaced by a concept of complementary specialization of the hemispheres, one for language functions (the **categorical hemisphere**) and one for spatiotemporal relations (the **representational hemisphere**).

Lesions in the categorical hemisphere produce

aphasia, whereas extensive lesions of the representational hemisphere do not. Instead, lesions in the representational hemisphere produce **astereognosis**— inability to identify objects by feeling them—and other agnosias. **Agnosia** is the general term used for the inability to recognize objects by a particular sensory modality even though the sensory modality itself is intact. Lesions producing these defects are generally in the parietal lobe.

Hemispheric specialization is related to handedness. Handedness appears to be genetically determined. In right-handed individuals, it is the left hemisphere which is the dominant or categorical hemisphere; in approximately 30% of left-handed individuals, the right hemisphere is the categorical hemisphere. However, in the remaining 70% of left-handers, the left hemisphere is the categorical hemisphere. In adults, the characteristic defects produced by lesions in either the categorical or the representational hemisphere are long-lasting. However, in young children subjected to hemispherectomy for brain tumors or other diseases, the functions of the missing hemisphere may be largely taken over by the remaining hemisphere no matter which hemisphere is removed.

The Frontal Lobes

Some insight into the other functions of the various parts of the cerebral cortex is gained by ablation studies. Bilateral removal of the neocortical portions of the frontal lobes in primates produces, after a period of apathy, hyperactivity and constant pacing back and forth. General intelligence is little affected, and tests involving immediate responses to environmental stimuli are normal. However, responses requiring the use of previously acquired information are abnormal. In humans, frontal lobectomy leads to deficiencies in the temporal ordering of events. For example, humans who have been lobectomized have difficulty remembering how long ago they saw a particular stimulus card. Interestingly, left frontal lobectomy causes the biggest deficit in tests involving word stimuli, while right frontal lobectomy causes the biggest deficit in tests involving picture stimuli. Frontal lobectomy also abolishes the experimental neurosis.

Experimental Neurosis

As noted above, animals can be conditioned to respond to one stimulus and not to another even when the 2 stimuli are very much alike. However, when the stimuli are so nearly identical that they cannot be distinguished, the animal becomes upset, whines, fails to cooperate, and tries to escape. Pavlov called these symptoms the **experimental neurosis.** One may quarrel about whether this reaction is a true neurosis in the psychiatric sense, but the term is convenient. In some species the experimental neurosis affects not only behavior in conditioning tests but general behavior as well.

Frontal lobectomized animals are still capable of discriminating between like stimuli up to a point; but when they can no longer discriminate, their failure does not upset them. As a result of these experiments in animals, **prefrontal lobotomy** and various other procedures aimed at cutting the connections between the frontal lobes and the deeper portions of the brain were introduced for the treatment of various mental diseases in humans.

In some mental patients, tensions resulting from real or imagined failures of performance and the tensions caused by delusions, compulsions, and phobias are so great as to be incapacitating. Successful lobotomy reduces the tension. The delusions and other symptoms are still there, but they no longer bother the patient. A similar lack of concern over severe pain has led to the use of lobotomy in treating patients with intractable pain (see Chapter 7). Unfortunately, this lack of concern often extends to other aspects of the environment, including relations with associates, social amenities, and even toilet habits. Furthermore, the relief from the suffering associated with pain usually lasts less than a year.

The effects which lobotomy can have on the personality were well described over 100 years ago by the physician who cared for a man named Phineas P. Gage. Gage was a construction foreman who was packing blasting powder into a hole with a tamping iron. The powder exploded, driving the tamping iron through his face and out the top of his skull, transecting his frontal lobes. After the accident, he became, in the words of his physician, ". . . fitful, irreverent, indulging at times in the grossest profanity (which was not previously his custom), manifesting but little deference to his fellows, impatient of restraint or advice when it conflicts with his desires, at times pertinaciously obstinate yet capricious and vacillating, devising many plans for future operation which are no sooner arranged than they are abandoned in turn for others appearing more feasible. . . .His mind was radically changed, so that his friends and acquaintances said he was no longer Gage."*

This description is classical, but it cannot be said to be typical. The effects of lobotomy in humans are highly variable from patient to patient. This variability has been attributed to variations in the milieu in which different patients are observed, and to differences in the extent and site of brain destruction. However, studies in which these variables were controlled make it clear that identical operations produce widely differ-

*From Harlow: Recovery from the passage of an iron bar through the head. Massachusetts Med Soc Publications 2:237, 1868.

ing results that depend upon each patient's preoperative personality and past experiences. Attempts have been made to reduce the variability and the incidence of undesirable effects by selective procedures such as lesions in the anterior portion of the cingulate gyrus. Nevertheless, the complications are frequent, and because the desirable effects of lobotomy can generally be achieved with tranquilizers and other drugs, lobotomies are rarely, if ever, performed for the treatment of mental disease.

Temporal Lobes

The effects of bilateral temporal lobectomy were first described by Klüver and Bucy. Temporal lobectomized monkeys ("Klüver-Bucy animals") are docile and hyperphagic and the males are hypersexual, all of which effects are due to the removal of limbic structures. The animals also demonstrate visual agnosia, and a remarkable increase in oral activity. The monkeys repeatedly pick up all movable objects in their environment. They manipulate each object in a compulsive way, mouth, lick, and bite it, and then, unless it is edible, discard it. However, discarded objects are picked up again in a few minutes as if the animal had never seen them before and subjected to the same manipulation and oral exploration. It has been suggested that the cause of this pattern of behavior may be an inability to identify objects. It could well be a manifestation of a memory loss due to hippocampal ablation. In addition, the animals are easily distracted. They heed every stimulus, whether it is novel or not, and usually approach, explore, manipulate, and, if possible, bite its source. This failure to ignore peripheral stimuli is called **hypermetamorphosis**.

Clinical Implications & Significance

Various parts of the syndrome described by Klüver and Bucy in monkeys are seen in humans with temporal lobe disease. Impaired recent memory follows bilateral damage to the hippocampus. Hypersexuality may develop in some individuals with bilateral damage in the amygdaloid nuclei and piriform cortex. It is obvious, however, that in the present state of our knowledge the abnormalities seen with temporal lobe lesions and, more generally, those produced by other neocortical lesions cannot be fitted into any general hypothesis of intellectual function. It is hoped that future research will provide such a synthesis and a better understanding of the neurophysiologic basis of mental phenomena.

• • •

17 . . .
Cerebral Circulation & Metabolism

The distribution of the cardiac output to various parts of the body at rest in a normal adult man is shown in Table 17—1. The general principles of cardiovascular physiology apply to the circulation of all these regions, but the vascular supplies of most organs have additional special features. The portal circulation of the anterior pituitary is discussed in Chapter 14. This chapter is concerned with the circulation of the brain, the nature and function of cerebrospinal fluid, and the metabolism of neural tissue.

ANATOMIC CONSIDERATIONS

Vessels

Except for a small contribution from the anterior spinal artery to the medulla, the entire arterial inflow to the brain in man is via 4 arteries: 2 internal carotids and 2 vertebrals. The vertebral arteries unite to form the basilar artery; and the circle of Willis, formed by the carotids and the basilar artery, is the origin of the 6 large vessels supplying the cerebral cortex. In some animals the vertebrals are large and the internal carotids small, but in humans a relatively small fraction of the total arterial flow is carried by the vertebral arteries. Substances injected into one carotid artery are distributed almost exclusively to the cerebral hemisphere

on that side. There is normally no crossing over, probably because the pressure is equal on both sides. Even when it is not, the anastomotic channels in the circle do not permit a very large flow. Occlusion of one carotid artery, particularly in older patients, often causes serious symptoms of cerebral ischemia. There are precapillary anastomoses between the cerebral arterioles in humans and some other species, but flow through these channels is generally insufficient to maintain the circulation and prevent infarction when a cerebral artery is occluded.

Venous drainage from the brain by way of the deep veins and dural sinuses empties principally into the internal jugular veins in humans, although a small amount of venous blood drains through the ophthalmic and pterygoid venous plexuses, through emissary veins to the scalp, and down the system of paravertebral veins in the spinal canal. In other species, the internal jugular veins are small and the venous blood from the brain mixes with blood from other structures.

The cerebral vessels have a number of unique anatomic features. In the choroid plexuses there are gaps between the endothelial cells of the capillary wall, but the choroid epithelial cells are densely intermeshed and interlocked. The capillaries in the brain substance resemble nonfenestrated capillaries in muscle and other parts of the body. However, the junctions between endothelial cells are tight from a functional point of view and do not permit the passage of substances that

Table 17—1. Blood flow and O_2 consumption of various organs in a 63 kg adult man with a mean arterial blood pressure of 90 mm Hg and an O_2 consumption of 250 ml/min. R units are pressure (mm Hg) divided by blood flow (ml/sec).*

Region	Mass (kg)	Blood Flow ml/min	Blood Flow ml/100 g/min	Arteriovenous Oxygen Difference (ml/liter)	Oxygen Consumption ml/min	Oxygen Consumption ml/100 g/min	Resistance in R units Absolute	Resistance in R units per kg	Percentage of Total Cardiac Output	Percentage of Total Oxygen Consumption
Liver	2.6	1500	57.7	34	51	2.0	3.6	9.4	27.8	20.4
Kidneys	0.3	1260	420.0	14	18	6.0	4.3	1.3	23.3	7.2
Brain	1.4	750	54.0	62	46	3.3	7.2	10.1	13.9	18.4
Skin	3.6	462	12.8	25	12	0.3	11.7	42.1	8.6	4.8
Skeletal muscle	31.0	840	2.7	60	50	0.2	6.4	198.4	15.6	20.0
Heart muscle	0.3	250	84.0	114	29	9.7	21.4	6.4	4.7	11.6
Rest of body	23.8	336	1.4	129	44	0.2	16.1	383.2	6.2	17.6
Whole body	63.0	5400	8.6	46	250	0.4	1.0	63.0	100.0	100.0

*Reproduced, with permission, from: *Medical Physiology*, 11th ed. Bard P (editor). Mosby, 1961.

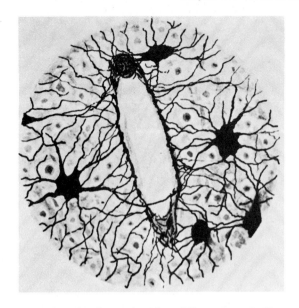

Figure 17—1. Membrane of end-feet of fibrous astrocytes (large dark cells) around a cerebral capillary. From occipital cortex of a monkey, silver carbonate stain. (Reproduced, with permission, from Glees: *Neuroglia, Morphology and Function.* Blackwell, 1955.)

pass through the junctions between endothelial cells in other tissues. There are relatively few vesicles in the endothelial cytoplasm, and presumably there is little vesicular transport. In addition, the brain capillaries are surrounded by a membrane made up of the end-feet of astrocytes (Fig 17—1). These end-feet are closely applied to the basal lamina of the capillary and cover most of the capillary wall. The protoplasm of astrocytes is also found around synapses, where it appears to be isolating the synapses in the brain from one another.

Innervation

There are numerous myelinated and unmyelinated nerve fibers on the cerebral vessels. The sympathetic fibers on the pial arteries and arterioles come from the cervical ganglia of the sympathetic ganglion chain. However, the vessels in brain tissue appear to be innervated by intracerebral noradrenergic neurons that have their cell bodies in the brain stem (see Chapter 15). The parasympathetic fibers pass to the cerebral vessels from the facial nerve via the greater superficial petrosal nerve. The myelinated fibers are probably sensory in function, since touching or pulling on the cerebral vessels is known to cause pain.

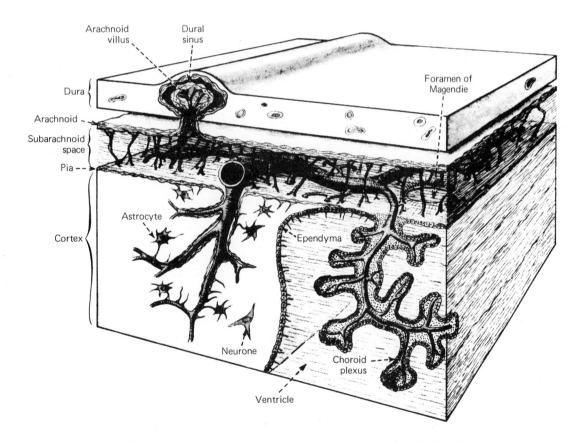

Figure 17—2. Section of the brain and investing membranes. (Reproduced, with permission, from Tschirgi in *Handbook of Physiology.* Field J, Magoun HW [editors]. Washington: The American Physiological Society, 1960. Section 1, pp 1865—1890.)

CEREBROSPINAL FLUID

Formation & Absorption

About 50% of the cerebrospinal fluid (CSF) that fills the cerebral ventricles and subarachnoid space is formed in the choroid plexuses (Fig 17–2); the remaining 50% is formed around the cerebral vessels and along the ventricular walls. The composition of the CSF depends on filtration and diffusion from the blood, along with facilitated diffusion and active transport, much of it across the choroid plexus. The composition (Table 17–2) is essentially the same as brain ECF, and there appears to be free communication between the brain extracellular space, the ventricles, and the subarachnoid space. The CSF flows out through the foramens of Magendie and Luschka and is absorbed through the arachnoid villi into the cerebral venus sinuses. Bulk flow via the villi is 500 ml/day in humans. Substances also leave the CSF by diffusion across adjacent membranes, and there is facilitated diffusion of glucose and active transport of cations and organic acids out of the CSF.

The rate of CSF formation is independent of intraventricular pressure, but the absorption, which takes place largely by bulk flow, is proportionate to the pressure (Fig 17–3). Below a pressure of approximately 68 mm CSF, absorption stops. Large amounts of fluid accumulate when the reabsorptive capacity of the arachnoid villi is decreased (**external, or communicating hydrocephalus**). Fluid also accumulates proximal to the block and distends the ventricles when the foramens of Luschka and Magendie are blocked or there is obstruction within the ventricular system (**internal hydrocephalus**).

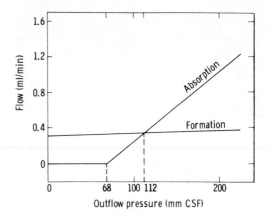

Figure 17–3. CSF formation and absorption in humans at various CSF pressures. Note that at 112 mm CSF, formation and absorption are equal, and at 68 mm CSF, absorption is zero. (Modified and reproduced, with permission, from Cutler & others: Formation and absorption of cerebrospinal fluid in man. Brain 91:707, 1968.)

Brain Extracellular Space

There has been considerable controversy about the size of the brain extracellular space. The sodium space in brain tissue is about 35% of brain volume and the chloride space is about 30%, but both ions are known to be present inside as well as outside of brain cells. Inulin and ferrocyanide, which do not enter cells, distribute in about 15% of brain volume. Under the electron microscope, brain cells appear very close together, and some electron microscopists have argued that the volume of the brain extracellular space could not be more than 4% of brain volume. However,

Table 17–2. Concentration of various substances in human CSF and plasma.*

Substance		CSF	Plasma	Ratio CSF/Plasma
Na⁺	(mEq/kg H_2O)	147.0	150.0	0.98
K⁺	(mEq/kg H_2O)	2.9	4.6	0.62
Mg⁺⁺	(mEq/kg H_2O)	2.2	1.6	1.39
Ca⁺⁺	(mEq/kg H_2O)	2.3	4.7	0.49
Cl⁻	(mEq/kg H_2O)	113.0	99.0	1.14
HCO_3^-	(mEq/liter)	25.1	24.8	1.01
P_{CO_2}	(mm Hg)	50.2	39.5	1.28
pH		7.33	7.40	...
Osmolality	(mOsm/kg H_2O)	289.0	289.0	1.00
Protein	(mg/dl)	20.0	6000.0	0.003
Glucose	(mg/dl)	64.0	100.0	0.64
Inorganic P	(mg/dl)	3.4	4.7	0.73
Urea	(mg/dl)	12.0	15.0	0.80
Creatinine	(mg/dl)	1.5	1.2	1.25
Uric acid	(mg/dl)	1.5	5.0	0.30
Lactic acid	(mg/dl)	18.0	21.0	0.86
Cholesterol	(mg/dl)	0.2	175.0	0.001

*Data partly from Davson: *Physiology of the Cerebrospinal Fluid,* Churchill, 1967; and partly courtesy of R Mitchell & associates.

asphyxia makes brain cells swell, and the brain extracellular space shrinks to 4% or less of brain volume when the brain is exposed to approximately the same amount of asphyxia as brain tissue prepared for electron photomicrography. These and other data indicate that the extracellular space in the living human makes up about 15% of brain volume.

Protective Function

The meninges and the CSF protect the brain. The dura is attached firmly to bone. There is normally no "subdural space," the arachnoid being held to the dura by the surface tension of the thin layer of fluid between the 2 membranes. The brain itself is supported within the arachnoid by the blood vessels and nerve roots and by the multiple, fine fibrous **arachnoid trabeculae** (Fig 17–2). The brain weighs about 1400 g in air, but in its "water bath" of CSF it has a net weight of only 50 g. The buoyancy of the brain in the CSF permits its relatively flimsy attachments to suspend it very effectively. When the head receives a blow, the arachnoid slides on the dura and the brain moves, but its motion is gently checked by the CSF cushion and by the arachnoid trabeculae.

The pain produced by spinal fluid deficiency illustrates the importance of spinal fluid in supporting the brain. As a diagnostic procedure in patients suspected of having brain tumors, spinal fluid is removed and replaced by air to make the outline of the ventricles visible by x-ray (**pneumoencephalography**). This procedure causes a severe headache after the fluid is removed because the brain hangs on the vessels and nerve roots, and traction on them stimulates pain fibers. The pain can be relieved by intrathecal injection of sterile isotonic saline.

Head Injuries

Without the protection of the spinal fluid and the meninges, the brain would probably be unable to withstand even the minor traumas of everyday living, but with the protection afforded it takes a fairly severe blow to produce cerebral damage. The brain is damaged most commonly when the skull is fractured and bone is driven into neural tissue (depressed skull fracture); when the brain moves far enough to tear the delicate bridging veins from the cortex to the bone; or when the brain is accelerated by a blow on the head and is driven against the skull or the tentorium at a point opposite where the blow was struck (**contrecoup injury**).

THE BLOOD-BRAIN BARRIER

Over 50 years ago, it was first demonstrated that when acidic dyes such as trypan blue are injected into living animals all the tissues are stained except most of the brain and spinal cord. To explain the failure of the neural tissue to stain, the existence of a **blood-brain barrier** was postulated. The work with dyes has been criticized, but subsequent research has established the fact that only water, CO_2, and O_2 cross the cerebral capillaries with ease, and the exchange of other substances is slow.

The general features of exchange across capillary walls between the plasma and the interstitial fluid are described elsewhere. There is considerable variation in capillary permeability from organ to organ in the body. However, the exchange across the cerebral vessels is so different from that in other capillary beds—and the rate of exchange of many physiologically important substances is so slow—that it seems justifiable to speak specifically of a blood-brain barrier.

Penetration of Substances Into Brain

As noted above, brain ECF is essentially identical to CSF, and substances enter the CSF by filtration, diffusion, facilitated diffusion, and active transport. There is an H^+ gradient between brain ECF and blood; the pH of brain ECF is 7.33, whereas that of blood is 7.40.

The rapidity with which substances penetrate brain tissue is inversely related to their molecular size and directly related to their lipid solubility; water-soluble polar compounds generally cross slowly. However, some substances are actively transported into the brain and some substances are transported out. Water, CO_2, and O_2 cross the blood-brain barrier readily, whereas glucose crosses more slowly. Na^+, K^+, and Mg^{++}, Cl^-, HCO_3^-, and $HPO_4^=$ in plasma require 3–30 times as long to equilibrate with spinal fluid as they do with other portions of the interstitial fluid. The relatively slow penetration of urea into brain and the cerebrospinal fluid is illustrated in Fig 17–4. Bile salts and catecholamines do not enter the adult brain in more than minute amounts. Proteins cross the barrier to a very limited extent, and it is because they are bound to

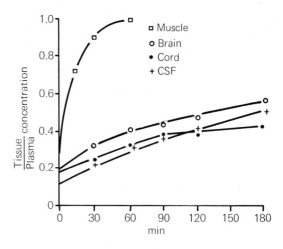

Figure 17–4. Penetration of urea into muscle, brain, spinal cord, and cerebrospinal fluid. (Modified and reproduced, with permission, from Kleeman, Davson, & Levin: Urea transport in the central nervous system. Am J Physiol 203:739, 1962.)

protein that acidic dyes fail to stain neural tissue. It is worth noting that no substance is completely excluded from the brain, and the important consideration is the rate of transfer of the substance. Certain compounds cross the blood-brain barrier slowly, whereas closely related compounds enter rapidly. For example, the amines dopamine and serotonin penetrate to a very limited degree, but their corresponding acids, L-dopa and 5-hydroxytryptophan, enter with relative ease (see Chapter 15).

Development of the Blood-Brain Barrier

The cerebral capillaries are much more permeable at birth than in adulthood, and the blood-brain barrier develops during the early years of life. In severely jaundiced infants, bile pigments penetrate into the nervous system and, in the presence of asphyxia, damage the basal ganglia (kernicterus). However, in jaundiced adults, the nervous system is unstained and not directly affected.

Circumventricular Organs

When an acidic dye is injected into an animal, 5 small areas in the brain stain like the tissues outside the brain. These areas are (1) the **subcommissural organ** and the adjacent **pineal,** (2) the **posterior pituitary** (neurohypophysis) and the adjacent ventral part of the median eminence of the hypothalamus, (3) the **area postrema,** (4) the **supraoptic crest** (organum vasculosum of the lamina terminalis, OVLT), and (5) the **subfornical organ** (intercolumnar tubercle).

These areas are referred to collectively as the **cir-

cumventricular organs** (Fig 17–5). All except the subcommissural organ have fenestrated capillaries, and because of their permeability they are said to be "outside the blood-brain barrier." Many appear to contain relatively large quantities of hypothalamic hormones. Most if not all of them appear to function as chemoreceptors of one sort or another. The area postrema is a chemoreceptor that initiates vomiting in response to chemical changes in the plasma (Chapter 14). The subfornical organ is a receptor for angiotensin II and plays a role in the regulation of thirst (Fig 14–8). Circulating sex hormones and cortisol may act on the median eminence region to regulate anterior pituitary secretion of gonadotropins and ACTH. However, the function of the subcommissural organ is uncertain, and no definite function has as yet been assigned to the supraoptic crest.

Function of the Blood-Brain Barrier

The blood-brain barrier probably functions to maintain the constancy of the environment of the neurons in the CNS. The neurons are so dependent upon the ionic composition of the fluid bathing them that even minor variations have far-reaching consequences. The constancy of the composition of the ECF in all parts of the body is maintained by multiple homeostatic mechanisms (see Chapter 1), but because of the sensitivity of the cortical neurons to ionic change it is not surprising that an additional defense has evolved to protect them.

Clinical Implications

The physician must know the permeability of the blood-brain barrier to drugs in order to treat diseases of the nervous system intelligently. For example, among the antibiotics, penicillin and chlortetracycline enter the brain to a very limited degree. Sulfadiazine and erythromycin, on the other hand, enter quite readily.

Another important clinical consideration is the fact that the blood-brain barrier breaks down in areas of the brain that are irradiated, infected, or the site of tumors. The breakdown makes it possible to localize tumors with considerable accuracy. Substances such as radioactive iodine-labeled albumin penetrate normal brain tissue very slowly but they enter rapidly into tumor tissue, making the tumor stand out as an island of radioactivity in the surrounding normal brain.

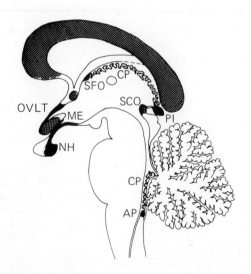

Figure 17–5. Circumventricular organs. The median eminence (ME), neurohypophysis (NH), organum vasculosum of the lamina terminalis (OVLT, supraoptic crest), subfornical organ (SFO), subcommissural organ (SCO), pineal (PI), and area postrema (AP) are shown projected on a sagittal section of the human brain. CP, choroid plexus. (Reproduced, with permission, from Weindl in: *Frontiers in Neuroendocrinology,* 1973. Ganong WF, Martini L [editors] . Oxford, 1973.)

CEREBRAL BLOOD FLOW

Kety Method

According to the **Fick principle,** the blood flow of any organ can be measured by determining the amount of a given substance (Q_X) removed from the blood stream by the organ per unit of time and dividing that value by the difference between the concentration of the substance in arterial blood and the concentration in the venous blood from the organ ($[A_X] - [V_X]$). Thus:

$$\text{Cerebral blood flow (CBF)} = \frac{Q_X}{[A_X] - [V_X]}$$

When an individual inhales small subanesthetic amounts of nitrous oxide (N_2O), this gas is taken up by the brain, and the brain N_2O equilibrates with the N_2O in blood in 9–11 minutes. After equilibration, the N_2O concentration in cerebral venous blood is equal to the concentration in the brain because the brain-blood partition coefficient for N_2O is 1. Therefore, the level in cerebral venous blood after equilibration divided by the mean A-V N_2O difference during equilibration equals the cerebral blood flow per unit of brain:

$$\text{CBF (ml/100 g brain/min)} = \frac{100\, V_u S}{\int_0^u (A-V)dt}$$

where V = Cerebral venous N_2O concentration (vol/100 g)
u = Time of equilibrium (minutes)
S = Partition coefficient of N_2O in blood and brain (= 1)
A = Arterial N_2O concentration (vol/100 g)

The mean A-V difference can also be estimated from a plot of the differences at various times during equilibration (Fig 17–6). When blood N_2O concentrations are expressed in volumes/100 ml of blood or, more accurately, in volumes/100 g of blood, the cerebral blood flow values obtained are in ml/100 g of brain/min. The value per unit of brain tissue can be con-

verted to an approximate value for total cerebral blood flow by multiplying by 1400 g, an average figure for brain weight in adult humans.

When the N_2O method (**Kety method**) is used to determine the cerebral blood flow in intact humans, arterial blood samples can be obtained from any convenient artery since the concentration of substances in systemic arterial blood is uniform throughout the body. Other inert gases such as krypton have also been used to measure cerebral blood flow. To obtain cerebral venous blood, a needle is inserted into the jugular bulb. This expansion of the internal jugular vein at its point of exit from the skull is readily penetrated if the needle is inserted in a slightly headward direction halfway between the mastoid process and the angle of the mandible. The subject inhales the gas for 10 minutes, and arterial and jugular venous blood samples are obtained repeatedly during this time. The gas content of the samples is determined, and the mean A-V gas difference is calculated.

Normal Values

The average value for cerebral blood flow (CBF) in young adults is 54 ml/100 g/min (750 ml/min for the whole brain), with a range of approximately 40–67 ml/100 g/min. In children, the value averages about 105 ml/100 g/min. It falls to adult levels at the time of puberty in normal individuals but remains high in prepuberal castrates, suggesting that the sex hormones are responsible for the drop at puberty. However, castration in adulthood does not lead to a rise in CBF, and CBF is unaffected by the administration of sex and adrenal steroid hormones.

Limitations

The accuracy of the Kety method depends upon obtaining cerebral venous blood that is not significantly diluted with blood from other structures with different N_2O uptakes. In humans, jugular venous blood is said to meet this requirement in over 95% of individuals, but it is not possible in most laboratory animals to obtain blood that comes only from the brain.

The value obtained with the Kety method is, of course, an average value for the flow during the 10 min equilibration period. Values for total CBF give no information about the relative blood flow in the various parts of the brain. Indeed, trying to draw conclusions about regional blood flow from total CBF measurements has been likened to trying to analyze the activity of individual tenants in a large apartment house by sampling the flow in the main water pipe and sewer pipe outside the apartment house. A reduction in flow to one part of the brain may be compensated by an increase in flow to another part, so that CBF remains unchanged (Fig 17–7). An uncompensated decrease in the blood flow to part of the brain results in decreased CBF, but the Kety method does not detect the decrease in total CBF produced by complete occlusion of the vessels supplying part of the brain. This is true because the method measures only the

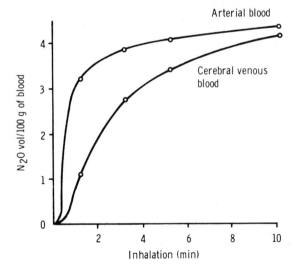

Figure 17–6. Arterial and cerebral venous blood N_2O levels while inhaling N_2O. (Redrawn and reproduced, with permission, from Kety, in: *Methods in Medical Research.* Vol I. Potter VR [editor]. Year Book, 1948.)

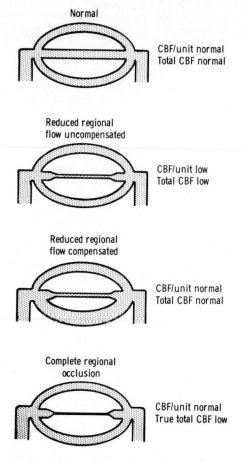

Figure 17—7. Variations in intracerebral circulation.

Table 17—3. Blood flow of representative areas of the brain of unanesthetized cats.*

Area	Mean Blood Flow (ml/g/min)
Inferior colliculus	1.80
Sensorimotor cortex	1.38
Auditory cortex	1.30
Visual cortex	1.25
Medial geniculate body	1.22
Lateral geniculate body	1.21
Superior colliculus	1.15
Caudate nucleus	1.10
Thalamus	1.03
Association cortex	0.88
Cerebellar nuclei	0.87
Cerebellar white matter	0.24
Cerebral white matter	0.23
Spinal cord white matter	0.14

*Data from Landau & others: The local circulation of the living brain: Values in the unanesthetized cat. Trans Am Neurol Assoc 80:125, 1955.

flow per unit of brain, and the nonperfused area takes up no N_2O. The remaining normal brain extracts normal amounts, so that the CBF per unit of brain tissue is unaffected.

Blood Flow in Various Parts of the Brain

By determining the distribution of an inert radioactive gas in frozen sections of the brains of experimental animals and comparing these values with the level of the gas in the blood, it is possible to measure regional blood flow in the brain. The flow in the cerebral and cerebellar cortex is large, but the part of the brain with the highest blood flow is the inferior colliculus (Table 17—3). The blood flow in gray matter is about 6 times the flow in white matter.

The blood flow of different regions of the brain has also been measured in conscious humans by injecting a radioactive gas such as ^{133}Xe dissolved in saline into one carotid artery. The arrival and clearance of the gas in various regions is then monitored by scintillation detectors placed over various parts of the head, and flow can be calculated from the clearance curves. In some studies, as many as 256 separate regions have been studied, but, not surprisingly, there is great overlap of the regions.

Cerebral Vascular Resistance

The cerebral vascular resistance (CVR) is equal to the cerebral perfusion pressure divided by the cerebral blood flow. The CVR in the supine position can be calculated on the basis of the mean brachial artery pressure (ignoring the relatively low cerebral venous pressure) without introducing a very large error. Calculated in this way, the normal CVR is approximately 100 "R units" (Table 17—1) per 100 g brain, or 7.2 R units for the whole brain.

REGULATION OF CEREBRAL CIRCULATION

Normal Flow

The cerebral circulation is regulated in such a way that a constant total CBF is generally maintained under varying conditions. For example, total cerebral blood flow is not increased by strenuous mental activity and is unchanged or even increased during sleep. However, when light is shone into the eyes of experimental animals, there is increased blood flow in the superior colliculi, lateral geniculate bodies, and occipital cortex, and there is evidence for increased regional blood flow in other parts of the brain when they become active.

The factors affecting the total CBF are the arterial pressure at brain level, the venous pressure at brain level, the intracranial pressure, the viscosity of the blood, and the degree of active constriction or dilatation of the cerebral arterioles (Fig 17—8). The caliber of the arterioles is in turn controlled by vasomotor nerves, cerebral metabolism, and autoregulation.

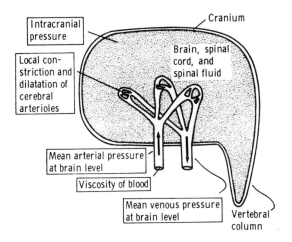

Figure 17–8. Diagrammatic summary of the factors affecting cerebral blood flow. (Modified from Patterson in: *Physiology and Biophysics,* 19th ed. Ruch TC, Patton HD [editors]. Saunders, 1965.)

Role of Intracranial Pressure

In adults, the brain, spinal cord, and spinal fluid are encased, along with the cerebral vessels, in a rigid bony enclosure. The cranial cavity normally contains a brain weighing approximately 1400 g, 75 ml of blood, and 75 ml of spinal fluid. Because brain tissue and spinal fluid are essentially incompressible, the volume of blood, spinal fluid, and brain in the cranium at any time must be relatively constant (**Monro-Kellie doctrine**). More importantly, the cerebral vessels are compressed whenever the intracranial pressure rises. Any change in venous pressure promptly causes a similar change in intracranial pressure. Thus, a rise in venous pressure decreases cerebral blood flow both by decreasing the effective perfusion pressure and by compressing the cerebral vessels. This relationship helps to compensate for changes in arterial blood pressure at the level of the head. For example, if the body is accelerated upward ("positive g"), blood moves toward the feet and arterial pressure at the level of the head decreases. However, venous pressure also falls and intracranial pressure falls, so that the pressure on the vessels decreases and blood flow is much less severely compromised that it would otherwise be. Conversely, during acceleration downward, force acting toward the head ("negative g") increases arterial pressure at head level, but intracranial pressure also rises, so that the vessels are supported and do not rupture. The cerebral vessels are protected during the straining associated with defecation or delivery in the same way.

Effect of Intracranial Pressure Changes on Systemic Blood Pressure

When intracranial pressure is elevated to more than 450 mm of water (33 mm Hg) over a short period of time, cerebral blood flow is significantly reduced. The resultant ischemia stimulates the vasomotor center, and systemic blood pressure rises. Stimulation of the cardioinhibitory center produces bradycardia, and respiration is slowed. The blood pressure rise, which was described by Cushing and is sometimes called the **Cushing reflex**, helps to maintain the cerebral blood flow. Over a considerable range, the rise in systemic blood pressure is proportionate to the rise in intracranial pressure, although eventually a point is reached where the intracranial pressure exceeds the arterial pressure, and cerebral circulation ceases.

Role of Vasomotor Nerves

The bulk of the evidence presently available indicates that even though cerebral vessels are innervated by adrenergic vasoconstrictor fibers and parasympathetic vasodilator fibers, vasomotor reflexes play little if any part in the regulation of cerebral blood flow in humans. Stimulation of the cerevical sympathetics does cause some constriction of pial vessels in animals, and injecting procaine into the stellate ganglion has had a considerable vogue in the treatment of cerebral thrombosis on the theory that the vasospasm associated with the thrombosis is mediated via vasoconstrictor nerves. However, careful measurements clearly show that blocking the stellate ganglion has no effect on cerebral blood flow, and the therapeutic value of stellate ganglion block is questionable. Of course, stellate ganglion block does not affect the intracerebral noradrenergic neurons that innervate the arterioles in the substance of the brain, but the functional role of this system is presently unknown.

Effects of Brain Metabolism on Cerebral Vessels

The arterioles in the brain, like those in other parts of the body, are directly affected by local changes in CO_2 and O_2 tension. A rise in P_{CO_2} exerts a particularly potent dilator effect on the cerebral vessels. A fall in P_{CO_2} has a constrictor effect, and cerebral vasoconstriction is an important factor in the production of the cerebral symptoms seen when the arterial P_{CO_2} falls during hyperventilation. Hydrogen ions also exert a vasodilator effect, and a fall in pH is associated with increased flow whereas a rise in pH is associated with decreased flow. Changes in P_{CO_2} lead to corresponding changes in hydrogen ion concentration in the brain, and current evidence indicates that the effects of CO_2 are mediated via changes in pH. The vasodilator effect of hydrogen ions appears to be due to a direct local action on the blood vessels.

Changes in local O_2 tension also affect the cerebral arterioles; a low P_{O_2} is associated with vasodilatation and a high P_{O_2} with mild vasoconstriction. In addition, adenosine and other vasoactive metabolites may produce local vasodilatation in active cerebral tissue.

Autoregulation

Autoregulation is prominent in the brain. This is a process by which the flow to many tissues is maintained at relatively constant levels despite variations in perfusion pressure. As in other tissues, cerebral autoregulation may depend upon an inherent capacity of vascular smooth muscle to contract when it is stretched or upon the washing away of CO_2 and other vasodilator metabolites when the perfusion pressure and hence the blood flow is increased—or upon both mechanisms.

Integrated Operation of Regulatory Mechanisms

The regulatory mechanisms discussed above maintain cerebral blood flow during changes in posture, exercise, acceleration, and a variety of other conditions. It is worth remembering that these mechanisms operate together to overcome such formidable challenges as the effect of gravity on the cerebral blood flow, not only in humans but also in giraffes when these animals stoop to drink water and when they raise their heads to nibble leaves from the tops of trees.

BRAIN METABOLISM
& OXYGEN REQUIREMENTS

Uptake & Release of Substances by the Brain

If the cerebral blood flow is known, it is possible to calculate the consumption or production by the brain of O_2, CO_2, glucose, or any other substance present in the blood stream by multiplying the cerebral blood flow by the difference between the concentration of the substance in arterial blood and its concentration in cerebral venous blood. When calculated in this fashion, a negative value indicates that the brain is producing the substance (Table 17—4).

Oxygen Consumption

The O_2 consumption of human brain, or **cerebral metabolic rate for O_2 (CMRO$_2$)**, averages about 3.5 ml/100 g brain/min, or 49 ml/min for the whole brain in an adult. This figure represents approximately 20% of the total resting O_2 consumption (Table 17—1). The

Table 17—4. Utilization and production of substances by adult human brain in vivo.*

	Uptake (+) or output (−) per 100 g brain/min	Total/min
Substances utilized		
Oxygen	+3.5 ml	+49 ml
Glucose	+5.5 mg	+77 mg
Glutamic acid	+0.4 mg	+ 5.6 mg
Substances produced		
Carbon dioxide	−3.5 ml	−49 ml
Glutamine	−0.6 mg	− 8.4 mg

Substances not utilized or produced in the fed state: lactic acid, pyruvic acid, total ketones, α-ketoglutarate.

*From data compiled by Sokoloff, in: *Handbook of Physiology.* Field J, Magoun HW (editors). Washington: The American Physiological Society, 1960. Section 1, pp 1843—1865.

Table 17—5. Oxygen consumption of parts of adult dog brain in vitro.*

	Oxygen Consumption (μl/100 mg/hour)
Caudate nucleus	136
Cerebral cortex	116
Cerebellum	107
Thalamus	101
Midbrain	92
Medulla	69
Spinal cord	50

*Data from Himwich & Fazekas: Comparative studies of the metabolism of the brain. Am J Physiol 132:454, 1941.

brain is extremely sensitive to hypoxia, and occlusion of its blood supply produces unconsciousness in as short a period as 10 sec. The vegetative structures in the brain stem are more resistant to hypoxia than the cerebral cortex, and patients may recover from accidents such as cardiac arrest and other conditions causing fairly prolonged hypoxia with normal vegetative functions but severe, permanent intellectual deficiencies. The basal ganglia also use O_2 at a very rapid rate. The values for in vitro O_2 consumption of various parts of the dog brain are shown in Table 17—5. The metabolic rate of the cerebral cortex relative to that of the basal ganglia may be higher in humans than in dogs, but it is well to remember that the basal ganglia are sensitive to hypoxia in humans and that symptoms of Parkinson's disease as well as intellectual deficits can be produced by chronic hypoxia. The thalamus and the inferior colliculus are also very susceptible to hypoxic damage.

Energy Sources

Glucose is the major ultimate source of energy for the brain under normal conditions. It is taken up from the blood in large amounts, and the RQ (respiratory quotient) of cerebral tissue is 0.95—0.99 in normal individuals. This does not mean that the total source of energy is always glucose. During prolonged starvation, there is appreciable utilization of other substances. Indeed, there is evidence that as much as 30% of the glucose taken up under normal conditions is converted to amino acids, lipids, and proteins, and that substances other than glucose are metabolized for energy during convulsions. There may also be some utilization of amino acids from the circulation even though the amino acid A-V difference across the brain is normally minute. Insulin is not required for most cerebral cells to utilize glucose.

Hypoglycemia

The symptoms of hypoglycemia are mental changes, ataxia, confusion, sweating, coma, and convulsions. The total glycogen content of the brain is about 1.6 mg/g in fasted animals, but the available glycogen and glucose are used up in 2 minutes if the blood supply is totally occluded. Thus, the brain can withstand hypoglycemia for somewhat longer periods than it can withstand hypoxia, but glucose and O_2 are both needed for survival. The cortical regions are more sensitive to hypoglycemia than the vegetative centers in the brain stem, and sublethal exposures to hypoglycemia, like similar exposures to hypoxia, may cause irreversible cortical changes.

Glutamic Acid & Ammonia Removal

The brain uptake of glutamic acid is approximately balanced by its output of glutamine. It is probable that the glutamic acid entering the brain takes up ammonia and leaves as glutamine. The glutamic acid-glutamine conversion in the brain—the opposite of the reaction in the kidney which produces some of the ammonia that enters the tubules—probably serves as a detoxifying mechanism to keep the brain free of ammonia. Ammonia is very toxic to nerve cells, and ammonia intoxication is believed to be a major cause of the bizarre neurologic symptoms in hepatic coma.

●   ●   ●

References: Section III.
Functions of the Nervous System

Beaven MA: Histamine. N Engl J Med 294:30, 1976.

Bonica JJ: *The Management of Pain,* 2nd ed. Lea & Febiger, 1974.

Bradshaw J, Geffen G, Nettleton N: Our two brains. New Scientist 54:62, 1972.

Brawley P, Duffield JC:The pharmacology of hallucinogens. Pharmacol Rev 24:31, 1972.

Bronisch FW: *The Clinically Important Reflexes.* Grune & Stratton, 1952.

Burnstock G, Costa M: *Adrenergic Neurons.* Wiley, 1975.

Capps JA: *An Experimental and Clinical Study of Pain in the Pleura, Pericardium and Peritoneum.* Macmillan, 1932.

Chusid JG: *Correlative Neuroanatomy & Functional Neurology,* 16th ed. Lange, 1976.

Davson H: *The Physiology of the Eye,* 3rd ed. Academic Press, 1972.

Eccles JC: *The Understanding of the Brain.* McGraw-Hill, 1973.

Elul R: The genesis of the EEG. Int Rev Neurobiol 15:1227, 1972.

Fitzsimons JT: Thirst. Physiol Rev 52:468, 1972.

Gaze RM, Kenting MJ: Development and regeneration of the nervous system. Br Med Bull 30:105, 1974.

Geschwind N: The apraxias: Neural mechanisms of disorders of learned movement. Am Sci 63:188, 1975.

Goldberg AM, Hanin I (editors): *Biology of Cholinergic Function.* Raven, 1975.

Granit R: *Mechanisms Regulating the Discharge of Motoneurons.* Thomas, 1972.

Greengard P, Kebabian JW: Role of cyclic AMP in synaptic transmission in the mammalian peripheral nervous system. Fed Proc 33:1059, 1974.

Guillemin R: Endorphins, brain peptides that act like opiates. (Editorial.) N Engl J Med 296:226, 1977.

Hensel H: Neural processes in thermoregulation. Physiol Rev 53:948, 1973.

Ingvar DH, Lassen NA (editors): *Brain Work.* Munksgoard, 1976.

Iverson LL: Dopamine receptors in the brain. Science 188:1084, 1975.

Jacobson M, Hunt RK: The origins of nerve cell specificity. Sci Am 228:26, Feb 1973.

Kales A, Kales JD: Sleep disorders. N Engl J Med 290:487, 1974.

Kontes HA: Mechanisms of regulation of the cerebral microcirculation. Curr Concepts Cerebrovasc Dis Stroke 10:7, 1975.

Kornhuber HH: Motor functions of the cerebellum and basal ganglia: The cerebellocortical saccadic (ballistic) clock, the cerebellonuclear hold regulator, and the basal ganglia ramp (voluntary speed smooth movement) generator. Kybernetik 8:157, 1971.

Krnjević K: Chemical nature of synaptic transmission in vertebrates. Physiol Rev 54:419, 1974.

Kuffler SW, Nicholls JG: *From Neuron to Brain.* Sinauer Associates, 1976.

Langitt TW & others (editors): *Cerebral Circulation and Metabolism.* Springer-Verlag, 1975.

Lefkowitz RJ: β-adrenergic receptors: Recognition and regulation. N Engl J Med 295:323, 1976.

Livett BG: Histochemical visualization of peripheral and central adrenergic neurons. Br Med Bull 29:93, 1973.

Llinás RR: The cortex of the cerebellum. Sci Am 232:56, Jan 1975.

Lowenstein OE (editor): *Mechanisms of Taste and Smell in Vertebrates.* Churchill, 1970.

Martini L, Ganong WF (editors): *Frontiers in Neuroendocrinology.* Vol 4. Raven, 1976.

Michael R: Determinants of primate reproductive behavior. In: *The Use of Nonhuman Primates in Research on Human Reproduction.* Diczfalusy E, Standley CG (editors). WHO Research and Training Centre on Human Reproduction, 1972.

Moulton DG: Spatial patterning of response to odors in the peripheral olfactory system. Physiol Rev 56:578, 1976.

Mountcastle VB: The world around us: Neural command functions for selective attention. Neurosci Res Program Bull 14:Suppl, 1976.

Naunton RF (editor): *The Vestibular System.* Academic Press, 1975.

Nicoll RA: Promising peptides. Neurosci Symposia 1:99, 1976.

Novin D, Wyrwicka W, Bray GA (editors): *Hunger: Clinical Implications and Basic Mechanisms.* Raven, 1975.

Oledendorf WH: Blood-brain barrier permeability to drugs. Annu Rev Pharmacol 14:239, 1974.

Pavlov IP: *Conditioned Reflexes.* Oxford Univ Press, 1928.

Penfield W: Engrams in the human brain. Proc R Soc Med 61:831, 1968.

Rapaport SI: *Blood-Brain Barrier in Physiology and Medicine.* Raven, 1976.

Rodieck RW: *The Vertebrate Retina.* Freeman, 1973.

Rushton WAH: Visual pigments and color blindness. Sci Am 232:64, March 1975.

Schmitt FO, Worden FG (editors): *The Neurosciences: Third Study Program.* MIT Press, 1974.

Schneider DJ (editor): *Proteins of the Nervous System.* Raven, 1973.

Schwartz GE: Biofeedback self-regulation and the patterning of physiological processes. Am Sci 63:314, 1975.

Sherrington CS: *The Integrative Action of the Nervous System.* Cambridge Univ Press, 1947.

Snyder SH: Opiate receptors in the brain. N Engl J Med 296:266, 1977.

Snyder SH, Bennett JP Jr: Neurotransmitter receptors in the brain: Biochemical identification. Annu Rev Physiol 38:153, 1976.

Snyder SH & others: Drugs, neurotransmitters, and schizophrenia. Science 184:1243, 1974.

Snyder SH & others: Synaptic biochemistry of amino acids. Fed Proc 32:2039, 1973.

Van Harreveld A: *Brain Tissue Electrolytes.* Butterworth, 1965.

Wightman FL, Green DM: The perception of pitch. Am Sci 62:208, 1974.

Wilson VJ: The labyrinth, the brain and posture. Am Sci 63:325, 1975.

Symposium: Alcoholism and the central nervous system. Ann NY Acad Sci 215:1, 1973.

Symposium: The cerebrospinal fluid and the extracellular fluid of the brain. Fed Proc 33:2061, 1974.

Symposium: Marijuana: Chemistry, pharmacology, and patterns of social use. Ann NY Acad Sci 191:3, 1971.

Symposium: Sound localization. Fed Proc 33:1899, 1974.

Symposium: Structure and function of the visual system. Fed Proc 35:36, 1976.

Appendix

NORMAL VALUES & THE STATISTICAL EVALUATION OF DATA

The approximate ranges of values in normal humans for some commonly measured plasma constituents are summarized in the table on the inside back cover. A worldwide attempt is currently being made to convert to a single standard nomenclature by using SI (Système International) units. However, there are a number of complexities involved in the use of these units, and they have not as yet come into general use. Consequently, they are not as yet used in this book. Values in SI units are listed beside values in more traditional units in the table on the inside back cover.

The accuracy of the methods used for laboratory measurements varies. It is important in evaluating any single measurement to know the possible errors in making the measurement. In the case of chemical determinations on body fluids, these include errors in obtaining the sample and the inherent error of the chemical method. However, the values obtained using even the most accurate methods vary from one normal individual to the next as a result of what is usually called **biologic variation.** This variation is due to the fact that in any system as complex as a living organism or tissue there are many variables that affect the particular measurement. Variables such as age, sex, time of day, time since last meal, etc can be controlled. Numerous other variables cannot, and for this reason the values obtained differ from individual to individual.

The magnitude of the normal range for any given physiologic or clinical measurement can be calculated by standard statistical technics if the measurement has been made on a suitable sample of the normal population (preferably more than 20 individuals). It is important to know not only the average value in this sample but also the extent of the deviation of the individual values from the average.

The average, or **arithmetic mean (M),** of the series of values is readily calculated:

$$M = \frac{\Sigma X}{n}$$

Where Σ = Sum of
X = The individual values
n = Number of individual values in the series

The average deviation is the mean of the deviations of each of the values from the mean. From a mathematical point of view, a better measure of the deviation is the **geometric mean** of the deviations from the mean. This is called the **standard deviation (σ):**

$$\sigma = \sqrt{\frac{\Sigma (M - X)^2}{n-1}}$$

The term $n-1$ rather than n is used in the denominator of this equation because the σ of a sample of the population rather than the σ of the whole population is being calculated. The following form of the equation for σ can be derived algebraically, and is convenient for those using a calculator to compute σ:

$$\sigma = \sqrt{\frac{\Sigma X^2 - \frac{(\Sigma X)^2}{n}}{n-1}}$$

Here, ΣX^2 is the sum of the squares of the individual values, and $(\Sigma X)^2$ is the square of the sum of the items, ie, the items added together and then squared.

Another commonly used index of the variation is the **standard error of the mean (SE, SEM):**

$$SE = \frac{\sigma}{\sqrt{n}}$$

Strictly speaking, the SE indicates the reliability of the sample mean as representative of the true mean of the general population from which the sample was drawn.

A **frequency distribution** curve can be constructed from the individual values in the sample by plotting the frequency with which any particular value occurs in the series against the values. If the group of individuals tested was homogeneous, the frequency distribution curve is usually symmetric (Fig 1) with the

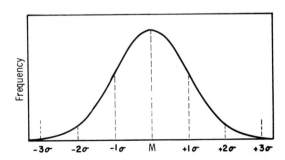

Figure 1. Curve of normal distribution (frequency distribution curve of values from a homogeneous sample of a population).

highest frequency corresponding to the mean and the width of the curve varying with σ (curve of **normal distribution**). Within an ideal curve of normal distribution, the percentage of observations which fall within various ranges are shown in Table 1. The mean and σ of a representative sample are approximately those of the whole population. It is therefore possible to pre-

Table 1. Percentage of values in a population which will fall within various ranges within an ideal curve of normal distribution.

Mean ± 1 σ	68.27%
Mean ± 1.96 σ	95.00%
Mean ± 2 σ	95.45%
Mean ± 3 σ	99.73%

dict from the mean and σ of the sample the probability that any particular value in the general population is normal. For example, if the difference between such a value and the mean is equal to 1.96 σ, the chances are 1 out of 20 (5 out of 100) that it is normal. Conversely, of course, the chances are 19 out of 20 that it is abnormal. It is unfortunate that data on normal means and σs are not more generally available for the important plasma and urinary constituents in humans.

Statistical analysis is also useful in evaluating the significance of the difference between 2 means. In physiologic and clinical research, measurements are often made on a group of animals or patients given a particular treatment. These measurements are compared with similar measurements made on a control group which ideally has been exposed to exactly the same conditions except that the treatment has not been given. If a particular mean value in the treated group is different from the corresponding mean for the control group, the question arises whether the difference is due to the treatment or to chance variation. The probability that the difference represents chance variation can be estimated by using **"Student's"** *t* **test.** The value *t* is the ratio of the difference in the means

of 2 series (M_a and M_b) to the uncertainty in these means. The formula used to calculate *t* is:

$$t = \frac{M_a - M_b}{\sqrt{\dfrac{(n_a + n_b)[(n_a - 1)\sigma_a^2 + (n_b - 1)\sigma_b^2]}{n_a n_b (n_a + n_b - 2)}}}$$

where n_a and n_b are the number of individual values in series a and b, respectively. When $n_a = n_b$, the equation for *t* becomes simplified to:

$$t = \frac{M_a - M_b}{\sqrt{(SE_a)^2 + (SE_b)^2}}$$

The higher the value of *t*, the less the probability that the difference represents chance variation. This probability also decreases as the number of individuals (n) in each group rises because the greater the number of measurements, the smaller the error in the measurements. A mathematical expression of the probability (*P*) for any value of *t* at different values of n can be found in tables in most texts on statistics. *P* is a fraction which expresses the probability that the difference between 2 means was due to chance variation. Thus, for example, if the *P* value is 0.10, the probability that the difference was due to chance is 10% (1 chance in 10). A *P* value of < 0.001 means that the chances that the difference was due to random variation are less than 1 in 1000. When the *P* value is < 0.05, most investigators call the difference "statistically significant," ie, it is concluded that the difference is due to the operation of some factor other than chance—presumably the treatment.

These elementary statistical methods and many others are available for analyzing data in the research laboratory and the clinic. They provide a valuable objective means of evaluation. Statistical significance does not arbitrarily mean physiologic significance, and the reverse may sometimes be true; but replacement of evaluation by subjective impression with analysis by statistical methods is certainly an important goal in the medical sciences.

•   •   •

References: Appendix

Colton T: *Statistics in Medicine.* Little, Brown, 1974.
Dybkaer R: Nomenclature of laboratory results in medicine. Fed Proc 34:2116, 1975.

Ipsen J, Feigl P: *Bancroft's Introduction to Biostatistics,* 2nd ed. Harper & Row, 1970.

Units of Measurement

Prefix	Abbreviation	Magnitude
tera-	T	10^{12}
giga-	G	10^{9}
mega-	M	10^{6}
kilo-	k	10^{3}
hecto-	h	10^{2}
deca-	da	10^{1}
deci-	d	10^{-1}
centi-	c	10^{-2}
milli-	m	10^{-3}
micro-	μ	10^{-6}
nano-	n, mμ	10^{-9}
pico-	p, $\mu\mu$	10^{-12}
femto-	f	10^{-15}
atto-	a	10^{-18}

These prefixes are applied to metric and other units. For example, a micrometer (μm) is 10^{-6} meter (also called a micron); a picoliter (pl) is 10^{-12} liter; and a kilogram (kg) is 10^{3} grams. Also applied to seconds, units, mols, hertz, volts, farads, ohms, curies, equivalents, osmols, etc.

Equivalents of Metric, United States, and English Measures
(Values rounded off to 2 decimal places.)

Length
1 kilometer = 0.62 mile
1 mile = 5280 feet = 1.61 kilometers
1 meter = 39.37 inches
1 inch = 1/12 foot = 2.54 centimeters

Volume
1 liter = 1.06 US liquid quart
1 US liquid quart = 32 fluid ounces = 1/4 US gallon = 0.95 liter
1 milliliter = 0.03 fluid ounce
1 fluid ounce = 29.57 milliliters
1 US gallon = 0.83 English (Imperial) gallon

Weight
1 kilogram = 2.20 pounds (avoirdupois) = 2.68 pounds (apothecaries')
1 pound (avoirdupois) = 16 ounces = 453.60 grams
1 grain = 65 milligrams

Energy
1 kilogram-meter = 7.25 foot-pounds
1 foot-pound = 0.14 kilogram-meters

Temperature
To convert centigrade degrees into Fahrenheit, multiply by 9/5 and add 32
To convert Fahrenheit degrees into centigrade, subtract 32 and multiply by 5/9

Greek Alphabet

Symbol		Name	Symbol		Name
A	α	alpha	N	ν	nu
B	β	beta	Ξ	ξ	xi
Γ	γ	gamma	O	o	omicron
Δ	δ	delta	Π	π	pi
E	ϵ	epsilon	P	ρ	rho
Z	ζ	zeta	Σ	σ, ς	sigma
H	η	eta	T	τ	tau
Θ	θ	theta	Υ	υ	upsilon
I	ι	iota	Φ	ϕ	phi
K	κ	kappa	X	χ	chi
Λ	λ	lambda	Ψ	ψ	psi
M	μ	mu	Ω	ω	omega

Index